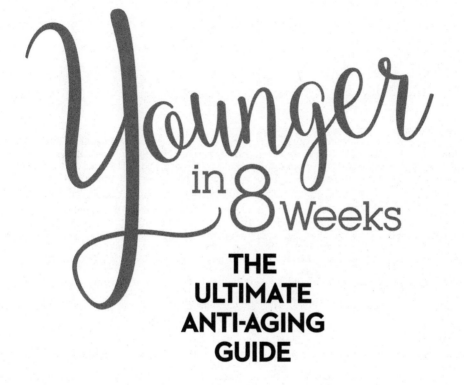

Younger in 8 Weeks

THE ULTIMATE ANTI-AGING GUIDE

THE EDITORS OF
Prevention.
WITH
Vonda Wright, MD

HEARST

© 2018 by Hearst Magazines, Inc.

Photographs © 2018 by Hearst Magazines, Inc.

Printed in the United States of America

All photos are by Mitch Mandel, except for the following: pages 10 and 121–124, Jeannette Graf, by Yolanda Perez; page 10, Suzanne Segerstrom, by Greer Photography; pages 11, 129, and 143, Eva Scrivo, by Stephen Murello; page 11, Andie Schwartz, by Jason Yokobosky; page 11, Michele Stanten, by Shannon Greer; pages 63, 117, 149, 233, 276–279, and 329, by Ari Michelson; and page 65, photo reprinted from the *Physician and SportsMedicine*.

Book design by Carol Angstadt

Library of Congress Cataloging-in-Publication Data is on file with the publisher

ISBN 978–1–62336–654–4 direct hardcover

4 6 8 10 9 7 5   hardcover

HEARST

CONTENTS

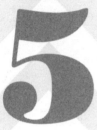

INTRODUCTION

As an orthopedic surgeon, researcher, and healthy aging expert, I've seen proof that we all have the power to transform our health—and, by extension, our lives. But I'm passionate about inspiring this potential in others because I have lived it.

I remember my 38th year vividly. I was in Pittsburgh, slogging through the 10th year of an 11-year journey through medical school and surgical training. I was exhausted, 20 pounds overweight, emotionally spent, and wondering where the last 10 years of my youth had gone. I'd been taught to work hard, and in that daily effort to care for sick people, I'd basically fallen into the habit of caring for everyone except myself. I had actually forgotten what it meant to prioritize my health and happiness. I hadn't taken the time to notice myself in years.

As my residency ended and I moved to New York for my final year of my orthopedic fellowship, I knew I wasn't happy. I finally paused to take notice of what was left of me. In a new city with a new job, I also wanted a new me. So I deliberately took steps toward getting the strong, healthy me back. I didn't know anyone in the city, so I joined one of the Taj Mahal–like, 7-story gyms on the Upper East Side as both a physical and social outlet. I harnessed my work ethic to sweat away the years of neglect, and I got into the best shape of my life. I became a New York foodie, seeking out only the freshest, most nourishing foods to rebuild my health and strength from the inside out. I wandered the streets, soaking up the sights and sounds, while stretching past my introverted comfort zone to connect with new people.

As I lost 20 pounds, became stronger than ever, and took time to truly engage with my life and the people in it, I started poring over the mounds of research I'd collected on healthy aging from masters athletes in the Senior Olympics. That data on these amazing individuals inspired me to believe I could change the way we age in this country. At that moment, I decided to write my first book, *Fitness after 40*. I also designed a series of research studies to prove that the view of aging as just a downward slope was a myth. I dedicated my academic career to proving that everything from our bones to our muscles to our brains will thrive if we challenge ourselves to live younger and not simply let gravity and aimless aging take over.

Today, after more than a decade of this work, I've witnessed the transformational power of making smart lifestyle choices exert itself again and again.

Often, big changes come from small steps. Like with my patient Linda, 55, who joined my first "Couch to 5K" class. She had never exercised regularly and was 30 pounds overweight. In just 8 weeks, she not only was able to walk 3.2 miles but literally changed her health from the inside out, shedding her chronically high blood pressure and prediabetes.

But sometimes even small steps can feel daunting when there's an enormous amount to fix.

I'm reminded of my friend Voni, a busy executive and mother in her fifties, who wanted to make major changes to her exercise habits, diet, and happiness. "The thought of changing everything about how I exercised and ate at once was overwhelming, but if I could just focus on making it to the next mailbox every day, I knew I could do it," she told me. And Voni did, one mailbox at a time. Gradually, she got into marathon-ready shape and started eating healthier, whole foods, and now she is one of the most happy and thankful people I know.

The future looks extremely bright for all of us. Every aspect of healthy aging—from enhancing mobility and improving our well-being through nutrition to boosting brainpower and happiness via social connection—is supported by mountains of research indicating that you can determine your future well-being by the choices you make today. In fact, a full 70 percent of your long-term health is determined by the decision you make every single day to invest time in moving, eating, and engaging.

The book you're holding is based on these data, giving you a sound and exciting way to purposefully face your future. This Younger in 8 Weeks Plan, packed with insights from top experts in different fields, will guide you to recommit to your health and rediscover "you." You'll also read about the successes of our 21 amazing test panelists, who in just 8 weeks on the plan dramatically changed their health from the inside out, learning new habits that will serve them for good.

They have learned to live younger. And so will you. I know it.

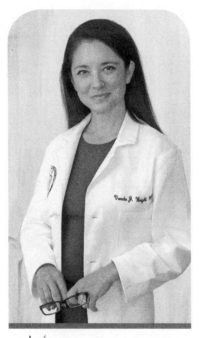

Vonda Wright, MD

PART

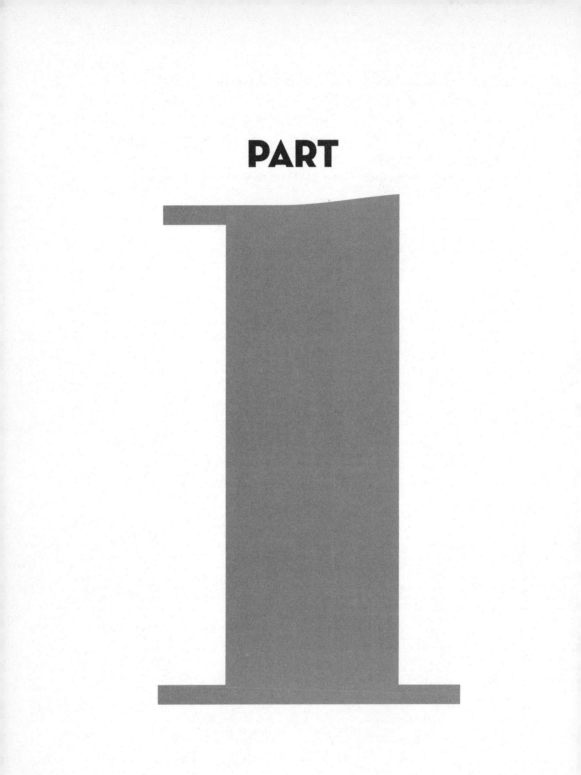

THE ART AND SCIENCE OF AGING

It's Never Too Late to Live Young

Think back (maybe even way back) for a second. Remember how you used to *want* to get older? As a teenager, you couldn't wait for the freedom of car keys and your own apartment. In your twenties, you envied the success and self-assuredness (and maybe the real estate) of your older peers. In your thirties, you figured that someday soon you'd actually have a chance to enjoy the life and home you were shaping and the friendships you'd made, if only you weren't so insanely busy all the time. And now, here you are—a little or a lot older than that. Be careful what you wish for, right? How did the years fly by? When did your body change, or start to hurt? Where did you misplace your energy? Your optimism? Your glow? Honestly, you feel a bit robbed.

Here's the thing: You can steal back those youthful qualities you're nostalgic for. Even better, you can regain your strength, your confidence, your vitality, and your positive outlook while also embracing all the amazing things you've accomplished on this earth so far (you wouldn't give back most of them!) and scheming about great things to come. To quote actress and activist

Jane Fonda (who knows a thing or two about self-reinvention), "It's never too late to start over, never too late to be happy."

All you need is 8 weeks.

That's how long it takes to complete our plan. At *Prevention* magazine, we've been helping women renew their lives and revive themselves—body, mind, and soul—for more than 65 years. We've brought this deep knowledge to you in the chapters that follow, while drawing on the latest breakthrough science about how our lifestyle choices affect us at the cellular level. We've also tapped the expertise of a dream team of advisors in fitness, nutrition, and beauty, led by orthopedic surgeon and healthy aging expert Vonda Wright, MD, to structure this plan, week by week.

Does the plan work? You bet. We road-tested it on 21 women from ages 36 to 66—who, just like you, had been struggling with weight gain, lack of energy, loss of luster, and other common age-related challenges. Two months later—well, check out their before-and-after photos (you'll find one in each chapter). Our test panelists lost as much as 25 pounds in 2 months, with an average weight loss of 10 pounds. Moreover, they gained strength, stamina, energy, a more positive attitude, and deeper connections with others, plus a whole new and more youthful look—including smoother skin, makeup that flatters their best features, and a killer haircut. "This plan has given me the code to healthy living," says homemaker Kate Pelham-Hambly.

That's the thing: Not only will you feel happier, fitter, glowier, and better rested week by week, but you'll also reap the benefits far into your future. That's because this plan *literally turns back the clock on the aging process* so that everything from your hair to your heart resembles that of a younger person. But more than that, we're giving you tools that you can use for the rest of your life.

Before we get to the plan, though, let's unpack the basics of aging to see what parts are inevitable and what parts can be controlled.

What's in an Age, Anyway?

"From the moment that we are two cells in the womb, we are aging," says Dr. Wright. We grow up, we grow old, and our cells continue to divide and refresh themselves, until they don't anymore (more on that in a sec).

But while aging is as fundamental as breathing, it's also as individual as a fingerprint. Much of what's known about the aging process comes from the

National Institute on Aging's (NIA) Baltimore Longitudinal Study of Aging (BLSA), which began in 1958 and has monitored the same subjects over time (totaling more than 3,100 people).

One major discovery from the BLSA is that the rate and progression of cellular aging varies dramatically from person to person. That's why some 60-year-olds can compete in triathlons while others decline into ill health and frailty. *Biological age* is a measure of how well your body and brain are holding up for your chronological age, and there's evidence that a healthy lifestyle can actually lower it.

While it's obvious how age takes its toll on the outside, a look under the hood would reveal that aging diminishes every single organ. Blood vessels in your heart accumulate fatty deposits and lose flexibility, resulting in atherosclerosis. The lenses of your eyes stiffen—making it harder to focus on close objects—and the number of nerve cells decreases, which impairs depth perception. In the gut, the production of digestive enzymes slows, inhibiting nutrient absorption. These may not be as visible as the crow's-feet you spot in the mirror, but they are no less problematic—and arguably more so, because we tend to wait too long to address them.

But just as the BLSA data shows that aging is different for everyone, it also makes very clear that much of the process is well within our control. Scientists believe that as little as 30 percent of aging is genetically determined, for better or for worse, while as much as 70 percent of how we age is related to lifestyle. In other words, the changes our bodies undergo over time do not inevitably lead to the diabetes, high blood pressure, or dementia of our parents. The way you live now and the choices you make today are the most important predictors of not only how long you'll live—but how well.

Your DNA Is Not Your Destiny

In recent years, a revolutionary new scientific insight has changed our understanding of aging from a process that can't be stopped to a process we ourselves can shape. This view, based on a Nobel Prize–winning discovery a few years back, holds that the bundles of DNA that cap the ends of our chromosomes, called *telomeres*, may be the key to the aging process.

As you may remember from high school biology, we have 23 pairs of chromosomes, which determine everything from our gender to our hair and eye color. Telomeres make it possible for cells to divide and—like the felt tip on a pool cue—buffer our genetic material from damage. Normally, cells divide a total of just 50 to 70 times; each time a cell divides, its telomeres shorten. Genetic research has linked shorter telomeres to a slew of age-related diseases, including cardiovascular disease, obesity, diabetes, dementia, and many forms of cancer. (Illness shortens them, too.) Eventually, when telomeres get too short, cells can no longer divide. And either they become inactive (senescent) or they die.

Telomere shortening is a natural consequence of aging. But here's the amazing thing: Although you can't change your DNA, you *can* change your telomere length.

Here's proof: In a groundbreaking study published in the *Lancet Oncology,* a team of researchers split 35 men with early-stage prostate cancer into two groups. They asked one group to make lifestyle changes that included a plant-based diet heavy in fruits, vegetables, and whole grains; 30 minutes of moderate daily exercise like walking; stress busters like meditation, yoga, or deep breathing; and weekly group therapy. The other group members just kept on with their less-than-healthy ways (lousy diet, sedentary lifestyle, little to no stress relief).

Among those who stuck with the new positive lifestyle changes, telomere length *increased 10 percent* after 5 years. And that's not all: The more closely the members of the lifestyle changes group followed the prescribed plan, the more their telomeres grew. (Scientists measure telomere length by looking at cells from blood samples under a microscope.) By contrast, during the same period, the telomeres of the control group shortened by 3 percent. While it's not clear exactly how much each of these lifestyle changes impacts health or longevity (is diet more influential than exercise, for instance?), the study's coauthor, noted cardiologist Dean Ornish, MD, has said it's likely that all of these changes work synergistically to boost telomere length and that *all* of them are part of the solution.

Other research supports the idea that telomere-protective lifestyle habits work effectively as a team. In a Harvard study that measured telomere length in 5,862 women, researchers zeroed in on five healthy practices that seemed to lengthen telomeres: a clean diet (more fruits, veggies, whole grains, and fish and less red meat and trans and saturated fats), maintaining a healthy weight, 150 minutes of moderate or vigorous exercise a week, moderate alcohol intake, and not smoking. Practiced alone, none of these habits significantly boosted telomere length, but together the effect was dramatic. Women who committed themselves to all five habits had a 31.2 percent increase in telomere length, while women who did four of the practices wound up with telomeres that were 22.6 percent longer.

You might be thinking, that's amazing for those women, but what does it have to do with me? Well, for our Younger in 8 Weeks Plan, we harnessed all of the latest scientific studies about the various habits that target telomere growth, from clean eating and exercise to other DNA-impacting habits like stress reduction. Then we translated them into a program that turns these positive behaviors into powerful antiaging weapons. No, we can't measure your telomeres for you. But just as all of our 21 panelists saw dramatic results—to their bodies, their looks, their strength, their energy levels, and other youth indicators—in just 2 months, we are confident that you will, too.

The Aging-Inflammation Connection

Telomere length is one key factor in genetic health and life span. Inflammation is another. Our plan tackles this age accelerator, too.

Let's back up. You've probably heard the word *inflammation* tossed around in a lot of different contexts. First off, it's important to know that inflammation is fundamentally a good and necessary function. Without the body's inflammatory response, you'd be toast—overrun by viruses, bacteria, fungi, and parasites that would finish you off long before you reached old age. Consider that when you sustain a paper cut or catch a cold, your immune system goes into combat mode, inflaming the area with an army of white blood cells that fight infection or a virus. In these cases, inflammation can show up in obvious ways—a swollen finger, a stuffy nose. But it can also happen inside you without outward signs. A healthy inflammatory response lasts a few hours or days and recedes when the threat is gone. But those white blood cells and potent virus-killing chemicals, called cytokines, can continue to proliferate long after their services are needed.

This longer-term version of inflammation, called chronic inflammation, wreaks havoc on your body, because cytokines don't just stay at the site of the insult. They can cruise through your bloodstream and, ultimately, damage tissue; an excessive buildup of cytokines can spur plaque formation in your arteries and may even promote tumor growth. Chronic inflammation is the common denominator of many age-related diseases, from arthritis and type 2 diabetes to Alzheimer's. But even in the absence of disease, inflammation can lead to serious loss of function throughout the body.

For example, excess weight can cause an inflammatory response within fat cells. Extra body fat isn't just baggage that slows us down; as people gain weight, their fat cells grow larger and begin to churn out cytokines. One such cytokine is interleukin-6 (IL-6), usually produced when the immune system fights an infection or tries to heal a burn. In one study, overweight people had 10 times as much of this substance in their body fat as people of normal weight. IL-6 and other inflammatory factors block insulin's ability to send signals within a cell, which is one way that insulin resistance, the precursor to diabetes, can develop.

Chronic stress can trigger inflammation, too. While the stress hormone cortisol plays a role in regulating the inflammatory response, stress that is severe and ongoing can mess with that hormone's ability to do so, which leaves inflammation unchecked. Constant stress also seems to increase the production of certain inflammatory white blood cells, increasing the risk of inflammation-related diseases.

Finally, because 70 percent of your immune cells reside in your intestines, the bacteria that live in your gut, or microbiota, can affect your immune system, too. These bacteria can either suppress or activate inflammation, depending on whether they're "good" or "bad." (We'll explain more about diet and gut health in the EAT chapter.) This is why there's so much interest among doctors to use probiotics to influence the gut's inflammatory response. Our Younger in 8 Weeks Plan includes a healthy dose of probiotic (as well as prebiotic) foods and offers other lifestyle changes to help combat inflammation.

Feel Amazing—Now and for Good

Some people talk about living forever. But what good is a long life if you aren't guaranteed to live well? Scientists refer to this as our *health span*—that is, the years we live in good health.

There's a huge difference between health span and life expectancy, or the average number of years people can expect to live. Life expectancy is higher than ever, due largely to advances in nutrition and disease prevention and treatment. (In the 20th century, average life expectancy jumped 30 years—the largest gain in the 5,000 years humans have been around!) And women tend to live longer than men, as you've no doubt heard: In 2012, life expectancy for American women was 81.2 years, compared to 76.4 years for men. The number of centenarians—or those who live until

100—has also spiked, having jumped 51 percent from 1990 to 2000.

But life expectancy isn't where it's at. Health span is. And the good news is that science is focusing on ways to increase it. The secret? Once again, it's telomere length. In one study, researchers analyzed DNA samples from centenarians and found that the telomeres of the healthy 100-plusers were significantly longer than those of their peers in ill health. That's great news, because it suggests that with every healthy choice we make, we can meaningfully extend our health span.

As we mentioned, science has shown that the majority of aging is related to lifestyle—your diet, exercise, and sleep habits; how you deal with stress; the quantity and quality of your relationships; your attitude toward life. Over time, these choices, habits, and learned responses can make a big difference in how your body ages from the inside out. For example, heart attack and stroke are top causes of death and disability as we age. In a bid to raise your health span, you can eat right, stay active, and make other choices scientifically shown to reduce the risk of those diseases and others. That's where this plan comes in.

Our Younger in 8 Weeks Plan: Road-Tested and Approved

We sifted through literally hundreds of studies and convened a team of experts (to learn more about them, see the box on pages 10–11) to help us formulate a plan that incorporates dozens of telomere-lengthening, inflammation-quenching practices. Then we put the plan to the test on our panel of 21 women, ages 36 to 66, who were at different weights and levels of fitness—and who presented us with a range of age-related challenges to overcome (from high blood pressure and lack of energy to aching joints). Meeting daily on a private Facebook page, our panelists swapped tips, brainstormed solutions, and helped us tweak the program to perfection.

At the end of nearly 2 months, we had our Younger in 8 Weeks Plan. And our panel got results.

- Eating often and well, they **lost belly and body fat**, dropping an average of 10 pounds and as much as 25.

- They **lowered their total blood cholesterol** by up to 39 points **and blood sugar** by as much as 14 points, improving their overall health.

- They **boosted their energy** by an average of 36 percent with clean eating and a simple at-home workout.

Meet the *Younger in 8 Weeks* Panel of Experts

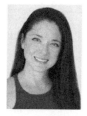

MEDICAL ADVISOR: VONDA WRIGHT, MD. Dr. Wright is an orthopedic surgeon, a researcher, and an internationally recognized authority on active aging. She's the director of the Performance and Research Initiative for Masters Athletes (PRIMA) at the University of Pittsburgh, medical director of UPMC Lemieux Sports Center, and author of *Fitness after 40* (among other books). Dr. Wright is an associate professor of orthopedic surgery at the University of Pittsburgh School of Medicine and head team physician for five University of Pittsburgh Panthers Olympic teams and the Pittsburgh Ballet Theatre. She oversaw the development of the Younger in 8 Weeks Plan every step of the way.

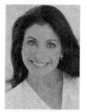

DERMATOLOGY/SKIN CARE: JEANNETTE GRAF, MD. A clinical assistant professor of dermatology at the Icahn School of Medicine at Mount Sinai in New York City, and a partner in Omni Aesthetics MD, Dr. Graf is the author of *Stop Aging, Start Living.* She created our skin-care regimen.

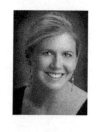

EMOTIONAL HEALTH: SUZANNE SEGERSTROM, PHD. A clinical professor of psychology at the University of Kentucky in Lexington, Dr. Segerstrom has conducted extensive research on the relationship between optimism and well-being. She is the author of *Breaking Murphy's Law: How Optimists Get What They Want from Life—And Pessimists Can Too.*

- They **slept soundly** and woke in the morning raring to go.
- They saw a 27 percent average **boost in confidence.**

These are just a few of dozens more changes, physical and emotional, that our panelists themselves will describe to you throughout the book. With their help, we broke down the biggest drivers of change into a daily schedule lasting 8 weeks. Each day's agenda incorporates strategies from the following four Stay-Young Steps.

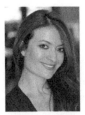

BEAUTY AND STYLE: EVA SCRIVO. A renowned hairstylist, colorist, and makeup artist, Scrivo is the owner of the eponymous Eva Scrivo Salons in New York City and the author of *Eva Scrivo on Beauty.* She created the beauty regimen and is responsible for our panelists' dramatic makeovers at the end of the book.

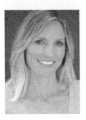

NUTRITION: ANDIE BERNARD SCHWARTZ, RD. A dietitian and certified personal trainer with a passion for plant-based diets, Schwartz provides nutritional counseling, personal training, and wellness coaching to both everyday people and professional athletes. She created our recipes and the Clean & Green eating plan.

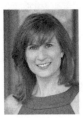

FITNESS: MICHELE STANTEN. An ACE-certified fitness instructor, the author of *Walk Off Weight*, and the former fitness director of *Prevention* magazine, Stanten helped develop the Younger in 8 Weeks Workout.

EAT. A dietitian-designed program can slow aging from the inside out by drenching your cells with key nutrients, fighting inflammation, supporting the gut, and promoting fat burn. Your tools: our delicious 2-week, clean-eating, plant-based menu (called Clean & Green) that includes 76 healthy recipes and a Meal Builder that lets you design your own meals with your favorite healthy foods.

MOVE. Our cardio and strength-training workouts will help you burn fat and build muscle as they lay the foundation for being active and physically adventurous for years. You'll start at your current fitness level and progress every week. (Don't worry—there are options, whether you are starting out in gym shape or if it's your first time off the couch in years.) Rounding out the workouts are no-sweat balance and flexibility routines, plus a mandate to get vertical: Simply being on your feet more can make a significant difference in your health.

ENGAGE. It's a fact: Adults who are open to new experiences, who are emotionally flexible and able to take life as it comes, tend to live longer, healthier, happier lives. Relationships matter, too; research has linked low levels of social support to shorter telomeres. Moreover, science has uncovered the connection between your mind-set and heart health. On our plan, you'll learn ways to tune in to life and wring more joy from each day—while also planning the new adventure of your Second Act.

GLOW. In as little as 4 weeks, the plan's skin-care routine, designed for us by a top licensed dermatologist, can help you restore lushness and luster to your skin and hair. And if you've been sporting the same look since the last millennium, you'll really love the hairstyling and makeup techniques from a renowned New York City salon owner. (If you don't use makeup, keep an open mind. A little bit of color can go a long way—and it can be empowering to make the changes to your look that you want to see.)

We know, that sounds like a lot of moving parts in one plan. But we break down the strategies in a daily, doable fashion so you'll start to see progress right away—and feel encouraged to keep going. Want more detail before you begin? Here's a closer look at each of the four pillars of the plan.

EAT

Nourish Your Body to Live Longer

If you saw the words *plant-based diet* a few paragraphs ago and are envisioning 2 months of choking down kale, you can relax. Basically, a plant-based diet means upping your intake of fruits and veggies, nuts and seeds, beans and whole grains—while cutting back on animal products and refined, processed carbohydrates. That's doable, right? Particularly when you consider that extremely strong evidence suggests that eating a plant-based diet is the master key to a healthy body and brain. And this isn't some crunchy-granola way of eating: In 2015, the Dietary Guidelines Advisory Committee—the ones who help come up with the government's official eating plan, like the graphic that we used to call the Food Pyramid and, more recently, MyPlate—recommended for the first time ever that Americans emphasize a plant-based approach to eating, while scaling back on their meat intake, for both health and environmental reasons.

Consider the evidence.

- A plant-based diet promotes longer telomeres and a longer life span, according to a study published in the *British Medical Journal.*

- The primarily plant-based MIND diet—or Mediterranean-DASH Intervention for Neurodegenerative Delay—reduced Alzheimer's risk by 53 percent among strict adherents and by 35 percent among those who followed it pretty closely. (Actually, it's similar to our plan.)

- Eating a plant-based diet may be the most effective way to lose weight, a study published in the journal *Nutrition* found.

- A diet that includes more plant-based foods and fewer animal-based foods is linked to a lower risk of death from heart disease and stroke, according to the American Heart Association.

- Fruit and veggie consumption may be the best and safest route to youthful-looking skin, reported an article in the journal *Dermato-Endocrinology.*

Our plan does allow for small amounts of dairy, red meat, poultry, and a few processed whole grain foods, like bread and pasta. But they're optional—and chances are you won't miss them much because our menu is high on the scrumptious scale. There'll be lots of fruits and veggies, of course. But add in

Turn-Back-the-Clock Breakthrough
LOSE WEIGHT, FIND 9 EXTRA YEARS

Obesity—the scourge that's been linked to so many diseases—can also make you age more rapidly. And even faster than cigarette smoking! In a study of 1,100 British women published in the *Lancet*, researchers found that the more women weighed, the older their cells appeared on a molecular level—with the heaviest women adding the equivalent of 9 years to their bodies. Meanwhile, even puffing a pack a day for 40 years caused less cellular aging (7.4 years) than being significantly overweight. ∎

hearty, unprocessed whole grains; plant proteins, like beans; plant-based milks; fish; yogurt; and healthy fats, like avocado. And let's not forget a glass of red wine with dinner, if you want one, in Week 3 and a smattering of sweet treats starting in Week 4. (Chocolate, of course.)

MOVE

Boost Energy and Build Strength

Dr. Wright studies the fitness and performance of masters athletes—men and women who played sports in their youth and have remained active into their fifties and beyond. She has seen how many changes in muscle mass and strength—once thought to be an inevitable result of aging—are actually caused by inactivity. "Sedentary living is the biggest deterrent to longevity," says Dr. Wright. But it's never too late to start being active. "There's no age where your body will not step up to the plate if you ask it to."

There are two main components to staying fit over time. Maybe you currently do one and not the other; maybe it's been a while since you've done more than take the occasional walk. That's totally all right. Our plan will ramp things up for you in a completely doable way.

Cardio. You know how good you feel when you walk, cycle, hike, or swim regularly—your weight drops, your mood brightens, and you've got stamina and energy to spare. All those benefits will come roaring back—fast—even if it's been a while since you last worked up a sweat. And as you reap cardio's mind/body benefits now, you'll set yourself up for peak health down the road. A study published in *JAMA* found that being fit at age 50 seems to stave off chronic conditions such as heart disease, stroke, diabetes, and Alzhei-

Turn-Back-the-Clock Breakthrough
WALK, SWIM, RUN OFF 6 TO 10 YEARS

In a study of 2,401 twins, published in the *Archives of Internal Medicine*, those who got a moderate amount of exercise—about 100 minutes a week—had telomeres that looked on average like they belonged to someone about 5 or 6 years younger than those who were least active (exercising about 16 minutes a week). Meanwhile, the most active subjects had telomeres about the same length as sedentary twins who were 10 years younger, the study found. ■

mer's. Cardio also improves bloodflow, which circulates more nutrients and other protective chemicals to all the body's organs.

Strength training. Use it or lose it is the name of the game with muscle strength—even more so as we age. "Loss of muscle mass increases markedly after age 50," says Dr. Wright. Start strength or resistance training at any point, though, and you can slow age-related muscle loss, strengthen muscles and connective tissues, increase bone density, reduce risk of injury, help ease aches and pains (back, shoulder, arthritis), and brighten mood and improve sleep quality in the bargain. If you have diabetes, strength training comes with an additional bonus, helping your body respond to the insulin you take or make by lowering your blood sugar.

Strength training is also the key to weight management as we age. The more muscle you have, the higher your metabolic rate. In fact, strength training can provide up to a 15 percent bump in your calorie-burning power—even when you're lying on the couch!

And you'll score benefits in only 30 minutes a day. Haven't exercised in a while? You'll be fine. "You were designed to move, and it's never too late to start," says Dr. Wright.

ENGAGE

Connect with Your Best Self—And the World around You

When you think of your younger self, there are probably a bunch of qualities you're glad to have left behind (indecision, impulsiveness, insanely bad judgment about romantic partners or hair). But you also possessed other positive traits that energized you and drove your enthusiasm for experiencing all that adult life had to offer: Positivity. Passion. Curiosity. Awe. Together, those qualities describe *engagement*—a tuning in to the people and the world around you. Science has linked these qualities and others you'll learn about to a long, healthy life and a sharper mind.

The ENGAGE chapter is packed with strategies that will help you step out of your comfort zone and reconnect, or connect more deeply, to life, as well as with yourself. You'll learn to think like an optimist (even if you're a knee-jerk pessimist), calm and clear your mind with simple meditation and breathing techniques, build emotional resilience to face inevitable challenges, and inject more passion, wonder, and purpose into your life.

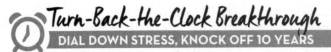

Turn-Back-the-Clock Breakthrough
DIAL DOWN STRESS, KNOCK OFF 10 YEARS

Stress that grinds on for weeks, months, or years may make us old before our time. In fact, such chronic stress is a pretty reliable predictor of shorter telomeres. Consider this outcome in a study of 647 women published in the journal *Cancer Epidemiology, Biomarkers & Prevention*. Researchers extracted DNA from the women's blood to gauge telomere length and measured their levels of stress hormones. The women also filled out a questionnaire that measured their levels of perceived stress.

Those who reported experiencing above-average stress levels had only slightly shorter telomeres than their low-stress sisters. But when researchers looked at perceived stress and telomere length in women with the highest levels of stress hormones, the difference in telomere length was similar to the effects of obesity, smoking, or 10 years of aging. ■

While all of this may sound rather pie-in-the-sky, the strategies couldn't be more practical. As you integrate them into your day, you'll start to create a vision for your future. That vision, Dr. Wright says, begins with a question: "What do I want, and where am I going?"

It's a question well worth asking. You have an amazing future ahead of you. It's yours to shape, and your attitude matters. One Yale study of adults over 50 found that, regardless of the state of their health, those with positive views of aging tended to live 7.5 years longer than those with less-positive outlooks. In fact, those perceptions had more of an impact on how long the participants lived than their blood pressure, cholesterol levels, or smoking status.

If life seems less purposeful or joyous than it used to be, this plan can help shake things up, and it starts with your vision. "It's not about dreaming the impossible dream," says Dr. Wright. "It's about painting a realistic picture of what you want your life to be. I've seen everyday people who were stuck—who had seemingly nowhere to go but old—go on to change their bodies and their feelings about themselves, their lives, and their future."

GLOW

Look as Good as You'll Feel

The effects of age on our looks need no introduction. Sun, pollution, a lousy diet, stress (frowning!), even gravity clobber us over time, while aging skin becomes uncooperative as the rate at which cells refresh themselves slows down. Still, much of this damage is not just preventable but reversible. Jeannette Graf, MD, a dermatologist at New York's Mount Sinai Hospital, has created a step-by-step skin-care routine that takes less than 5 minutes in the morning and at night and requires only six products. If you've been a soap-and-water type for years, prepare for visible changes in your skin's brightness and luster—and lots of unsolicited compliments.

And beauty expert Eva Scrivo has designed cosmetic solutions for the most common age-related beauty challenges. For example, you'll learn to use makeup to camouflage lines and wrinkles, even a sagging neck, and to plump up skimpy brows and lashes. And you'll find out how to give thinning hair a volume boost.

However, these techniques are the icing on the look-younger cake. The cornerstone of healthy skin and hair is the healthy habits rooted in the plan itself, including a better diet, more exercise, and sound sleep.

Don't Wish for Success—Plan for It!

Dr. Wright has a favorite quote: "A goal without a plan is just a wish." No doubt you've wished countless times to improve your health, lose weight, and get fit. But as the saying goes, you can wish in one hand—and, well, you can guess the rest. To make this time different, you've got to plan ahead.

You know how life goes: a late start, a snag in your schedule, a sick pet or flat tire—all of these bummers can derail your day, and your good intentions along with it. If you have a Plan A *and* a Plan B—workout clothes in your car, healthy staples in your pantry and freezer—you'll be more likely to navigate around speed bumps and stay on plan.

Take it from our panelists. Their lives were as busy as yours no doubt is, packed with long workdays, caring for family and aging parents, volunteer commitments, and laundry that doesn't wash itself. To succeed, they had to plan for the inevitable obstacles and temptations.

Panelist Ann Raines, an organizational development consultant, tells her clients that great ideas or intentions aren't enough. They need a solid plan—what Ann calls "wheels"—to move them forward. "For me, this plan has wheels," Ann says—and wishes with "wheels" come true. Where they take you may surprise you.

Less than a week into the plan, Lisa Boland, an administrative assistant, had an epiphany: "I realized that one of the biggest reasons I didn't make better choices for my health in the past was my belief that I wasn't strong enough to resist temptation or make myself exercise." She learned otherwise during a night out, when she was able to resist the offer of dessert not once but many times. "That proved to me that I *am* strong enough," she says. "I also learned that when I make a plan and stick to it, I'm less frazzled and more successful."

Above all, believe you can succeed. That conviction will sustain you on days where obstacles pop up faster than the critters in a whack-a-mole game. To get there, set small goals you know you can hit, achieve them, and then move on to bigger goals. In our plan, we've done that for you over 8 weeks so that you can build on your progress in ways that you can see and feel, without feeling lost or overwhelmed.

Perhaps panelist Kate Pelham-Hambly says it best. "I've had a goal weight for 20 years. I kept saying to myself, 'If I could just get down to X pounds, I would be happy.' For the first time in my life, I feel like I have a guided plan that could turn all this wishing into planning and achieving."

It's time to begin. Your recharged and revitalized self awaits! The first step on your journey to younger: to assess where you are right now.

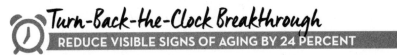

Turn-Back-the-Clock Breakthrough
REDUCE VISIBLE SIGNS OF AGING BY 24 PERCENT

On our plan, you'll use a broad-spectrum sunscreen every day—not just on your face but on your neck and hands, too. Here's why: In a study of 903 adults younger than 55, published in the *Annals of Internal Medicine*, those who used a broad-spectrum sunscreen—which protects against both ultraviolet B and ultraviolet A rays—every day were 24 percent less likely to show increased wrinkling over 4.5 years compared to those who used sunscreen less often. ■

Self-Assessment: How "Old" Are You Today?

You know how sometimes you'll see someone who is aging enviably well? She seems confident in her skin (which has a distinctly healthy glow); she's got a certain stylish flair; she displays the energy and spirit of someone half her age. Speaking of which—how old is she, anyway? It can be hard to tell. The fact is, her chronological age matters less than her *perceptual age*—the number she feels and the image she projects to the world.

Our goal for this book is to help you bring down your perceptual age (how old you feel)—as well as your biological age (how old your body is, right down to your DNA). Both are utterly within your control, based on lifestyle choices you make each day.

To begin your journey to a younger-feeling self, it will help a lot to know where you are right now. How are you aging compared to others? What are you doing right? What are your less-than-healthy habits that accelerate aging? Once you identify these habits, it becomes much easier to target them for change, upgrading your present and future health and well-being.

In this section, you'll complete a detailed quiz and then fill out a worksheet that identifies some vital info about your starting point (such as weight, resting heart rate, and blood-cholesterol profile). The purpose: to establish your own "before" and "after" and create a record of your gains. We even encourage you to take before-and-after selfies, if you're into that (the proof is always in the picture!).

And if you don't want to write in the book itself, go ahead and use a journal. There will be a few other exercises in the following chapters that will call for written reflection, so be sure to take notes in a format that's comfortable.

Here's how this section works.

1. **Complete the quiz**. The 40 questions below are designed to gauge whether you're aging slowly, on schedule, or a little too quickly. Once you finish the quiz, use the key to score and interpret your answers.

2. **Fill out the worksheet**. This is all about the numbers. Some of these you can fill in yourself (your weight and measurements, for example). Others will require input from a health-care provider—cholesterol, blood pressure, fasting blood sugar, and the like. You can use recent test results if you have them or request testing from your doctor. (Generally, you can do this as part of a wellness visit.)

The "How Old Are You Today?" Quiz

Give yourself two points for every (a) answer, one point for every (b) answer, and zero points for every (c) answer.

1. **WHICH OF THE BELOW BEST DESCRIBES YOUR DAILY DIET?**
   a. Whole foods—veggies and fruits, nuts and beans, brown rice and other whole grains, plain yogurt.
   b. A mix of whole and processed/packaged foods.
   c. Mostly processed/takeout/convenience foods.

2. **HOW WOULD YOU ASSESS YOUR FITNESS LEVEL?**
   a. I'm not as fit as I was when I was 20—I'm fitter!
   b. I feel slower and stiffer than I used to, but I'm still pretty active.
   c. I have a bad back (or bum knee/shoulder/foot), but doesn't everyone slow down as they get older?

3. **BY NATURE, DO YOU CONSIDER YOURSELF:**
   a. More of an optimist.
   b. Mostly an optimist, with occasional bouts of pessimism.
   c. More of a pessimist.

4. **HOW HAS YOUR WEIGHT CHANGED SINCE YOUR EARLY TWENTIES?**
   a. I can still fit into the same jeans.
   b. I've gained a few pounds, but my weight stays mostly consistent.
   c. My weight has gone up and down over the years.

5. **OUT OF 21 MEALS A WEEK—BREAKFAST, LUNCH, AND DINNER—HOW MANY DO YOU COOK?**
   a. Half or more. I prep and cook meals ahead of time, so there's usually a healthy meal or snack option.
   b. At least half, but I get takeout or dine out a few times each week.
   c. Less than half.

6. **IF A FRIEND ASKED YOU TO HELP HER MOVE, YOU'D BE ABLE TO:**
   a. Lift and carry boxes and even move heavy furniture with little problem.
   b. Lift and carry boxes, but hope that my back doesn't go out.
   c. Pack boxes or cook food for those helping out, but that's about it.

7. **HOW PURPOSEFUL DOES LIFE FEEL RIGHT NOW?**
   a. Very—I enjoy my daily work/job, and I take part in several activities and organizations.
   b. Somewhat—I know my family needs me, but life sometimes seems a little *been there, done that*.
   c. Not very—these days, I feel adrift and unsure of my purpose in life.

8. **YOUR MOM'S APPEARANCE CAN GIVE YOU A CLUE ABOUT HOW GENETICS WILL AFFECT YOUR SKIN OVER TIME. HOW DOES YOUR MOM LOOK FOR HER AGE?**
   a. She looks younger than her age.
   b. She looks her age.
   c. She looks older than her age.

9. WHAT ARE YOUR GO-TO BEVERAGES MOST DAYS?

a. Morning coffee or tea with a splash of regular or plant-based milk, and water throughout the day.

b. Coffee with half-and-half and sugar or Splenda in the a.m., and diet soda or bottled teas throughout the day.

c. A sweet-and-frothy coffee-shop coffee drink in the morning, and then bottled teas and soda, diet or sugared.

10. WHEN YOU LOOK FOR A PARKING SPACE, YOUR RULE IS:

a. Park at the far end of the lot and walk.

b. Walk if I can't find a choice spot.

c. Circle the lot until I find a spot close to the entrance.

11. HOW WOULD YOU DESCRIBE YOUR SOCIAL NETWORK—FRIENDS, FAMILY, COLLEAGUES, AND ACTIVITY-BASED RELATIONSHIPS?

a. Full—I have many people in my life, and they're a source of support and pleasure.

b. Half-full—I have one or two close friends or family members, but I could stand to have a wider social circle.

c. Small—I haven't made much time for friends lately, and I'm feeling lonely these days.

12. THE PIGMENT IN NATURALLY DARKER SKIN OFFERS SOME UV-RAY PROTECTION THAT CAN SLOW THE AGING PROCESS. DESCRIBE YOUR NATURAL SKIN COLOR.

a. Dark

b. Medium

c. Fair

13. WHAT KINDS OF VEGETABLES DO YOU EAT?

a. I eat pretty much all of them, raw and cooked.

b. I have a couple that I like (broccoli, green beans, romaine) and tend to stick with those.

c. The few my family will eat—canned peas or corn, baked potatoes, the occasional salad.

14. HOW OFTEN DO YOU WORK OUT?

a. At least five times a week.

b. At least twice a week, but sometimes life gets in the way.

c. It's been quite a while since my last workout.

15. **HOW WELL DO YOU BOUNCE BACK FROM ADVERSITY, SETBACKS, OR EVEN TRAGEDY?**
    a. Very well—I'm good at asking for support and staying focused on the future.
    b. Somewhat well—I may fall apart for a time, but ultimately I rally.
    c. Not very well—I recover slowly, if ever, from setbacks or tragedy.

16. **DESCRIBE YOUR LEVEL OF ACTIVITY OTHER THAN EXERCISE.**
    a. I have an active job, so I'm constantly on the move.
    b. I look for opportunities to get up from my desk or the couch.
    c. I spend a good part of my day sitting down.

17. **DO YOU WATCH YOUR INTAKE OF ADDED SUGARS?**
    a. Most of the sugar in my diet comes from whole foods like fruit, but I do have some chocolate or a dessert once in a while.
    b. I try, but it's tough to give up some of my favorite treats—not to mention packaged foods like fruity yogurt and sandwich bread.
    c. No, it's too hard to avoid—when I go without sugar, I feel cranky and deprived.

18. **HOW WOULD YOU DESCRIBE YOUR EXERCISE ROUTINE?**
    a. Well-rounded—cardio, strength training, and stretching or yoga.
    b. I mostly stick to one type of exercise, like cardio (walking, running) or lifting weights.
    c. Pretty much nonexistent—I just can't seem to get motivated.

19. **WOULD YOU AGREE WITH THIS STATEMENT: "I USUALLY EXPRESS MY FEELINGS RATHER THAN BOTTLE THEM UP"?**
    a. Yes, I'm not shy about expressing my feelings.
    b. Mostly yes, though I occasionally resort to the silent treatment or passive-aggression when I'm angry or hurt.
    c. I rarely express how I feel to others.

20. **PINCH THE FLESHY PART OF YOUR HAND BETWEEN YOUR THUMB AND INDEX FINGER. HOW MANY SECONDS DOES IT TAKE FOR THE SKIN TO SPRING BACK?**
    a. Less than a second
    b. Two to 5 seconds
    c. More than 5 seconds

21. **HOW OFTEN DO YOU EAT RED MEAT (BEEF, LAMB, PORK—YES, PORK COUNTS AS "RED")?**
    a. Twice a week or less, and if I do it's a small amount, like in a stir-fry or salad.
    b. At least three times a week, with fish, chicken, or beans as healthy alternatives.
    c. Nearly every day; I also rotate in hot dogs, sausage, and deli meats.

22. **HOW WOULD YOU DESCRIBE YOUR ENERGY LEVEL DURING AND AFTER YOUR WORKOUT?**
    a. High—I work hard and feel great when I'm done.
    b. So-so—some days I'm in the zone, and some days I feel achy or out of breath.
    c. Low—I'm typically tired when I start and exhausted when I'm finished.

23. **HOW WOULD YOU DESCRIBE YOUR OVERALL VIEW OF AGING?**
    a. Mostly positive—we may grow older, but life is meant to be enjoyed.
    b. Mixed feelings—sometimes I'm fine, but other times I fret about my health, energy level, or appearance.
    c. Mostly negative—I worry about my future health, finances, and memory.

24. **WHICH OF THE STATEMENTS BELOW BEST DESCRIBES YOUR SUNNING HABITS?**
    a. I've protected myself from the sun for years. I've rarely been burned, and tanning isn't a priority.
    b. I've had a few sunburns in my life, but typically I remember to use sunscreen.
    c. I use (or have used) a tanning bed and get sunburned at least once every year.

25. **WHAT'S YOUR FAVORITE TYPE OF YOGURT?**
    a. 2% plain or full-fat Greek or regular yogurt, maybe with a bit of fresh fruit.
    b. Low-fat plain yogurt.
    c. Fruited yogurt, either blended or fruit-at-the-bottom, or yogurt with artificial sweeteners.

26. WHAT DO YOU KNOW ABOUT INTERVAL TRAINING?
   a. It's been part of my workout for a while now.
   b. I've tried it but am not regularly doing it.
   c. I don't do it—sounds too hard.

27. DO YOU HAVE A PET?
   a. Yes, more than one!
   b. Yes, my dog (or cat) is a loyal companion.
   c. Nope, no pets.

28. WHICH BEST DESCRIBES YOUR SKIN TYPE?
   a. Oily
   b. Oily in some parts, dry in others
   c. Dry

29. HOW OFTEN DO YOU BUY ORGANIC FOODS?
   a. More than half of my foods—including produce, meat, and dairy—are certified organic.
   b. When I can afford to, and especially in the summer, I buy organic or locally grown fruits and veggies at the farmers' market.
   c. I'd love to buy organic foods, but they seem unreasonably expensive.

30. DO YOU STRETCH EVERY DAY?
   a. Yes, as soon as I get out of bed and especially anytime I work out.
   b. No, except maybe after a particularly long car ride or workday.
   c. Never; it hurts too much to stretch.

31. WOULD YOU DESCRIBE YOURSELF AS A CURIOUS PERSON?
   a. Yes—I love learning and have taken classes just for fun.
   b. I'll try new things on occasion, but it has to be something that interests me personally.
   c. I've spent years just doing the same activities and not venturing out of my comfort zone.

32. WHICH OF THE BELOW BEST DESCRIBES YOUR REGULAR SKIN-CARE ROUTINE?
   a. Cleanser, antioxidant serum, broad-spectrum sunscreen, retinoid cream, moisturizer, eye cream
   b. Two or more of the above
   c. One or none of the above

33. WHICH OF THE BELOW BEST DESCRIBES HOW YOU FEEL WHEN YOU FINISH A MEAL?

a. I mostly or always feel satisfied—I eat pretty slowly and watch servings and portion sizes.

b. I mostly feel satisfied, but occasionally I overeat and feel stuffed or crave more.

c. I mostly feel uncomfortably stuffed—it's hard to say no to seconds of foods I love.

34. WHEN I THINK OF MY JOB OR CAREER, THE FIRST WORD THAT POPS INTO MY MIND IS:

a. Fulfilled. I love what I do.

b. Neutral. There are good and bad days, but overall I'm content.

c. Stuck. I've been dreaming of a career change or retirement.

35. DO YOU PRACTICE ANY TYPE OF MEDITATION?

a. Yes, at least once or twice a week—it really helps me manage my stress.

b. I've tried it and liked it, but I fell out of practice and can't find the time.

c. I've never tried it—I'm not the yogi type.

36. BECAUSE SKIN CANCER IS MOST PREVALENT IN SUNNIER STATES, WHERE IN THE COUNTRY HAVE YOU LIVED LONGEST?

a. Northwest

b. Northeast and Midwest

c. Sunny Southern states

37. HOW WOULD YOU DESCRIBE YOUR WEIGHT?

a. I'm at a healthy weight.

b. I'm about 10 to 20 pounds heavier than is healthy.

c. I'm about 20 or more pounds over a healthy weight.

38. WEEKENDS ARE FOR . . .

a. 5Ks, fun runs, or hikes.

b. Home projects, errands, or the garden.

c. Netflix, naps, and snacks.

39. HOW MANY HOURS A DAY DO YOU WATCH TV?

 a. An hour or less a day—I'm just too busy to watch more.

 b. Two hours at night, just to unwind from the day.

 c. At least 2 hours a day—more when I can't get to sleep.

40. WHEN WAS THE LAST TIME YOU UPDATED YOUR SKIN-CARE ROUTINE?

 a. Six months ago.

 b. Two to 3 years ago.

 c. I've used the same routine for as long as I can remember.

60–80 POINTS: YOU'RE AGING SMART. A practitioner of a bunch of cutting-edge health trends and on the lookout for new and practical ways to age successfully, you're very motivated to preserve your strength, energy, and mental resilience. You're likely at a healthy weight or within a few pounds of it, physically active, and continuing to milk fun out of life. You may also look younger than your age. Still, you know there's always something new to learn, particularly about health and longevity. Our program is sure to deliver a few surprises, even to someone as age-savvy as you.

40–59 POINTS: YOU'RE AGING ON SCHEDULE. While you may have more than a few pounds to lose or may even be grappling with a weight-related health issue (high cholesterol, high blood sugar), you're still relatively active and in good health. Even so, you may be missing out on some aspects of a healthy lifestyle that could give you more and higher-quality years, and you could do with less stress and more energy. A younger appearance wouldn't hurt, either. Whether the pieces are related to diet, physical activity, appearance, or attitude, you're sure to find them in this plan.

0–39 POINTS: YOU NEED THIS BOOK. Your weight and health have been ongoing concerns; you may even be at risk for type 2 diabetes, heart disease, or other age-related health conditions. You might carry around certain attitudes or beliefs about life, youth, and age that make you look and feel older than you are, and that may impact your future health in less-than-desirable ways. Fortunately, our program is loaded with simple ways to regain your health, energy, and positive outlook. They're all still there, waiting for you to claim them. And we'll be there every step of the way!

Next, it's time to complete the worksheet. If the prospect makes you anxious, take a deep breath. By Week 4, you'll be psyched about how much progress you've made. By Week 8, you'll be positively amazed! Your results before and after the program will stand as proof that small steps, taken one day at a time, can lead to a dramatic transformation in your health, your appearance—and your life.

The "Before" and "After" Worksheets

Fill out the first section only. You'll return to these pages to record your progress at 4 and 8 weeks. (Don't worry—we'll remind you!)

Your "Before" Profile

MEASURE THIS	HOW TO MEASURE	MY RESULTS
Weight	Weigh yourself in the morning after using the bathroom.	
Waist measurement	Measure just below your belly button. (The risk of developing weight-related health problems rises with a waistline of 35+ inches for women or 40+ inches for men.)	
Hip measurement	Measure just below your hip bones.	
Waist–hip ratio	Divide your waist measurement by your hip measurement. (A number above 0.8 suggests unhealthy levels of abdominal fat.)	
Resting heart rate	After sitting quietly for 10 minutes or first thing in the a.m., place your index and middle fingers across the inside of your opposite wrist, below the thumb's base. Press with flat fingers until you feel a pulse. Once you do, count the beats for 30 seconds, and then multiply by 2 to calculate beats per minute.	
Optional: Body-fat percentage	You can use a home scale with a body-fat calculator, but these are typically a little inaccurate (though you can monitor changes in body fat). Or call around to local gyms; many offer body-fat percentage tests.	

Your Numbers

If you have recently gone to the doctor and had a fasting glucose tolerance test, a blood pressure reading, and a complete fasting lipoprotein profile (which includes total cholesterol, "good" HDL cholesterol, "bad" LDL cholesterol, and triglycerides), feel free to use those results. If you don't have these numbers, no worries—this part is optional.

WHAT TO MEASURE	OPTIMAL NUMBER	MY RESULTS
Total cholesterol	Less than 180 mg/dL.	
Triglycerides	Less than 150 mg/dL.	
HDL cholesterol	60 mg/dL and higher.	
LDL cholesterol	Less than 100 mg/dL.	
Fasting blood glucose	70–100 mg/dL. Impaired fasting glucose (a type of prediabetes): 101–125 mg/dL. Full-blown type 2 diabetes: 126 mg/dL and higher.	
Blood pressure	119/79 or lower. Prehypertension: 120–139/80–89 (prehypertension means you may develop high blood pressure unless you take steps to prevent it). High blood pressure: 140/90 or higher.	

So What's Next?

Now that you've completed the quiz and profile, you know much more about your perceptual and biological ages (and whether one is "younger" than the other). Whatever your results, you've taken a huge step forward; you have a baseline for your "after," which means that you're ready to start your journey to younger.

Part 2 presents the research that supports our Stay-Young Steps—EAT, MOVE, ENGAGE, and GLOW—and our experts' insights into those findings. Although we were amazed by how dramatically a healthy lifestyle can help roll back the years, we were even more blown away when we saw the vivid effects of this science at work in our panelists. When you begin the 8-week program in Part 3, you'll know the "why" behind every aspect of our plan. You'll also feel confident that this isn't a plan with results that fade but a lifestyle that delivers long-lasting benefits to every aspect of your life.

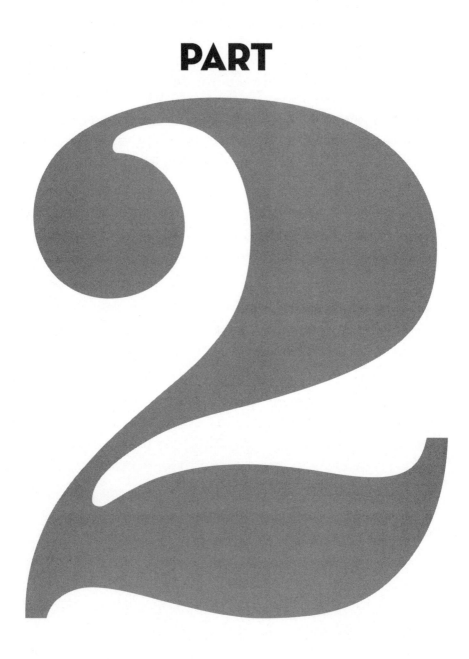

PART

2

HOW TO
TURN BACK
THE CLOCK

EAT

Nourish Your Body to Live Longer

If you take away only one thing from this book, let it be this: Shifting to a whole-foods, plant-based approach to eating (what we call Clean & Green) is the most impactful change you can make to turn back the clock and extend your health span.

A healthy diet is a force multiplier—that is, it intensifies a bunch of other positive outcomes. These include weight loss (which can lower your risk of obesity-related diseases, from diabetes to heart disease), more energy (so you'll have the fuel to exercise and be out and about with friends and family), a balanced mood (giving you the resilience necessary to deal with stress and challenges when they strike), and more radiant skin and hair. "We literally are what we eat, from what we see in the mirror down to the very way our genes express themselves to build our bodies, our brain, and our bliss," says our medical advisor, Dr. Vonda Wright. "If women only have time to make a few changes that will profoundly impact their health, we start with food."

By eating clean and green, we mean sticking to a plant-based diet that's low in sugar and processed ingredients and high in cell-nourishing nutrition. "Compared to a meat-centered diet, plant-based eating offers far more nutritional value—more fiber and antioxidants, with less saturated fat and cholesterol," says Andie Bernard Schwartz, RD, the dietitian who created our eating plan. And a mounting pile of research demonstrates incontrovertibly that a plant-based approach to eating has numerous health benefits, from lower blood pressure and cholesterol levels to a reduced risk of heart attack and even cancer. The Greek medical pioneer Hippocrates said that we should let food be our medicine—and in this case, it's like swallowing an entire vial of youth serum.

A plant-based diet may even help you eat your way to longer telomeres and a longer life. Recently, researchers from Harvard Medical School and Brigham and Women's Hospital in Boston wondered whether people who follow the Mediterranean diet—characterized by liberal amounts of veggies, fruits, nuts, beans, unrefined grains, olive oil, and fish as well as wine with meals—have longer telomeres than people who don't. So they scored the diets of nearly 5,000 healthy women on a scale from zero to nine—the higher the number, the more strictly they followed the diet—and then measured the women's telomere length from blood samples. Indeed, women with higher scores tended to have longer telomeres than those who scored lower. For every point higher that a woman's diet scored, her telomeres appeared about 1.5 years younger. Researchers surmise that all of the antioxidants and anti-inflammatory compounds in the Mediterranean diet may protect against telomere shortening.

Our Clean & Green eating plan is similar to the Mediterranean diet but goes beyond it to include powerful gut-boosting foods, while reducing added sugars and unhealthy chemicals. It's also anything but restrictive (which is why we refuse to call it a diet). You'll be able to keep enjoying so many of your favorite foods while discovering new and delicious flavors, from aromatic veggies to nutty-flavored grains. And don't forget your glass of red wine and chunk of chocolate with dinner, if you so choose.

In this chapter, with Schwartz's help, we've laid out the basic principles and the science behind our eating plan. Then turn to page 157 to get started on planning your daily menus.

Go Pro-Plant

When you make plants the centerpiece of your plate, you're not just doing your health a solid; you're beginning a love affair with real food that processed and convenience foods just can't match.

You're skeptical. Okay, consider this: Mac 'n' cheese and macarons—*love*, right? But the romance is fleeting. Open box or bag. Chew or gulp. Done. Then the pleasure quickly turns to pain when you feel bloated, fatigued, and full of remorse. It may be hard to believe, but you will come to crave the feeling of eating foods that nourish your organs and supercharge your cells—and, even better, when you know that those berries or broccoli come from nutrient-rich soil just a few miles away. Bottom line: These healthy foods love you back.

Of course, farmers' markets aren't always practical or accessible, so thank goodness for the supermarket produce aisle and frozen food section. (Frozen veggies and fruits are as nutritious as fresh, provided they aren't sugared or sauced.) Taking even the smallest step toward a plant-based diet, as organic and local as possible, connects you to the source of life and deep, lasting health in a way that can't happen when you consume mostly processed food. As some Internet wit once said, "Give peas a chance."

Along with its potential to boost telomere length, a plant-based diet can set you up for:

Weight loss. In an analysis of 15 studies, people on a vegan or mostly vegan diet lost an average of 10 pounds over 44 weeks—with no workout changes or portion control required. What's more, those who were heavier to start with lost more weight. This is in part because a plant-centered diet tends to be low in calories and high in fiber, which fills you up but not out. And when you eat mostly plants, *your after-meal metabolism revs up by about 16 percent*. Yes, it happens after every single meal and lasts about 3 hours, which represents a significant calorie burn over time.

Lowered risk of diabetes and heart disease. Compared to vegetarians, meat eaters were 74 percent more likely to develop type 2 diabetes over a 17-year period, one study found. By comparison, a low-fat, plant-based diet appears to improve insulin sensitivity and reduce insulin resistance. And in yet another study of nearly half a million adults, those whose diets were about 70 percent plant-based were 20 percent less likely to die from heart disease than people whose diets consisted of more than 50 percent meat, dairy, eggs, and fish.

Potential immortality. Okay, just kidding. But when a team of scientists analyzed the eating habits of more than 65,000 Brits over more than a decade, those who ate 7 or more servings of fruits and vegetables a day had a *42 percent lower risk of death at any point in time*. The risk of death from any cause fell by 14 percent for 1 to 3 servings, 29 percent for 3 to 5 servings, and 36 percent for 5 to 7 servings. For the super fruit-and-veggie eaters, we're talking a 25 percent lower risk of death by cancer and a 31 percent lower risk of death by heart disease. Score another for peas.

In Part 3, we'll tell you exactly how to adapt every meal to a plant-centric approach to eating. If you want to see a preview, turn to the How to Eat Clean & Green chapter on page 157, which details the foods you'll be putting at the center of your plate and those that you'll be eating less of or cutting out entirely. Then proceed to the Meal Builder (page 173), which gives you an easy formula for DIYing your day of eating, followed by the Food Shopping Guide (page 403), with helpful tips on brands to look out for. We even have 76 easy and delicious recipes for you, starting on page 333.

Eat Organic When You Can

At some point you've likely been told not to believe the hype about organic food. You grew up eating conventionally farmed, pesticide-sprayed produce and you don't have two heads, right? Right—but your parents probably didn't always eat this way.

Since World War II, the use of chemical pesticides has increased roughly tenfold as a result of the introduction of monoculture farming (growing single crops on a huge scale). While 90 percent of these chemicals haven't been tested for long-term health effects before being considered "safe," according to the National Academy of Sciences, in the long run we now know that many of them can be harmful. Synthetic pesticides have been associated with a variety of health problems, from skin, lung, and eye irritation to certain cancers. Not to mention the fact that chemical pesticides and fertilizers foul our water, deplete the soil, and pollute the environment.

Fruits and veggies are most likely to be contaminated by these agricultural chemicals, but animal foods—meat, poultry, eggs, dairy, even fish—aren't off the hook. Cows, chickens, and pigs are fed chemical-laden animal parts, fish meal, and grains. Big fish in polluted waters eat smaller fish, accumulating all of those toxins in the food chain. Also passed into meat and dairy foods are the growth hormones that big-scale US farmers give to cattle to increase the amount of meat and milk they produce. Because these hormones don't break down, they pass directly into our diets and have been linked to everything from early onset of puberty to tumor growth. And antibiotic use in animals is yet another unhealthy practice that has been blamed for the explosion of antibiotic-resistant bacteria.

But we don't have to eat this way. Sustainable farming methods have been shown to produce plenty of food—no toxic chemicals needed. You see, eating organic isn't a snobbery thing. It's a good health practice.

Organic is cleaner. Crops that are USDA Certified Organic are sprayed

Which Veggies Are Best for You?

THE QUESTION INVITES PLENTY OF SPECULATION. Lately, kale and spinach have been duking it out across the Internet for the top spot. (Team Spinach edges Team Kale out with more calcium.) But recently, a surprising upstart has entered the ring: watercress. When a researcher at William Paterson University in New Jersey assembled a list of 41 "powerhouse fruits and vegetables" ranked by their nutrient content, including fiber, calcium, folate, vitamin B_{12}, and vitamin D, this tangy, spicy green—kin to kale and collard greens—emerged as #1. (Try to add it to salads, sandwiches, or soups anytime you can.)

But asking which vegetables are the healthiest is a bit like wondering which type of exercise is the best. They're all good. The point is to try a range of them. The healthiest and tastiest diet looks like an artist's palette—plenty of red, blue, orange, purple, yellow, orange, even white. In fact, the pigments that give fruits and veggies their Crayola hues—called phytonutrients—are largely what make them so healthy (the fiber's good, too). The deeper the color, the higher the phytonutrients and the bigger the potential benefit to your well-being. Not only do brightly colored plant foods protect your health, they guard against cancer and other diseases. The upshot: Aim to eat at least one veggie or fruit (or legume) from each color group every day. Here's some inspiration for your next trip to the supermarket.

RED: Strawberries, tomatoes, apples, cranberries, watermelon, radishes, pomegranate

YELLOW/ORANGE: Squash, sweet potatoes, carrots, apricots, cantaloupe, oranges, corn, pineapple, lemons

GREEN: Lettuce, spinach, zucchini, broccoli, green beans, Brussels sprouts, soybeans

BLUE/PURPLE: Grapes, figs, blueberries, red cabbage, black currants, eggplant, black beans, plums

WHITE: Garlic, onions, pears, black-eyed peas, cauliflower

with natural pesticides, which don't mess with your health.

Organic is more nutritious. Yup! Organic produce is slightly higher in antioxidants than the regular kind. And a major analysis of 343 peer-reviewed studies, published in the *British Journal of Nutrition*, found that *switching to organic fruits, vegetables, and cereals would provide a whopping 20 to 40 percent* *more telomere-friendly antioxidants*, the equivalent of 1 to 2 extra servings of fruits and veggies a day. The study concluded that organic fruits and veggies can significantly boost your overall health.

Admittedly, organic does tend to cost more. That's because the cost of farming organically is higher for growers and producers. (By the way, if more people bought organic, the cost would likely come down—basic economics.) Here are a few ways to help you shop smart and ease the squeeze on your wallet.

- **Look for the USDA Certified Organic label.** This guarantees that you're buying produce or a food product that wasn't sprayed with toxic fertilizers or pesticides; if it's meat or dairy, it means the animals weren't given antibiotics or growth hormones and were fed a 100 percent organic diet. You'll find that the term *organic* is thrown around loosely at the supermarket (and words like *natural* or *clean* aren't regulated), so at least spend your money on bona fide organics.

- **Use the "Dirty Dozen" list.** If you don't want to pony up for organic across the board, at least do it for those fruits and vegetables with the highest pesticide levels, named the Dirty Dozen by the Environmental Working Group. Buying organic versions of these fruits and veggies will right away reduce your family's pesticide exposure by up to 90 percent, according to the EWG. You can look the list up at ewg.org (or download the handy app for iPhone or Android).

- **Eat local.** Food grown locally on small farms tends to be less heavily sprayed with harmful chemicals, even if it's not certified organic. Local produce also tends to be fresher—and therefore more delicious and nutritious—since shipping food across country (and then letting it sit on supermarket shelves for up to a week) diminishes certain nutrients. And during bumper-crop season—think piles of tomatoes, corn, and zucchini at the local farm stand—produce will be more affordable, as well.

- **Embrace frozen organics.** Typically, frozen organic fruits and veggies are less expensive than the conventionally grown items in the produce aisle.

- **Go for the store brand.** Whether you shop at Publix or Wegman's, Trader Joe's or Kroger, all store brands labeled "organic" are required to stick to the guidelines set by the USDA organic certification program (look for the official organic seal). Chances are that store brands will taste just as good as the spendier options.

Our bottom line: Opt for organic foods when you can. If you can't, don't feel bad about it. It's far better to munch lots of regular produce prepared at home than feast on a craptastic diet of processed foods.

Turn-Back-the-Clock Breakthrough
THE DIET THAT DEFEATS ALZHEIMER'S

Stick to greens and whole grains, nuts and berries, wine and fish and you can slash Alzheimer's risk by as much as 53 percent.

That's the conclusion of a study on a diet called MIND (short for Mediterranean-DASH Intervention for Neurodegenerative Delay). Developed using years of research on nutrients that help and hurt brain function over time, MIND is a cross between two well-researched and ultra-healthy plant-based ways to eat: the Mediterranean diet and DASH (Dietary Approaches to Stop Hypertension). Both older diets are proven to reduce the risk of high blood pressure, heart attack, and stroke. Now, scientists from Rush University Medical Center in Chicago found that they—as well as the new MIND hybrid—protect against Alzheimer's-related dementia, too. In the study, the eating patterns of nearly 1,000 older adults were tracked for an average of 4.5 years. Those who ate most often from a list of 15 brain-healthy foods—and limited red meats, butter and stick margarine, sweets, and fried food—slashed their risk of Alzheimer's by more than half. Even those who followed the diet only moderately well got a hefty 35 percent risk reduction. Good news: The foods on the MIND diet— beans and whole grains, salads and veggies, nuts and berries, and poultry and fish—are the very same as those on our plan. ■

Reclaim Your Kitchen

Nearly one-third of Americans say they cook just four out of 21 possible meals a week. It's totally understandable—you're busy, you're tired after work, you barely have time to make a piece of toast, let alone create a menu. But there's good reason to get reacquainted with that box in your kitchen that makes fire.

For one, home cooks eat better. Researchers from the Johns Hopkins Bloomberg School of Public Health analyzed the eating habits of more than 9,000 people and found that those who made dinner 6 or 7 nights a week ate

Renew Right Now

Why did you eat that sleeve of saltines when you knew there were apples in the crisper? Why did you have seconds at dinner when that wasn't the plan? Actually, there's a scientific explanation for it—and, even better, there are science-tested fixes for stupid food choices that knock you off plan.

Brian Wansink, PhD, director of the Cornell University Food and Brand Lab, has studied how people make decisions about food for decades. Consider just this one study (and there are dozens). Dr. Wansink and his team already knew that multiple portions (or "refills") can lead people to overeat. So he conducted an experiment to find out whether people would eat less if they kept the food on the stove or counter, rather than on the table. This simple "dish over here, dine over there" technique slashed the amount men ate by 29 percent and the amount women ate by 10 percent.

Want in on this action? Fix your kitchen with the quick makeover below, courtesy of Dr. Wansink.

CLEAR OUT THE KITCHEN CLUTTER. When you keep the table clear, it's more likely you'll actually sit down to eat, which encourages

---

an average of 137 fewer calories, 3 grams less fat, and 16 grams less sugar daily than those who cooked once weekly or not at all. Cutting 100 calories a day is 10 pounds lost in a year. Cooler still: In that same study, home cooks also ate fewer calories even when they *did* dine out, which suggests that healthy tastes formed at the stove carry over to restaurant meals. That's a great trade-off for a bunch of dirty dishes.

Not only will you eat less when you cook, but you'll save money (buying in bulk really does put money in your pocket and is way cheaper than buying prepared foods). You'll also take back control of what you put into your body and nourish it with more whole foods, which give your cells the nutrients they need for energy, repair, and peak health.

To help you get back into the kitchen, you need to rethink your experience of eating out. Remember when you were a kid and a restaurant meal, or even a trip to the local burger palace, was an event? Not anymore, thanks to drive-thrus, takeout, and wing night at Applebee's. To make it special again, you to munch mindfully. Both adults and kids tend to have lower BMIs if they eat meals together around the table. The camaraderie and chatter—and maybe a little peer pressure to not overindulge—seems to trump the desire to overeat.

LOAD UP YOUR FRUIT BOWL. People with fruit bowls on their counters weigh an average of 8 pounds less than their neighbors. (Make room for those super-healthy avocados!)

DESIGN YOUR FRIDGE FOR SUCCESS. When you put healthy food at eye level in clear containers, you're about three times more likely to eat the first thing you see, rather than an item you have to dig out. (Be sure to use BPA-free plastic containers or glass.)

RETHINK YOUR PLATES . . . People serve 18 percent more on dishes that match the food's color and 22 percent more on large plates, regardless of hunger, so opt for small (10-inch) plates that present a pleasing contrast to your food.

. . . AND SERVING UTENSILS. Scoop out food with regular tableware so you don't dish out oversize portions.

reframe your experience as a treat that you get to indulge in once a week, or even just twice a month.

This will mean one thing: more cooking. But take a deep breath; you can do it. Just follow this simple three-step routine.

Step 1: Declare a weekly Batch Day. Pick one day or time to get the bulk of your cooking done for the week. How about Sunday afternoons? On this typically quiet, restful day, cooking takes on a meditative quality if you crank up some tunes or stream a podcast you've been meaning to listen to. Or recruit a family member to help make it fun. Refrigerate or freeze a couple of extra dishes and the reward is tangible: fresh, healthy meals ready to go when you arrive home tired and hungry after work. (Not to mention the delicious scent of a pot of soup or roasted chicken filling your house all afternoon.)

Step 2: Decide on your menu. A couple days before Batch Day, choose three simple plant-based mains and sides to cook the following week. (For the next 8 weeks, you can break in the habit by choosing from among our

Clean & Green recipes or by using our Meal Builder.) As your culinary confidence grows, you can expand your repertoire of dishes. Just wait to see what happens when you plug watercress into the Internet!

Step 3: Make a list. Once you've planned your meals, make a list and hit the market—ideally, the same day and time each week.

Repeat these steps every week. Before long, you'll get in the swing of planning, shopping, and cooking, and you may actually—yes—learn to enjoy preparing nutritious, wholesome food.

Give Added Sugars the Axe

After decades of mounting sugar consumption in this country—last time we checked, the typical American allegedly sucks up anywhere from ¼ to ½ pound of sugar a day—we're finally witnessing a pushback against added sugar. While some of it is easy to target, the tricky part is that much of the sugar in our diets is hidden in healthy-sounding foods, from things like flavored yogurt to wheat crackers.

Regardless of its source, that extra sweetness is taking a bitter toll on our health and longevity. Excess sugar consumption is linked to a wide variety of age-related diseases, like high blood pressure, type 2 diabetes, kidney disease, and fatty liver disease. Sugar may also stir up trouble in the liver, which can lead to higher levels of cholesterol and other blood contaminants. And sugary drinks have been directly implicated in cell aging: In a University of California at San Francisco study, telomeres were found to be shorter in the white blood cells of participants who reported drinking more soda. In fact, drinking one 20-ounce soda a day equated to roughly 4.6 years of telomere shortening. Yikes!

The American Heart Association advises that **women should consume no more than 6 teaspoons (24 grams) of added sugar a day,** while the figure is slightly higher for men at 9 teaspoons, or 36 grams. (How much is that? See "Sugar Math: How to Ace It," page 44.)

Happily, a low-sugar life can be surprisingly sweet—and we'll help you start yours. Before you begin the 8-week plan, we'll tell you which sugar-laced foods to toss or give away (some will definitely surprise you). And in Week 4, when you'll have the green light to eat small amounts of sweet treats if you want them, we'll help you choose better options. For now, the tips

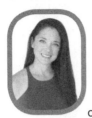

Dr. Vonda Wright says . . .
BE A LEADER IN THE KITCHEN

We women are the "chief health officers" of our homes—the key influencers of not only our own health but that of every person in our families. And food is the cornerstone of good health. As the CHO, you are in the position to choose what you and your family eat, and how much of it.

In my busy household—a blended family of six kids, with three still at home—I have aced the simple-but-healthy meal routine. Our weekday meals are basic: a healthy protein (say, grilled salmon), roasted or grilled veggies, and a simple starch (wild rice). While we don't deprive ourselves of the bounty of great food all around us, I stick to these healthy guidelines.

1. **NO FRIED FOODS.** I sauté, roast, or bake to limit the calories we consume from oil.

2. **WHOLE FOODS, THE BRIGHTER THE BETTER.** If you were to peek into my refrigerator, you'd see lots of color—broccoli crowns, baby carrots, grape tomatoes. And you couldn't miss the orchard of fresh fruit in the huge crystal bowl on my counter. Neon hues—that is, processed foods—aren't in nature's color palette, or in my house.

3. **LIMITED JUICE.** My family and I almost never drink juice. It's packed with sugar, and whole fruit offers fiber and nutrients that juice doesn't. If you are a juice family, I suggest fresh, no-sugar-added, 100 percent juice varieties.

4. **PLANT FATS OVER ANIMAL FATS.** That means olive oil, natural nut butters, and avocado, although I do use some organic butter. But because even healthy, plant-based fats are high in calories, when cooking, I put my olive oil in a spritz bottle (available in the kitchen-gadget section of any big-box store) and spray a thin film over food rather than pour directly from the bottle.

5. **NO ADDED SUGAR—PERIOD.** I choose to avoid it completely. You can choose not to. But when I cut it out of my diet, my health and energy improved, and I rarely miss it.

6. **READ FOOD LABELS.** It takes mere seconds but clues me in to what unhealthy ingredients may lurk within a bottle, box, or carton, and therefore what I'm putting into my body or the bodies of the people I love. Label reading also helps me understand what a portion is and whether an item is as healthy as I think it is.

Sugar Math: How to Ace It

WHEN YOU SCAN THE NUTRITION LABEL on a drink or box of cereal, you'll find that the amount of sugar is listed in grams. How exactly are you supposed to know if it's a lot or a little?

Here's a quick trick: **4 grams of sugar equals 1 teaspoon.**

With this simple equation, you'll know how much added sugar 1 serving of a processed food contains. It's a powerful formula that helps you make smarter choices about what you eat and how much.

Let's say you're looking at a bottle of barbecue sauce. Its nutrition facts label says:

Serving size: 2 tablespoons

Calories: 70

Sugars: 16 grams

Once you divide 16 grams by 4, you know that 1 serving (2 tablespoons) of that sauce contains 4 teaspoons of sugar. This plan allows for 6 teaspoons of sugar per day. Do you want to spend two-thirds of your sugar allotment on barbecue sauce? If you do, that's your call— just stick to 2 teaspoons for the rest of the day.

below can help you feel more satisfied eating less added sugar.

Swap out soda. This is probably the most impactful change you can make if you're still a soda or sweet tea drinker. (Careful, too, of so-called nutrition waters and sports drinks, which tend to harbor high amounts of sugar.) Choose sugar-free black or green tea, hot or iced, as well as club soda or water. Go ahead and doctor your drink with natural flavor blasts—a wedge of lemon or lime, slices of cucumber, a sprig of fresh basil—or sample our flavored waters on page 170.

Seek flavor, not sugar. Enhance foods with spices that are naturally sweet—such as cinnamon, vanilla extract, and ginger—rather than sugar or even sugar substitutes. An always-defensible splurge: fresh vanilla-bean pods and cinnamon sticks.

Do dessert in style. Try a few fresh, fat berries dipped in dark chocolate. Or microwave a serving of your favorite fruit and then stir in vanilla extract, cinnamon, a tablespoon or two of 2% plain Greek yogurt, and a tablespoon of your favorite nuts. Sweet and sensational.

Repurpose your sugar bowl. Too tempted? Pack it with your favorite tea. Store your keys in it—or fill it with dog or kitty treats! The switch can help you skip the spoonfuls you might otherwise be itching to add to cereal, coffee, or tea.

Renew Right Now

INDULGE YOUR CHOCOLATE CRAVING

It's a superfood, it's a treat—yes, it's a little bit sweet, but dark chocolate rocks! According to research, around two small squares per day— make sure it's at least 70 percent cocoa—can help your . . .

MOOD. Cocoa butter fats can trigger natural endorphins and tiny amounts of anandamide, a marijuana-like brain chemical. (The name anandamide comes from ananda, the Sanskrit word for *bliss*.) Not to worry—chocolate makes you happy, not high.

ENERGY. Epicatechin, one of the compounds that gives cocoa its bitter taste, can amplify your cells' mitochondrial function. That's the scientific way of saying that it recharges your batteries.

WEIGHT. Regular chocolate eaters are slimmer than those who abstain altogether, research has found. Just don't plow through your sweet stash all at once.

HEALTH. The credit goes to flavanols, a powerful antioxidant in cocoa beans (as well as berries, tea, onions, and other plant foods), which can do everything from boost heart health to prevent cancer. It also seems that good belly bugs, such as *Bifidobacterium* and lactic acid bacteria, love dark chocolate. As they feast, they ferment the bittersweet morsel, producing anti-inflammatory compounds that the body absorbs—ultimately reducing inflammation in cardiovascular tissue and lowering the risk of stroke. One study found that the arteries of men who ate 70 grams of dark chocolate a day (almost 2.5 ounces) became more flexible and supple. Researchers also observed that dark chocolate helped to keep white blood cells from sticking to artery walls.

LEARNING AND MEMORY. Flavanols increase bloodflow to the brain, promote the formation of new brain cells (neurons), improve brain-cell function, and protect brain cells from free-radical damage.

Bottom line? Savor it regularly, just a square or two at a time, to keep your mood bright, your cardiovascular system clean, and your mind sharp. That's a pretty sweet deal.

Power Up Your Gut

Do you like thick, creamy Greek yogurt? So does the colony of beasties that lives in your intestinal tract, called the gut microbiota. A growing body of research suggests that this microscopic universe plays a critical role in our overall health, helping the digestive system perform at its peak, boosting immune function, and helping to regulate metabolism. Over time, these microscopic crusaders form colonies to battle obesity, type 2 diabetes, heart disease, autoimmune disease, and even certain cancers.

Your gut microbiota is composed of tens of *trillions* of microorganisms—ten times more cells than in the rest of your body. And what you eat plays a key role in the bacterial "richness" of your gut. In a study of 153 men and women, those who adhered closely to a Mediterranean diet (again, plant and whole-grains based) were found to have higher levels of beneficial short-chain fatty acids (SCFAs) produced by gut bacteria. Research suggests that some SCFAs play a protective role against diseases like type 2 diabetes, cancer, and heart disease.

Our Clean & Green plan goes beyond a basic Mediterranean diet by helping you integrate even more types of gut power foods. Here's a breakdown.

- **Prebiotics** are various types of fibers that bacteria munch on. You don't fully digest them; rather, they hang out in the large intestine to "feed" healthy bacteria. (Although all prebiotics are fiber, not all fiber is prebiotic.) Prebiotics are naturally a part of whole foods like vegetables (especially, for some reason, garlic, onions, and asparagus), oats, and soybeans. You'll be eating your fill of these over the next 8 weeks.

- **Probiotics** are the bugs themselves that are contained in certain foods—various bacterial species that are capable of rebalancing the healthy population of gut bacteria. Probiotic-rich fare often begins as whole foods; then, with the help of microorganisms, their sugars and carbs are converted into compounds like lactic acid—the stuff that gives sauerkraut and pickles their signature sour taste. Yogurt and tempeh (fermented soybeans) are also probiotic foods. Fermentation converts these foods into probiotic powerhouses that boost levels of good bacteria in your digestive tract, thereby improving the health and balance of your body's collective bacterial community. A healthier microbiome, in turn, has been shown to aid in digestion, crank up immunity, and—some preliminary studies report—reduce blood pressure and help you lose weight. (People with large colonies of some microbes, like those that help the body absorb sugar, are more likely to struggle with weight gain, scientists have found.)

Our panelists reported that eating Clean & Green settled some gut issues, like indigestion and gas; one panelist even experienced a dramatic reduction in her IBS (irritable bowel syndrome) symptoms. Even if you don't suffer from digestive woes, supercharging your gut health by regularly incorporating

Yogurt: Your Ally against Aging

FERMENT MILK WITH BACTERIAL CULTURES and you get yogurt. But there's "yogurt" and then there's the kind that nutrition researchers get excited about. Your job: to hack your way through the yogurt jungle in your supermarket's dairy case and score the healthiest variety. There's reason to be picky.

- PLAIN YOGURT IS ÜBERNUTRITIOUS. Schwartz likes 2% or even full-fat Greek or regular, which boosts satiety more than low-fat; bonus health points if it's grass-fed and/or organic. Compared with milk, yogurt's got 20 to 100 percent more protein, B vitamins, and minerals. Yogurt's acidity also helps the body absorb calcium, zinc, and magnesium. (Many people with mild lactose intolerance find they do just fine on yogurt.)

- YOGURT REDUCES THE RISK FOR TYPE 2 DIABETES AND HIGH BLOOD PRESSURE. Using health data from 100,000-plus participants in three long-running studies, Harvard researchers linked 1 serving of yogurt a day—just cow's milk yogurt, no other dairy products—to an 18 percent lower risk of type 2 diabetes. (The probiotics in yogurt improve insulin sensitivity and reduce inflammation.) In another study, those who ate 1 or more 6-ounce servings of yogurt twice a week over 14 years were about 31 percent less likely to develop high blood pressure than those who didn't.

- IT PROMOTES WEIGHT LOSS. Never mind that scoop of cottage cheese. A recent study by the Jean Mayer USDA Human Nutrition Research Center on Aging at Tufts University found that people who consumed more than 3 weekly servings of yogurt gained less weight over a 1-year period than those who ate less than 1 serving a week. This is probably due to the diversity of gut bugs mentioned above, which can rev the metabolism.

pre- and probiotics into your diet is a great health practice. On our plan, you'll aim to include a few gut-friendly foods on your plate each day. Below is a list of 20 power foods for gut bugs. Come back to it each time you strategize your daily menu.

10 Prebiotic Powerhouses

Prebiotic foods contain fiber that gut bacteria feed on, producing fermentation by-products that benefit health. Here are some of the most potent types.

- Almonds
- Asparagus
- Garlic
- Leafy greens
- Leeks
- Legumes
- Kiwifruit
- Mushrooms
- Oats
- Onions

10 Probiotic Powerhouses

Probiotic-rich foods are fermented by common bacteria, like lactobacilli, that break down the sugars into acids that both preserve the food and impart a salty or tangy flavor. Potent probiotics include:

- Cultured dairy products: yogurt and buttermilk

- Fermented vegetables: sauerkraut, kimchi, beets, lacto-fermented pickles, and traditional cured Greek olives

- Fermented beverages: kefirs and kombuchas

- Raw apple cider vinegar

Pack Protein (Mostly Meatless) into Every Meal

Protein is your body's repair service. It is the building block of every cell, tissue, and organ in your body. Your body gets this nutrient from food, and then uses it to repair tissue, muscle, and bone. It's especially important to get enough protein as you age, when cellular damage becomes an ongoing thing.

You don't need to eat like a caveman to get plenty of protein. But you do need to make sure you're eating the right kinds, in the right portions, particularly as you cut back on the amount of protein-rich red meat in your diet.

Consider this trio of protein-packed foods.

- **3 ounces broiled porterhouse:** 20 g protein, 6 g saturated fat, 0 g fiber

- **3 ounces wild salmon:** 17 g protein, 1 g saturated fat, 0 g fiber

- **½ cup cooked lentils:** 9 g protein, < 1 g saturated fat, 7.5 g fiber

Look beyond the protein and consider the whole package. Unlike the salmon (an excellent source of heart-healthy omega-3 fats) or the lentils (which offer tons of fiber and only a trace of saturated fat), the porterhouse contains calorie-dense saturated fat, also found in animal products like milk and butter.

If you're feeling confused about how bad saturated fat really is, you're not alone. A recent scientific review that got a lot of media play suggested that, contrary to longstanding nutritional wisdom, saturated fats may not contribute to heart disease or early death. But does that mean we can all start eating our red meat like Fred Flintstone? Not quite—the study couldn't rule out the possibility that saturated fat *does* raise the risk of premature death from heart disease. And besides, as you've heard us say, there's a ton of evidence that a plant-based approach to eating (with animal fat in smaller portions) is the proven route to combating heart disease, obesity, and diabetes and to lengthening your telomeres. So for now, Schwartz advises, particularly if you're looking to lose weight, continue to limit saturated fat and get most of your fats from healthy monounsaturated and polyunsaturated fats, like those found in fish, nuts, olives, and avocado.

Back to choosing healthy protein sources. There's even more to weigh, like evidence suggesting that animal protein causes health-threatening inflammation and the fact that conventionally raised red meat tends to contain antibiotics and growth hormones. (Poultry, pork, and even fish may contain antibiotics, too.) A recent study found that people on high-animal-protein diets during middle age were four times more likely to die of cancer than people on low-protein diets—a mortality risk factor comparable to smoking.

Plant proteins—such as beans and lentils, tofu and seitan, quinoa and edamame—simply offer a healthier overall package and are proven to lower heart disease risk. Plant-based proteins also help you in the weight department. One study that followed more than 120,000 Americans for up to 20 years revealed that meat eaters gained an extra pound every 4 years, versus just ½ pound for those who ate a lot of nut proteins.

What's the Right Amount of Protein?

In the United States, the Recommended Dietary Allowance of protein is 46 grams for women and 56 grams for men. (This translates to 0.8 gram per every 2.2 pounds of body weight.) Getting an adequate amount of protein is important to keeping hunger at bay and maintaining lean muscle mass. To find out how much is right for you, multiply your weight by 0.36. For example, if you're 150 pounds, you'd want to consume 54 grams of protein per day—and slightly more if you're super-active or over 65.

Here's a quick overview of the proteins you'll be making friends with on the Younger in 8 Weeks Plan.

Beans. They're similar to meat, poultry, and fish in their contribution of protein; 1 cup packs as much as 17 grams of protein, more than half of the daily 24 grams recommended for women. But they offer what animal proteins can't. First, lots of fiber. Beans also brim with plant chemicals associated with health benefits, such as cancer- and heart disease–fighting anthocyanins and saponins. With so many varieties and flavors to try, you'll want to enjoy them all—common types, such as black beans, chickpeas, and black-eyed peas, as well as more exotic varieties, such as red lentils (popular in Indian cuisine) and flageolets (immature kidney beans), a favorite in France.

Don't let worries about gas keep you away. In one study, less than half of participants who ate a half-cup of beans every day for 3 weeks reported increased flatulence in the first week, and most pronounced it gone by Week 3. The study's conclusion: Our concerns about excessive gas from eating beans may be exaggerated.

Nuts and seeds. Good things come in these small packages—protein, fiber, heart-healthy monounsaturated fats, and vitamins and minerals (B vitamins, vitamin E, iron, zinc, and magnesium). Choose raw nuts and seeds, and skip varieties roasted in oil or slathered in sugar or salt. Watch portions, too—a 1-ounce serving of nuts or ½-ounce serving of seeds packs 160 to 200 calories—so use them to replace other protein foods, like meat or poultry, rather than add them to what you already eat. (You can actually count out how many nuts make up a 1-ounce serving; see page 172.)

Nut and seed butters are also good sources of vegetable protein—for example, a serving of natural almond butter (2 tablespoons) contains almost 7 grams of protein and over 3 grams of fiber. Opt for natural varieties without added sugar. Again, stick to no more than that 2-tablespoon serving size,

Renew Right Now

which contains roughly 100 calories per tablespoon. Stray from tasty but common nut butters made from almonds or peanuts to try more unusual varieties—say, sunflower-seed butter, or tahini, a key ingredient in hummus. Or mix a tablespoon or so of tahini with extra virgin olive oil, apple cider vinegar, and herbs and spices, and enjoy it as a creamy, flavorful salad dressing.

Eggs. New science has exonerated the humble egg. Noting that "cholesterol is not a nutrient of concern for overconsumption," the new federal dietary guidelines recently dropkicked the limit on egg consumption. Go ahead and have an egg a day—or a two-egg meal for breakfast or lunch. Each large egg will score you 6 grams of protein. Opt for organic eggs if you can. And if you can find them, go for free-range or pasture-raised eggs that come from chickens raised outdoors—where they roam free and eat grass and insects, along with certified organic feed—and therefore contain the most healthy omega-3s and vitamin E.

Dairy. A rich source of protein, dairy keeps you full because your body digests it slowly. But full-fat dairy, while it boosts satiety, is quite caloric. If you're interested in weight loss and upping your intake of good-for-you plant nutrients, Schwartz recommends opting for plant-based milks over regular milk (except in cooking). If you do love a splash of regular milk in your coffee or oatmeal, choose 2% or full fat, and always organic over regular (which can expose you to growth hormones used in some conventional dairy operations). Ease up on the cheese, which is super calorie-dense. But calcium- and probiotic-rich yogurt is an exception! See page 47 for more on yogurt's nutritional goodness.

Chicken/poultry. It's an excellent source of protein and B vitamins and leaner than red meat. Once again, seek out organic free-range or pastured birds if you can; they're more nutritious and contain none of the antibiotics of factory-farm-raised birds. Schwartz's recommendation: 3- to 4-ounce servings of poultry two or three times a week.

Red meat (beef, pork, lamb). It's optional on this plan (and discouraged if you want the full telomere-lengthening benefits of a plant-based diet). But if you really miss it, Schwartz recommends grass-fed beef and lamb and pasture-raised pork (which means the pigs were given access to fields and

Renew Right Now

HEALTHY UP TONIGHT'S BURGER

Nearly one-third of us are low in vitamin D, especially in the winter, when we're housebound and get less of the "sunshine vitamin." Vitamin D helps the body to absorb calcium, which is important for strong bones. It also plays a role in healthy immune function and reducing inflammation. And since a recent study published in *JAMA Neurology* suggests that mental function may decline faster in older adults with low levels of vitamin D, it's smart to up your intake. An easy way to do it: Add more mushrooms to your menu.

Mushrooms are the only natural source of vitamin D in the produce aisle and one of the few nonfortified food sources. These flavorful fungi are also rich in the B vitamins riboflavin, niacin, and pantothenic acid, and they break down proteins, fats, and carbohydrates to help fuel our bodies.

Mushrooms can make meat-based dishes like burgers, meatballs, and tacos more flavorful, while slashing unhealthy fats.

. Before you wrinkle your nose, a taste test sponsored by the Mushroom Council showed that people generally preferred meat-mushroom ate a mostly natural diet that may have been supplemented with grain). Grass-fed or pasture-raised meat is worth the price: Studies have shown that it contains higher levels of brain- and heart-healthy omega-3 fatty acids, is typically leaner than its corn-fattened counterpart, and is free of hormones, antibiotics, and other substances (like ammonia gas and food dyes). Also, because red meat is a once-a-week treat, you can buy smaller amounts of higher quality.

Fish. "Fish has fewer calories than chicken but packs more protein and beneficial omega-3 fatty acids," Schwartz says. A 3-ounce serving of salmon contains 17 grams of protein, while the same amount of tuna packs a whopping 25 grams. Schwartz recommends 3- to 4-ounce servings of fish two or three times a week. (For more info on this protein powerhouse, keep reading.)

Go Fish for Better Health

The evidence couldn't be clearer: Fish is amazing for your heart. Low in saturated fat, fish is an excellent source of lean protein. And fatty fish like mackerel, lake trout, and salmon are packed with EPA and DHA, powerful

blends in tacos over 100 percent beef; the taste-test participants said they liked the aromas, flavors, and moisture. They might be tasting what the Japanese call umami—the fifth taste—which elicits savory, brothy, rich, and meaty taste sensations.

To give this tip a try, experiment with the humble button mushroom, the meaty portobello, or the crimini variety, often called baby bellas. Store unwashed mushrooms in the refrigerator for up to 3 days.

When you're ready to make your healthier burgers, be sure to use the right ratio of mushrooms to beef. In the Mushroom Council taste test, people liked a 50-50 blend. Some chefs, however, advise a ratio of 80 percent beef to 20 percent mushrooms, or 4 ounces of 'shrooms per pound of ground beef. Whichever ratio you use, chop the mushrooms and sauté them for up to 5 minutes to release all the liquid. Add your favorite taco/burger spices—Worcestershire sauce, oregano, chopped dried chile pepper, cumin, whatever—and combine the mushroom mixture with the ground beef.

omega-3 fatty acids that help cool the chronic inflammation linked to age-related frailty and disability. Our plan includes fish early and often, so if you're not a huge fan, let these facts persuade you.

Fish boosts brain performance. Researchers at the University of Pittsburgh School of Medicine analyzed the eating habits and brain MRI scans of study volunteers with normal brain health. Those who ate baked or broiled fish at least once a week had greater volumes of gray matter in areas of the brain responsible for memory (4.3 percent) and cognition (14 percent) compared to fish-phobes. (Fish prepared this way contains higher levels of omega-3s than fried, because the heat of frying destroys the fatty acids.)

Fish may save your hearing. A team at Brigham and Women's Hospital tracked 65,215 women for nearly 18 years. Those who ate 2 or more servings a week of fish—fresh, canned, finfish or shellfish, it didn't matter—had a 20 percent lower risk of hearing loss. The more fish they ate, the sharper their hearing stayed. (Researchers speculate there may be something about how omega-3s boost cochlear bloodflow.)

A plant-based diet that includes fish may help prevent colorectal cancer. Compared to omnivores, fish-eating vegetarians (aka pescatarians) had a 43 percent lower chance of colorectal cancer, a study of 77,659 subjects found. Again, thank those omega-3s. Previous research has found that omega-3s have anticancer properties and may help prevent and treat colorectal cancer.

While eating fish is a no-brainer, buying it can be tough. Which fish is more nutritious—wild or farmed? You've heard that some fish are polluted with mercury, which can harm developing nervous systems, so which ones have the lowest levels? And how do you ensure that the fish you buy is "sustainable"—that is, caught or farmed responsibly, to help preserve the long-term health of the planet?

The short answer: It's complicated.

WILD-CAUGHT FISH can contain pesticides, fertilizers, and polychlorinated biphenyls (PCBs) as well as mercury, released into the air through pollution (which becomes methylmercury when it accumulates in streams and oceans). Fish feed on and absorb the methylmercury, which builds up in their bodies—more so in big predator fish, like tuna or swordfish, than in smaller fry. And fishing practices like bottom trawling (in which large, weighted nets are dragged along sea floors, destroying habitats) affect both marine ecosystems and fish populations.

FARMED FISH has seen a boom in demand, but most of the farmed fish we eat comes from other countries. (In fact, the United States imports up to 90 percent of our seafood, half of which is farmed.) Aquaculture has its own drawbacks. Some pens built in open water threaten the surrounding coastlines, reefs, trees, and swamps. Some chemicals used in aquaculture can be toxic to wildlife, and the farmed fish themselves are often given antibiotics and vaccines. Finally, the huge amounts of organic waste fish farms create can contaminate water in the surrounding environment.

If it sounds like there's no clear answer on wild-caught versus farm-raised, you're right. But the benefits of eating seafood outweigh its potential risks. When Schwartz shops for fish, she relies on the following system.

- **Look for wild-caught salmon.** Some studies have found wild salmon to contain more healthy omega-3s than farmed—or wild cod, Schwartz says. If she can't find wild, she'll opt for wild-caught frozen fish, with farm-raised fish as her second option. (Bonus: "Frozen fish is usually cheaper than fresh," says Schwartz.)

- **Only buy fish from the United States.** Unlike some other countries, the United States has strict environmental and food safety laws. Schwartz also checks packages for sustainability labels. These include the Aquaculture Stewardship Council logo on farmed seafood, which indicates that it's free of antibiotic residue and grown under decent environmental and labor conditions. And the Marine Stewardship Council's designation indicates sustainably caught wild fish.

- **Be a "bottom-feeder."** Fish that live near the ocean floor generally contain fewer contaminants than those that live closer to the surface. These include anchovies and sardines as well as some larger fish, such as wild pink salmon and sockeye salmon.

- **Select shellfish.** Not only are clams, mussels, and oysters high in nutrients, they also clean their environment; these "filter feeders" eat what they find as they filter the water around them. This clean-up-as-you-eat trait makes the oceans healthier for other seafood species that we're in danger of losing.

- **Be tuna-smart.** Love canned tuna? Look for brands like Wild Planet that source younger fish—which are lower in mercury—and cook them just once, in the can, to preserve omega-3s.

- **Don't freak out over mercury.** As scary as it sounds, it's a caution aimed mostly at pregnant women, women who are breastfeeding, and young children, who should avoid the four types of fish highest in mercury: tilefish from the Gulf of Mexico, shark, swordfish, and king mackerel. They should also limit their consumption of white albacore tuna—which typically contains three times as much methylmercury on average as canned light tuna—to 6 ounces a week.

- **Let the experts fish for you.** The Monterey Bay Aquarium's "Super Green" list of seafood highlights fish that are both healthy and sustainable. Every fish on the list is a good source of omega-3s, low in mercury, and currently on the aquarium's Seafood Watch "Best Choices" list. Bookmark the site (seafoodwatch.org/consumers/seafood-and-your-health), and check back often, since it's updated regularly.

Drink to Your Health

What you sip can be just as important as what you chew. From dewy skin to disease prevention, healthy bowels to a high-performance brain, the following healthy libations have numerous antiaging benefits. So fill your glass or cup (not plastic! never plastic!)—though, of course, coffee, tea, and wine are optional.

Water

For millions of years, this was the only beverage in town. It met our health needs then, and it still does. Water provides everything your body requires to replace fluids lost through metabolism, breathing, sweating, and waste removal. And when you're low, your body reacts. As little as a 2 percent reduction in your body's normal water volume can give you a headache, cause fatigue, and make it hard to focus, a study published in the *Journal of Nutrition* found. Here are a few of the benefits you'll reap from steady water sipping.

Water promotes weight loss. Dieters who drank two 8-ounce glasses of water before each meal shed 5 pounds more over the course of a year than those who didn't increase their water intake, according to a Virginia Tech study. It's a small change with a big impact that can help prevent weight creep as you age. One of the reasons those extra sips make a difference is because they increase the weight of your meal so you feel fuller and, ergo, eat less.

It gooses your workout. Muscle cells that are low on fluids don't perform as well. The American College of Sports Medicine recommends drinking 8 to 12 fluid ounces of water 10 to 15 minutes before exercise and an additional 3 to 8 fluid ounces of water every 15 to 20 minutes when you work out for less than an hour. (That's a lot of math; basically, just keep sipping when you sweat.)

It protects against cancer. Higher water intake has been linked to a 45 percent lower risk of colon cancer in women. Further, another study found a 53 percent lower risk of bladder cancer in people who consumed 47 ounces (just under six 8-ounce glasses) of water per day, compared with those who consumed less than 14 ounces daily.

It boosts glow. One of the best antiaging "cosmetics" comes straight from your tap. Six to eight glasses of water each day helps skin stay elastic and supple. When your skin is adequately hydrated, it looks healthier and more vibrant, and some wrinkles seem less visible.

It helps you go. It's tough to feel like you can attack your day when your bowels have gone on strike. The more water you drink, the more regular you'll get—and stay.

Green tea

Hot or cold, it may be the healthiest beverage next to water; research has uncovered benefits from protection of brain cells to lowered risk of cancer and stroke.

Green tea's antioxidant polyphenols battle free radicals in your system, which—as you know by now—contribute to age-related degenerative diseases. One of these polyphenols, epigallocatechin-3-gallate (EGCG for short), has been shown to be a powerful antioxidant. Much of the research conducted on humans has been done in Japan, where green tea is a traditional beverage, especially popular among the older generation. While some studies used extracts of green tea (or matcha, which is now turning up in bottled drinks and snack foods and is equally potent), experts say that you can reap similar benefits by the cup.

Green tea revs your memory. A drink with 250 milliliters of green tea extract increased the brain connections that process and store information.

It staves off stroke. Three cups of green tea a day could reduce the risk of stroke by up to 20 percent.

It's bad news for cancer. Digestive cancer risk was 17 percent lower in women who drank at least 3 cups a week.

It may fend off brain drain. Flavonoids—concentrated in berries and tea—may reduce the risk of neurodegenerative conditions and may even help to keep the brain healthy. In a Japanese study of more than 1,000 people over 70, those who drank more than 2 cups of green tea a day reduced the effects of cognitive impairment by 64 percent.

Coffee

If you know you get jittery when you imbibe more than your morning mug, no need to sip more. This plan offers plenty of other ways to boost your energy and benefit your health. But if you kick back daily with a cup or two of your favorite caffeinated brew, you're less likely to die of—well, a lot of things. A study of 229,119 men and 173,141 women ages 50 to 71, published in the *New England Journal of Medicine,* found that drinking 2 or more cups a day equated to a 15 percent reduction in overall death for women and a 10 percent reduction for men versus drinking no coffee. Although the study didn't demonstrate cause and effect, there's definitely a link between drinking coffee and living longer.

What gives this little bean its big benefits? A bunch of virtues: "Coffee contains more than 1,000 compounds that might affect the risk of death," the *New England Journal of Medicine* study helpfully notes—but it calls out antioxidants and caffeine as potentially the two most potent qualities. Here are a few other perks of coffee.

Coffee protects your liver. Coffee is emerging as a therapy to treat the liver, especially nonalcoholic fatty liver disease. The drink seems to counter liver inflammation and improve fat storage as it reduces the risk of liver disease. And a review that combined the results of 16 different studies found that those who drank more than 3 cups of coffee a day seemed to cut their risk of liver cancer by as much as half.

It powers up memory. Researchers at the University of South Florida found that caffeinated coffee increases the levels of a hormone that helps produce new neurons, which may reduce Alzheimer's risk.

It chases away the blues. Depression risk was 20 percent lower in women who drank four 8-ounce cups of coffee a day, a study conducted by the Harvard T.H. Chan School of Public Health found. It's likely that caffeine's effect on the brain chemicals serotonin and dopamine is at work.

It helps you push through a workout. In a University of Illinois study of 25 people, consuming the caffeine equivalent of 2 to 3 cups of coffee an hour before a 30-minute, high-intensity workout reduced perceived muscle pain.

Red wine

A nightly glass of red wine with dinner is a pleasure with health perks, research suggests, with some of the benefits attributed to the plant compound resveratrol. Found in red wine and grapes as well as dark chocolate, this potent antioxidant seems to have heart-protective effects, including shielding cells from oxidative stress and relaxing the coronary arteries.

Despite a recent finding that resveratrol did not reduce disease risk, there's still ample evidence that moderate drinkers—those who consume no more than 1 serving of alcohol a day—have a lower risk of heart trouble and death from any cause. There was even a 2-year study of people on the Mediterranean diet that found that those who drank a nightly glass of red wine (versus water) had significantly higher levels of "good" HDL cholesterol, a healthier cholesterol ratio, and better glycemic control (which affects diabetes). Sleep quality even improved among wine drinkers.

Previous studies of red wine have shown other benefits.

Red wine boosts brainpower. Resveratrol has been shown to hamper the formation of beta-amyloid protein, a key ingredient in the plaque found in the brains of people with Alzheimer's.

It protects against cancer. The resveratrol you get from drinking one glass of red wine three or four times a week may be enough to starve nascent cancer cells. When researchers dosed human cancer cells with resveratrol, they found that the compound inhibited the key action of a cancer-feeding protein.

Our Younger in 8 Weeks Plan cuts alcohol consumption during the first 2 weeks, mainly because it's calories you don't need and it lowers inhibitions, so you're more easily derailed. It's allowed back (a drink a night) in Week 3, though Schwartz encourages skipping it during the entire plan if possible—again, unnecessary calories.

Spice Up Your Life

A staple of East Indian cuisine, curry is a rich blend of spices that includes turmeric, the spice that gives curry its distinctive golden hue. Population studies in India suggest that the country has one of the lowest rates of Alzheimer's disease in the world, possibly because they eat a lot of turmeric. This tangy spice with a gorgeous deep-yellow hue is packed with curcumin, a chemical with potent antioxidant and anti-inflammatory properties.

Research backs up the link between curcumin and lower rates of Alzheimer's. In a recent small study, Japanese researchers gave people with Alzheimer's (who displayed classic symptoms like irritability, anxiety, and agitation) doses of turmeric in capsule form (equivalent to 100 milligrams of curcumin). After 3 months, their symptoms improved significantly, the study found.

You'll find turmeric (via curry powder) in a few of our Clean & Green recipes. Here are a couple of other ways to get your daily dose.

Get to love Indian cuisine. Hugely flavorful and heavy on beans, veggies, fish, and spice blends, it's perfect for your slow cooker. Don't know your *biryani* from your *vindaloo*? Check out Indian food made easy at prevention.com/food/cook/healthy-indian-food-recipes.

Brew up some spicy brain protection. Turmeric tea is simple to make. Bring 1 cup of water to a boil. Add ¼ teaspoon ground turmeric. Reduce the heat to a simmer for 10 minutes. Strain the tea through a mesh strainer or a cheesecloth into a cup, and add a dash of ginger or a squeeze of fresh lemon to taste.

Give knee arthritis a shot of relief. You can do this by sipping a (virgin) Bloody Mary spiked with turmeric. A study of people with knee osteoarthritis showed that the spice was as effective as ibuprofen at relieving the ache, with less stomach irritation. Roxanne B. Sukol, MD, a preventive medicine specialist at the Cleveland Clinic, has her osteoarthritis patients make this pain-relieving cocktail with tomato juice, a few drops of olive oil, a dash or two of ground black pepper, and the contents of two capsules of curcumin/turmeric. Don't neglect the olive oil and black pepper—both help the body absorb turmeric.

There's another spice that research suggests can help jumpstart weight loss, reduce body fat, and improve unhealthy cholesterol levels naturally: cumin.

Iranian researchers randomly split 88 overweight women into two groups.

For 3 months, both groups received nutrition counseling and ate 500 fewer calories a day. But one group consumed 3 grams (a bit less than 1 teaspoon) of cumin powder daily mixed into 5 ounces of yogurt. A control group got the same amount of yogurt minus the cumin. At the end of the trial, the cumin group lost 13 pounds, 3 more than those in the control group. But that wasn't all. The cumin group reduced body fat percentage by 14.64 percent—almost *triple* the 4.91 percent loss posted by the control group—apparently due to the addition of the fat-burning spice.

There were internal benefits, too. The cumin group's levels of harmful blood fats, or triglycerides, dropped by 23 points, while the control group's levels fell only by 5. Cumin eaters also knocked an average of nearly 10 points off their "bad" LDL cholesterol, compared to the control group average of just ½ point.

Cumin is rich in phytosterols, plant chemicals known to inhibit the absorption of cholesterol in the body. Since this is the first research to show the spice has weight-loss benefits, the study authors also speculate that cumin, like other hot spices, temporarily increases metabolic rate.

Cumin has a distinctive earthy, nutlike flavor. Since cumin mixed into plain yogurt isn't the most enticing snack idea, here are some tastier ways to use this spice.

- Sprinkle it over your favorite roasted veggie recipe.

- Add a dash to mayo or hummus for sandwiches and dips.

- Sprinkle it into a batch of roasted chickpeas or nuts.

Now it's time to MOVE into a fitter body that looks—and feels—years younger.

SUCCESS!

Kate Pelham-Hambly, 41

MY STORY Usually it's the kids in the household who complain about having to eat their vegetables. But at Kate Pelham-Hambly's house, she was the veggie hater. "I love plants; they're beautiful," she said before starting the Younger in 8 Weeks Plan. "The problem is that I hate eating them. I don't like the way they smell. I don't like the way they taste. I don't like the way they feel in my mouth."

Fast-forward a week or two, and Kate is eating an entire head of broccoli in one sitting. What changed? One of her fellow test panelists suggested that she roast her veggies. "I liked how the broccoli became kind of crispy. It really transformed the flavor. Roasting makes them sweeter."

Kate now shops, cooks, and eats completely differently. She does the bulk of her shopping in the produce and natural food sections, skipping the soda and junk food aisles. And her ordinarily picky family isn't complaining.

Instead of red meat, now they almost exclusively use turkey or chicken. "My 10-year-old son says turkey bacon is meatier than the regular kind," she said. Pasta is now whole

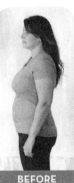

BEFORE

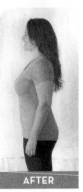

AFTER

grain, and rice is either brown or wild. In place of chips, they snack on roasted garbanzo beans, steamed edamame, low-fat mozzarella sticks, blanched almonds, apples, and clementines. "My 13-year-old daughter has taken to looking up clean eating recipes on Pinterest," she said. And her husband ordered a portobello mushroom cheesesteak instead of a burger when he was out with colleagues. "He said that he feels great since we've been eating lighter and didn't want to stuff his face with fattening food!"

Kate is feeling the payoff, too. She no longer mindlessly eats in front of the television, in the car, or standing over the sink. Now she sits down and enjoys meals without any distractions. "I really focus on the food and savor it," she said. "When I slow down, I eat less."

"I feel like I've been given the code to healthy living," she added. "I'm shopping, cooking, and eating with the knowledge of what is good for my body and why. I'm consistently exercising 5 or 6 days a week. So many other programs seem like finite plans—30 days to a better you. This one teaches you what you need to live your life in the healthiest way possible."

LOOK AT ME

- Increased
  energy level
  23 percent

- Lowered high
  blood pressure

- Eliminated
  migraines

- Boosted
  confidence
  17 percent

- Weight lost:
  11.4 pounds

- Inches lost: **4.25**

Tip TRY USING
TECHNOLOGY
TO STAY ON TRACK.
Kate used the app
MyFitnessPal to scan
food labels and easily
track calories and
other nutrients, which
helped her manage
portion sizes. A Fitbit
activity monitor moti-
vated her to move
more by creating chal-
lenges with friends
and family to see who
could take more steps.

MOVE

Boost Energy and Build New Strength

Sweat really is the ultimate youth serum. Frequent exercise—and more time spent on your feet, in general—can ratchet up your energy while giving you the speed and endurance needed to torch that hiking trail or finish that road race. You'll also have more strength and stamina to crush it at work—and to do more of the things you love to do (garden) or need to do (clean out the basement).

Exercise literally makes you younger—right down to your DNA. When researchers examined the genetics and lifestyle habits of more than 2,400 twins, they found that the telomeres (those caps on the end of your DNA that correlate with age) of regular exercisers looked 10 years younger than those of their sedentary peers. Working out also reduces the effects of age-stoking inflammation. In one study, researchers tracked the exercise habits and inflammation markers of more than 4,000 middle-aged subjects for more than 10 years and found that those who got 2.5 hours of moderate exercise each week—about 20 minutes a day—reduced inflammation by at least 12 percent.

"Living the life you want starts from the inside out, and the key is exercise," says Dr. Vonda Wright, who helped design our Younger in 8 Weeks Workout with ACE-certified fitness instructor Michele Stanten.

The benefits kick in quickly, and they go beyond weight loss. "My joints don't hurt, I'm not stiff in the morning, I sleep better, and my skin looks great," said test panelist Lisa Boland a little more than halfway through the program. If a sit-down lifestyle has robbed you of muscle, vitality, and mobility, our workouts can help you steal them back.

Use It or Lose It

What is "it"? Breath. Strength. Muscle. Agility. Your body—that exquisitely engineered temple of tissue, blood, and bone—was designed to *move*. And age doesn't change that. In fact, remarkable studies coauthored by Dr. Wright show that losing "it" is related more to inactivity than age. And she has the pictures to prove it.

In one study, Dr. Wright and her colleagues gathered 40 competitive runners, swimmers, cyclists, and triathletes. All the participants, ages 40 to 81, trained 4 or 5 days a week. The research team measured the athletes' lean muscle mass—for example, leg strength and intramuscular fat tissue. Take a look at the results.

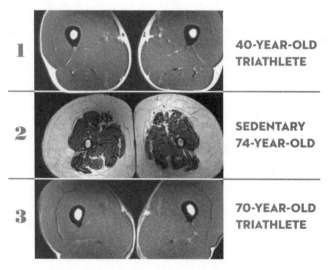

1   **40-YEAR-OLD TRIATHLETE**

2   **SEDENTARY 74-YEAR-OLD**

3   **70-YEAR-OLD TRIATHLETE**

Image 1 is the cross-section of the thigh of a 40-year-old triathlete; you'll see very little white peripheral fat. Image 2 is the thigh of a sedentary 74-year-old, with thick fat and loose muscle architecture—"like a fatty rump roast," Dr. Wright says—and Image 3 is the thigh of a 70-year-old triathlete—lean and fit. Those scans are dramatic evidence of the use-it-or-lose-it principle of exercise. The athletes in their seventies and eighties had almost as much lean muscle mass in their thighs as their 40-year-old counterparts, and very little fat tissue. "You want your muscle to look like lean flank steak," Dr. Wright says.

Why is that? Because lean muscle—the kind low in fat and packed with mitochondria (mitos for short)—has a powerful influence on weight, energy level, and risk of diabetes and heart disease. Even your chances of surviving a hospital stay or of beating cancer are affected by the health of your muscle.

A healthy, lean muscle contains tons of efficient mitos, which serve as the energy producers of cells, converting glucose and fat into fuel. They increase in number the more that we move. Stop exercising, however, and your body notices that it doesn't need as many mitos and tells the extras to take a hike. Over time, this key internal power source dwindles. Your energy plummets, and so does your capacity to burn fat. So muscle tissue grows marbled, raising your risk of some chronic diseases and making physical activity even more challenging. Quite a vicious cycle.

Bottom line: The more you exercise, the more mitos you make, and the more efficient your muscles get at burning fat and providing energy. Regular strength training is one proven way to reverse this process, but aerobic workouts have an effect, too, sparking the cellular system that creates new mitochondria. And this reversal can happen quickly! In one study of sedentary men and women in their late sixties, participants who walked on a treadmill or rode an exercise bike for 30 to 40 minutes 4 to 6 days a week increased their mitochondria volume by as much as 68 percent in just 12 weeks.

The Younger in 8 Weeks Workout

You'll be using "it" over the next 8 weeks—and hopefully beyond—so you don't lose it. Our workouts promote the essential qualities you need—endurance, strength, flexibility, and balance—to turn your muscles into lean, mito-making machines. Here's a snapshot of the routines, which begin on page 287.

- Endurance (aerobic) exercise—also called cardiovascular exercise or cardio—increases your respiration and heart rate. Our cardio workouts keep your heart, lungs, and circulatory system healthy and improve your overall fitness.

- Strength training, aka lifting weights, not only firms your muscles and strengthens your bones, but it also does wonders for your mood and self-confidence. Our strength workout starts in Week 4, and there's an Advanced Strength Workout to step up to when you're ready.

- Flexibility—the ability of muscle to lengthen and allow your joints to move through their full range of motion—is the hallmark of a youthful body. Our Sunrise Stretch, Dynamic Warmup, flexibility stretches, and foam-roller routine help keep your muscles limber and increase range of motion, which can help reduce pain, relieve stiffness, and prevent injury.

- Balance exercises help keep you steady on your feet and will guard against falls. Our optional balance moves are so simple you can do them anytime, anywhere.

If you're thinking, "Whoa, that sounds like a lot!" rest assured that we don't throw all of these things at you at once. Instead, we step them up gradually, starting with a daily stretch in Week 1 and introducing basic cardio in

Turn-Back-the-Clock Breakthrough
A BRIGHT IDEA FOR WEIGHT LOSS (IN 20 MINUTES A DAY)

One unlikely weapon against weight gain? Morning sun. In a recent study, people who got most of their daily exposure to even moderately bright light in the a.m. had significantly lower BMIs (that stands for body mass index, or weight-to-height ratio) than those who got most of their exposure later in the day.

In the study, researchers from Northwestern University recruited 54 people to wear wrist monitors, which kept tabs on their light exposure, activity, and sleep patterns for 7 days. They also had the participants fill out food logs to track their eating patterns. After factoring in other possible influences, such as age, gender, and sleep, researchers found that the impact of morning light on weight accounted for roughly 20 percent of the subjects' BMIs. In other words, those with earlier light exposure weighed less. We're not talking a ton of light, either: The minimum threshold for a lower BMI was just 500 lux. Consider that outdoor light measures more than 1,000 lux, even on a cloudy day. On a day with clear blue skies? It's more like 100,000 lux. The thinking is that light could have an impact on metabolism, hunger, and satiety.

To take advantage, you just need 20 to 30 minutes of morning light every day between 8 a.m. and noon, the study said. Exercising outdoors fills this quota, even in the winter. And sunscreen—which you should always wear—won't dampen the outcome; researchers believe sunlight's effects go directly from the eye to the brain. ■

Week 2. As noted, strength comes in at Week 4, and we'll keep nudging up the duration and intensity as the weeks progress. In all, you'll never spend more than 30 to 45 minutes daily on the exercise portion of the program (unless you want to add on the optional moves—up to you!). Turn to page 304 to check out sample weekly schedules.

Build Endurance with Cardio

Imagine two friends on a hike. They approach a steep hill and start to climb. Minutes later, one is breathless; her heart pounds, her lungs burn. The other takes that hill like a boss. Her heart and blood vessels, which make up the cardiovascular system, can supply the oxygen her body demands.

This scenario illustrates why we need cardio. It builds *endurance*, your body's ability to deliver "vitamin O"—oxygen—to your muscles, which allows them to work hard. A stronger heart doesn't need to beat as fast. It also pumps blood more efficiently, which improves flow to all parts of your body. So cardio conditions your heart and blood vessels so they can deliver oxygen to your muscle cells quickly and efficiently.

This conditioning becomes more important as you age. With every beat of your heart, a volume of blood (called stroke volume), nutrients, and oxygen whooshes through your body. The maximum volume of oxygen your working muscles can extract from your blood is called max VO_2.

Beginning when we're 25 to 30 years old, max VO_2 declines 5 to 15 percent every 10 years. One reason for that: As we grow older, we're typically less active. We lose it rather than use it. But regular exercise can deliver a dramatic turnaround. In fact, it can give older adults the same 10 to 30 percent increase in max VO_2 that young adults get.

An increase in max VO_2 means your cardiovascular system is working to capacity. And the fitter you are, the more efficiently your muscles consume oxygen. Translation: Your endurance increases, and suddenly, you can take the stairs without stopping to rest.

To really boost your endurance—and to prevent and reduce high blood pressure, diabetes, high cholesterol, and belly fat—fast bursts of high-intensity aerobic exercise followed by short rest periods are far more effective than continuous moderate-intensity exercise, says Dr. Wright. That's why our cardio routine includes *intervals*. When you do intervals, you alternate between short bursts of higher-intensity activity and short recovery periods—like if

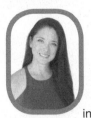

Dr. Vonda Wright says . . .
YOU REALLY CAN "JUST DO IT"

No matter what your age or fitness level, your body remembers how to move toward better health. To give in to the myth that you can be too old or too out of shape to exercise is to expect too little out of life.

Growing up in Kansas, I recall a woman in our town; she was around 60. Like my dad, she was a runner. Now, this was back in the 1970s. They'd say, "Look at Milly, running at her age." But it wasn't meanness. The town celebrated her for that.

Here in Pittsburgh, where I live, there's a race called the Liberty Mile—a 1-mile run straight down one of our streets. I sponsor the masters age heat. Last year, as the pack raced toward the finish line, there was one runner far ahead of the rest. As I watched them come into focus, I realized that the runner in front was Sonia, 46, an everyday woman like you and me. Strong, lean, and powerful, she finished the race in 4 minutes and 45 seconds—a full 10 yards in front of the men trailing her. It was such a joy to watch her cross that finish line.

As an orthopedic surgeon, I know that mobility saves lives. There are so many excuses you can make not to exercise, but there's always a way to fit it into your busy day. I run with my husky; I practice ballet with my daughter (or in the summer, while she swims, I run in the water instead of sitting poolside); and I'm so physically active in the operating room that I can burn about 2,000 calories. I've seen so many of my patients come to live healthy, vital, active, joyful lives—competing in races, even climbing to Everest basecamp. Once, some of them thought they were too old and too out of shape to exercise. Don't believe it for a second. If they can, so can you.

you ran a block for a bus, and then slowed to a walk once it stopped for you. Burst and recover. Burst and recover. That's interval training. Intervals also deliver a powerful metabolic punch, meaning that you burn calories at rest even hours after you finish working out.

If you have or are at risk for type 2 diabetes, the benefits of adding interval training are huge. One study found that interval training while walking—specifically, walking 3 minutes briskly followed by 3 minutes at an easier pace, repeated for an hour—can help control blood sugar. Researchers suspect that during high-intensity bursts, your muscles gobble more glucose (or

Six Great Reasons to Get Moving—Today

1. An active lifestyle can **cut your risk of age-related macular degeneration** by up to 70 percent, according to a study of 4,000 adults. This incurable eye disease makes it difficult to read and drive, and it's the most common cause of blindness after age 60.

2. Women ages 50 to 75 who did 45 minutes of moderate-intensity cardio 5 days a week had one-third as many colds as those who did once-weekly stretch sessions, one study found.

3. Women ages 60 and older who walked or danced for at least an hour four times a week woke up half as often and slept an average 48 minutes more a night than sedentary women, a study in the journal *Sleep Medicine* found.

4. In another study, walking 2 miles five times a week prevented diabetes better than running nearly twice as much. Because fat is the primary fuel for moderate exercise, walking may better improve the body's ability to release insulin and control blood sugar.

5. Exercise is linked to a lower risk of Alzheimer's disease among older people; research now shows it can prevent brain fog at a much younger age.

6. Sedentary, overweight women ages 50 and older who took up exercise lowered their levels of C-reactive protein—an inflammatory blood marker linked to heart disease—by 10 percent after 1 year, a recent study found.

blood sugar) for fuel. Remember, you tailor those short explosions of effort to your current level of fitness. And anyone—no matter your size or the shape you're in—can do it.

Starting in Week 2, you'll perform a cardio workout 3 to 5 days a week. You'll do your first cardio session at a nice steady pace, moving to intervals in Week 3. You can walk outdoors or use any type of cardio machine, and you can do cardio and lift weights on the same day once weight training starts in Week 4.

The only real rule: Get your heart pumping. *Intensity* is a measure of how hard your body is working. You can precisely measure your target heart rate—the level at which your heart is being exercised but not overworked—by using a heart rate monitor (some fitness trackers also measure heart rate). But a far easier option—and totally sufficient for the purposes of our workout plan—is to use Rate of Perceived Exertion (RPE), a simple, gadget-free scale for gauging your exercise intensity. While the scale is not as precise as a heart rate monitor, studies show that perceived exertion correlates well with heart rate. In other words, if you think you're working hard, your heart rate is probably elevated.

The RPE scale runs from 0 to 10, and the numbers correspond to how challenging you find an activity. For example, 0 would be how you feel as you watch TV; 10, how you would likely feel at the end of an exercise stress test. Keep the following in mind, as we'll be using the RPE scale in our cardio workout.

0–1 Little or no exertion; you're at your desk or crashed on the couch

2–3 You're walking slowly, at a stroll; this pace is how you warm up your body before exercise and cool it down afterward

4–5 Your muscles are warm and you're starting to break a sweat; your breathing rate is slightly elevated but you can still hold a conversation while you exercise

6–7 You're working harder but can still utter a full sentence without gasping

8–9 You're breathing hard and getting close to your maximum limit; you can only say a few words

10 You're at the absolute limit of what you can do; you can't waste a breath on a single word

Lift Weights to Maximize Muscle

To be strong, healthy, and feel 10 years younger, you have to hit the weights. Strength training is as vital to your health as mammograms, and it becomes even more critical after age 50, says Dr. Wright. That's because, starting in their thirties, women who don't do strengthening activities lose up to 5 percent of their lean muscle tissue per decade—and that percentage increases after age 65.

There's a direct correlation between your health and your muscle mass. The more muscle you build, the faster your metabolism hums, which makes it easier to lose weight and keep it off. In fact, strength training can rev metabolic rate by up to 15 percent. That's above and beyond its other proven benefits, which include reducing your risk for diabetes, stroke, and heart disease and cutting your risk for falls. Not to mention that muscle has the effect of shrink-wrapping your body so you look firmer and more toned.

As you've learned, age-related declines in muscle reduce the activity and number of mitochondria in cells. Strength training, a key part of the mito revival, helps you keep the muscle you have while building more as a buffer against natural loss. Moreover, strength training stresses muscles in a good way, causing tiny tears to the tissue, which in turn jumpstarts your body's muscle-building process.

A substantial body of research links strength training to a host of other benefits.

It builds bone. Strength training is what's called a weight-bearing exercise—one that pits your body against the force of gravity—and as such, it promotes bone strength. In a yearlong study of postmenopausal women, those who trained with weights just 2 days a week had 1 percent gains in hip and spine bone density, 75 percent increases in strength, and 13 percent increases in balance. Those who didn't train lost bone, strength, and balance.

It helps you sleep. People who exercise regularly (both cardio and strength training) doze off more quickly, sleep more deeply, awaken less often, and sleep longer. The sleep benefits are comparable to treatment with sleep medications, but without the morning-after grogginess.

It reduces joint pain. In a Tufts University study, older men and women with moderate to severe knee osteoarthritis who lifted weights reduced their pain by 43 percent. Even better, strength training worked just as well as, if not better than, medications.

It sharpens your mind. In one study, 62 men between the ages of 65 and 75 were put through a 6-month strength-training routine. One group lifted at a moderate intensity, while the other lifted at a high intensity. Before and at the end of the study, researchers tested the participants' concentration skills and short-term and long-term memories. Both the moderate- and high-intensity groups significantly improved their scores on the neurological tests, reported a higher quality of life, and showed much higher levels of the protein IGF-1, a growth factor that promotes the survival of brain neurons. It may be that lifting weights increases bloodflow to your brain—which brings more oxygen and nutrients to your nervous system—or promotes higher levels of the brain-boosting IGF-1. Or that strength training lifts your mood, and research has shown that for older adults, a better mood is linked with sharper cognitive performance. Whatever the reason, it's time to grab the weights.

You'll begin the strength workout in Week 4 and continue with it 2 to

Renew Right Now

HOTWIRE YOUR WORKOUT WITH CAFFEINE

It happens—exercise time rolls around, and you're less than pumped. Findings from one study offer a simple way to jack up your get-up-and-go: Sip caffeine before your workout.

Researchers from Coventry University in England had 13 people do a typical strength-training workout on two separate occasions, 2 days apart. An hour before one workout, the participants drank a caffeinated beverage. An hour before the other, they had a caffeine-free placebo drink. The results? The group completed an average of 38 percent more repetitions of each exercise during the caffeinated workout. Participants also reported feeling less tired during the caffeinated session and more enthusiasm about working out again soon.

Here's why caffeine helps. When you put your muscles to work, a molecule called adenosine builds up in your muscle cells. Adenosine muddles communication within your central nervous system, which hinders muscle activity and limits your workout potential. However, caffeine appears to curb adenosine buildup. (Other studies have shown that caffeine can enhance performance during cardiovascular exercise, too.)

To experience the benefit found in the study, you need to consume 10 to 15 milligrams of caffeine per 10 pounds of body weight. For a 130-pound woman, that's about 175 milligrams of caffeine, found in one cup of coffee (depending on the strength of the brew). *Note:* If you have heart disease, high blood pressure, or other heart problems, talk to your doctor before you combine caffeine and exercise. And if caffeine gives you the jitters, skip it and drink water instead. Here are a few other things to keep in mind.

DON'T GET OVERLY PERKED. Avoid sipping more than the recommended daily amount of caffeine—400 milligrams for healthy adults. That's about four cups of coffee, 10 cans of soda, or two energy drinks (though Schwartz recommends two or three 8-ounce cups). Consume more than that maximum and you may feel heart-poundingly anxious or irritable.

KEEP THAT WATER BOTTLE FULL. While caffeine can goose your workout, you'll run out of gas if you're not properly hydrated. So sip water before and after your workout, and throughout the day.

SIP YOUR LAST CUP WAAAY BEFORE BED. Consuming caffeine as long as 6 hours before bedtime can significantly disrupt sleep, according to a study published in the *Journal of Clinical Sleep Medicine*.

3 days a week through Week 8 (and hopefully way beyond that!). If it becomes too easy at any point, graduate to our Advanced Workout. (Or start this more challenging workout after Week 8, whenever you're ready.)

If you're new to lifting weights, don't sweat it. It's not as difficult as you think. In the strength-training section of the Younger in 8 Weeks Workout, we've got some guidelines to cover proper form and help you learn the ropes. Keep in mind that it's normal to experience slight muscle soreness or fatigue afterward. It should fade after a week or two. Also be sure to take a day of rest between workouts so that your muscles have time to repair themselves.

Focus on Flexibility

For many of us, stretching is like flossing. You know it's important, but it's all too easy to let it slide. Besides, why stretch when you could spend those minutes on the parts of your workout that burn calories and build muscle?

This attitude sends fitness experts into face-palm mode. Stretching is as important to overall fitness as cardio and strength training because it increases *flexibility*. Right now, you may not value flexibility the way you do a slimmer waistline and a firmer butt. But it's the foundation of your future health, mobility, and independence.

Flexibility is a matter of muscle. Stretching a muscle lengthens the tendons that attach it to the bone. Flexible muscles have give; stiff muscles and tendons don't. Think of those old, dry rubber bands you find in the back of your desk drawer. Try to use them, and they snap. Try to use stiff muscles, and they may "snap," too. Bingo—you're laid up with an injured back, shoulder, or leg.

Besides, flexibility isn't just for your future health; it can improve your life right now. It'll be easier to tie your shoes, clip your toenails, make love (in whatever order of priority you wish). You'll also be less likely to get injured when you work out or tackle everyday tasks, and pliable muscles significantly reduce the likelihood of back pain.

Stretching also improves circulation, which helps protect against chronic age-related ills like type 2 diabetes and kidney disease. Further, the easier it is for you to touch your toes, the lower your blood pressure and heart disease risk are likely to be. In a Japanese study, the most limber over-40 women had about 7 percent less arterial stiffness (a marker of heart disease) than their less-flexible peers. Increased bloodflow from stretching may expand arteries, which helps keep them pliable.

Renew Right Now

STRENGTHEN BONES IN 2 MINUTES

Throughout our lives, new bone cells grow and old bone cells break down to make way for new, stronger bone. Between the ages of 18 and 25, we reach *peak bone mass*, which means we're in possession of the greatest amount of bone we'll ever have. As we grow older, however, we have to work to maintain that thick, solid bone.

Weight-bearing exercise promotes the mineralization that keeps bones strong. Here's another way to strengthen your bones in a minute a day: Hop to it.

Jumping up and down 10 times twice a day provides greater bone-building benefits than running or jogging, a study of 60 women ages 25 to 50 found. In this study, researchers had volunteers—all osteoporosis-free—jump as high as they could 10 times a day with 30-second pauses between each jump. In 4 months, the volunteers increased their hip bone mineral density by 0.5 percent. If that doesn't sound like much, consider this: The nonjumping group members *lost* about 1.3 percent of their bone density over the same period.

How can such a simple action be better for bones than a regular run? It seems that the repeated stress of running desensitizes bone; it just doesn't react as much. But when you jump with at least 30 seconds between jumps, bone can get stressed without becoming desensitized. And that means it continues to respond to the impact by building more bone mass. Twice a day, jump up and down 10 to 20 times, pausing 30 seconds between each jump. Be consistent—you have to do the jumps daily to get the benefits.

As with all forms of exercise, flexibility is a use-it-or-lose-it proposition. Also, it's vital to keep it up. While you're likely to feel the benefits of regular stretching sessions in 6 weeks, stop and you'll lose them all within a month.

Persuaded yet? We're confident that once you start stretching daily, you'll want to stick with it. Stretch sessions, with their focus on slow, deliberate movements and deep breathing, can become the oasis of calm in an otherwise crazy day.

You'll begin stretching during your first week on the program (our panelists found it quite pleasurable). Our fast, three-move Sunrise Stretch is designed to unkink muscles, reduce stiffness, and rev you up for the day. If you can't fit it into your morning, do it to melt away stress during the day or to relax at day's end.

In Week 2 and beyond, you'll incorporate other types of stretching. Before workouts, do our Dynamic Warmup (page 291) to wake up your muscles so they're ready for action. When you're done, perform our flexibility stretches (page 298) to increase your flexibility and range of motion.

Keep Your Balance

When you're young, it's no big deal to stay firmly on your feet; balance is an automatic reflex. Your muscles work together with three of your body's sensory systems: visual; the sensations received constantly from nerves in your skin, muscles, limbs, and joints (proprioception); and nerve signals from the inner ear (vestibular). These systems give your brain information about your position in space and the pull of gravity. Your brain's sensory cortex processes this intel and coordinates your body's response.

Voilà: You take the stairs and don't look down; recover quickly when you trip on a crack in the sidewalk; dodge, dip, duck, and dive just like the Average Joes in the film *DodgeBall*. With your brain and body working together, you'll walk with confidence and without any conscious thought.

With age, however, you're on shakier ground—literally. After age 25, the connections between our brains and muscles become less accurate, says Dr. Wright. Age-related changes like weak muscles, slowed reflexes, and vision problems affect balance. Certain health issues, such as inner ear disorders or nerve damage do, too. When balance falters, so does the drive to stay active. After older people fall once, they may begin to limit their activities. As they move less, their muscles weaken further and falls become a real possibility. In fact, one-third of Americans 65 or older falls each year, but less than half tell their doctors.

Regular exercise seems to help preserve balance and prevent falls, a review of multiple studies concluded. Strength training is particularly beneficial; it helps muscles react more quickly when you're thrown off balance.

You can retrain your neuromuscular pathways and improve your balance in less than 5 minutes a day with the three Antiaging Balance Exercises found on page 316 (they're introduced in Week 5, but feel free to start them anytime). As you reduce your risk of future falls, you reap an immediate benefit—a greater capacity to push yourself harder when you work out, which raises your overall level of fitness.

How's your balance right now? Get off the couch and test yourself. It's helpful to have someone time you.

- Stand with your feet together, anklebones touching, and your arms folded across your chest. Close your eyes. Though it's normal to sway a little, you should be able to stand for 60 seconds without moving your feet.

- Place one foot directly in front of the other and close your eyes. You should be able to stand for at least 38 seconds on both sides.

- Stand on one foot and bend your other knee, lifting that foot off the floor without letting it touch your standing leg. (Do this in a doorway so you can grab the sides if you start to fall.) Repeat with your eyes closed. People age 60 and younger can typically hold the pose for about 29 seconds with their eyes open, 21 seconds with their eyes closed. People age 61 and older: 22 seconds with eyes open, 10 seconds with eyes closed.

If you find you aren't able to hold these poses for the minimum length of time, consider integrating our balance moves into your day—as you chat on the phone, do the dishes, or brush your teeth. You can also flick them into your workouts as you rest between sets. If you feel unsteady, do these moves with a sturdy chair next to you or nearby so you can grab it if needed.

Take a Stand against Sitting

You walk 30 minutes a day and sleep 8 hours a night. How do you spend the rest of those 15.5 hours? On your rear if you're the typical American. At work, we sit. We come home and sit. No study we've ever heard about links sitting to longevity. In fact, researchers have begun to suspect that exercise—even daily exercise—may not counteract the effects of the park-it American lifestyle.

Here's proof in stark numbers: A study of 7,744 men ages 20 to 89 examined the relationship between cardiovascular disease and two sedentary behaviors, driving and watching TV. Those who reported being sedentary more than 23 hours a week had a 64 percent greater risk of dying from heart disease than those who reported being inactive less than 11 hours a week, according to the study.

How do you counteract the insidious effects of our sit-down culture? Build motion into your day—every day. Get up and move for just 1 minute as often as possible during the day.

Renew Right Now

EASE SORENESS WITH A PILL (NOT THE ONE YOU THINK)

You feel great during your spin class or strength-training workout. It's afterward that your muscles feel sore. If that sounds like you, consider adding a fishy fix to your foam-roller routine: omega-3 fatty acids. In one Indiana University study, taking an omega-3 fish oil supplement before exercise was found to significantly reduce muscle soreness afterward.

In the study, half the participants took 400 milligrams of fish oil for 26 days; the other half took a placebo. After that time period, all the participants were put through a 20-minute downhill running workout on the treadmill, shown to cause muscle damage (as anyone who's tried downhill running can tell you). Over the next 4 days, the participants kept taking the supplement (or the placebo) and were asked to rate muscle soreness in their legs on a scale from 0 to 10, or "no soreness" to "unbearably painful." They also had their blood tested for markers of inflammation.

Compared to the placebo group, the fish oil group reported significantly less soreness in their legs and had lower levels of inflammation markers in their blood. The omega-3 fatty acids in fish oil have anti-inflammatory properties. If you'd rather not take a fish oil supplement, you can always add more fish to your diet.

Why would we suggest this? Because there's a study that links "breaks in sedentary time" to better scores on several measures of metabolic health. In this study of 168 middle-aged people, researchers measured their volunteers' waist circumference and other health indicators. Then they gave participants gadgets called accelerometers—which measure physical activity—and instructed them to wear these for 7 days in a row while they were awake.

The accelerometer data let researchers see how much time participants spent sedentary and physically active, as well as how intense their activity was. The results? Overall, the total number of breaks in sedentary time, even when they lasted a minute, was associated with significantly lower waist circumference, BMI, triglycerides, and blood sugar. In other words, if the volunteers were vertical, it helped.

Use these move-more, sit-less tips as a starting point; feel free to substitute strategies that work for you.

- Buy one of the many fitness-tracking apps or wearable monitors on the market and challenge yourself to hit a daily step count (set a baseline goal, then aim for an additional 2,000 a week until you hit 10,000). You'll start marching in place just to boost your number!

- At your desk, hop up and down for a minute. If you own an old weighted jump rope, bring it to the office and loop it over a chair as a visual reminder—finally, a use for it.

- If you're pressed for time, head for the nearest flight of stairs and trot up and back.

- Hold or suggest a "moving meeting." An outdoor walk-and-talk not only gives you the benefit of exercise but may also spur creative solutions.

- When you get a call on your cell phone, stand up to take it. Before long, you'll get to your feet automatically.

Turn-Back-the-Clock Breakthrough
SWEAT: THE DO-IT-NOW ANTI-ALZHEIMER'S STRATEGY

If you have a family history of Alzheimer's disease, one of the most dreaded diseases of aging, you have even more reason to get moving. Moderate physical activity may stave off shrinkage of the hippocampus, the brain region attacked first in Alzheimer's, a recent study suggests.

People who carry a variant of a gene known as APOE e4 are at increased risk of Alzheimer's, but not everyone who has the gene will develop the disease, suggesting that lifestyle factors may help protect against it. In this study of nearly 100 people ages 65 to 89, half the volunteers carried the APOE e4 gene. These gene carriers were divided into two groups: the exercisers (a minimum of 3 days a week) and nonexercisers. For comparison, there were also two groups of exercisers and nonexercisers who did not carry the gene.

Fast-forward 18 months, and brain scans revealed that the hippocampus of the nonexercising gene carriers had shrunk—3 percent, on average—while the exercisers showed almost no shrinkage. (The other groups who did not carry the gene saw little change to their brains, whether or not they exercised.) Amazing, right? Researchers don't know exactly how exercise can guard the hippocampus, but another study found that 3 hours of physical activity a week improved brain function and memory, perhaps by increasing bloodflow in certain regions of the brain, including the hippocampus. ∎

- Download an audiobook and listen as you garden or clean instead of sitting and reading a book.

- Boot up your favorite playlist on Spotify or your phone and dance for a minute or two while nobody's looking (and even if someone is).

- Do a few pushups. The on-your-knees version is perfectly okay. If you don't want to get down on the floor, place your hands on a desk or counter and knock out 10.

- Get off the couch and fill your water glass (remember, hydration equates to energy). And then you'll have to get up again to go to the bathroom.

- Take your dog out for an unscheduled potty break. Add a ball toss if you like.

Get Rolling

As you age, your joints and connective tissue lose elasticity—and suddenly you can feel pain in the simplest of tasks, like getting out of the car. Even if you exercise regularly, it's still possible to wake up with an achy neck or back; wince over tight, sore hips or legs after a day on your feet or at your desk; or grit your teeth as you work out.

You probably feel too young for such discomfort. So what's going on? It's likely that you have "knots" in the connective tissue surrounding your muscles (or fascia) called *myofascial adhesions*, which develop from a variety of causes, such as inactivity, past injuries, and the aging process. The solution: a DIY technique called foam rolling. Similar to a deep-tissue massage, this combination of stretching and massage breaks up fibrous tissue and boosts circulation so you're less sore. It also helps hydrate the fascia, which can become dry and brittle over time.

Foam rolling involves rolling tight, tender areas of your body across a log of dense foam. The pressure massages the fascia, the connective tissue that surrounds muscles, nerves, and blood vessels from the top of your head to the soles of your feet. Rolling out the fascia can help increase range of motion, reduce muscle fatigue from exercise, and ease muscle soreness. Dr. Wright is a fan, as are trainers, physical therapists, and our own test panelists.

Use the roller before exercise on problem spots, and you can reduce muscle fatigue and soreness dramatically enough that workouts feel easier. Or use it after workouts, as part of your cooldown, to reduce postexercise discomfort. You can also do a whole-body routine a few times a week to keep aches and pains at bay.

Many of our panelists were amazed by the difference foam rolling made—not only to their particular pain points but also to their well-being. For example, panelist Sandy Fromknecht's daily headaches vanished once she started rolling her upper back and shoulders—and if she misses a day, they return. "It's heavenly and free," she said. Panelist Cindy Hafner pulls out the roller to loosen her muscles—and mind—when she gets home from work or before bed: "It's a nice way to relax."

While foam rolling is optional on our plan, Dr. Wright highly recommends it. "It's a marvelous way to stretch tight tendons and muscles," she says. All you need is floor space and a roller. (Foam rollers come in different lengths, firmnesses, and diameters and can be purchased at big-box and sporting-goods stores for $20 and up.)

- To break up tightness in your muscles and make your workout a bit easier, roll your pain points as part of your Dynamic Warmup.

- To reduce pain and stiffness in tight, injury-prone areas, such as the upper back and IT band, tack on a roll session of those target areas to your flexibility stretches.

- To boost your workout performance and stay pain-free, try our 15-minute full-body routine two or three times a week.

One thing to note: The firmer the roller, the more aggressive the massage. You might want to start with a softer foam roller and experiment with the amount of pressure you apply; in the beginning, minimal pressure may feel better. Once you get the rolling part down, administer pressure to sensitive areas for 20 to 30 seconds. As you become more familiar with the practice, you can go shorter or longer as needed.

Over the next 8 weeks, whether you stick mainly to the cardio, strength, and flexibility exercises or rotate in some of the optional (but highly beneficial!) balance and foam-roller workouts, you'll be doing your body and mind a huge favor. You'll have more youthful energy and get-up-and-go to really rock the next section of the book: ENGAGE. Turn the page to find out how you can shape your next chapter to live the life you've been waiting for.

SUCCESS!

Sandy Fromknecht, 53

MY STORY When Sandy turned 40, a switch flipped. "And it wasn't a good switch," she said. "I didn't like the way I looked, my joints were starting to hurt, I didn't have energy, and I had little mental clarity." Like many women, she blamed it all on menopause. "I thought it was out of my control," Sandy said. "But since this program, I've realized that isn't true."

Now at 53, Sandy feels better than she did in her forties. Eating healthy, stretching, and exercising has more than tripled her energy levels and completely eliminated her brain fog. Sure, she's lost weight along the way, but that doesn't matter to Sandy. "I didn't want to be a certain size. I don't care much about that," she said. "But I care about having energy and mental clarity."

After completing the Younger in 8 Weeks Plan, Sandy started singing again, something she hadn't done since junior high school. "My husband is in a choir at church, and he always encouraged me to try out," she said. "Before, I was just too tired. Now, singing is a lot more enjoyable! I'm not out of breath and I have stronger control."

Sandy has regained control over not only her voice but also her lifestyle choices. She said eliminating her three major food groups—sugar, caffeine, and wine—was the hardest part. And she's thankful that for the first time in her life, she has skin-care and beauty routines. With her fabulous antiaging haircut and new nightly skin-care regimen, Sandy was surprised at how great she felt after making a few simple changes. "I always had little bumps under my skin and slight rosacea," Sandy said. "My skin looks and feels so much healthier!"

Along with a skin transformation, Sandy noticed a drastic change in her taste buds. "I thought eating healthy would take too much time and cost too much money. But that wasn't the case," she said. "It doesn't take any time at all to roast vegetables and cook a piece of fish. My husband and I started eating tons of fish like trout and haddock, which I didn't know about before. Plus, I noticed my taste buds change after a few weeks of eating the fresh, clean foods on the plan. Now I look forward to a big salad with vegetables and homemade balsamic vinaigrette!"

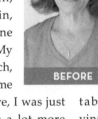
BEFORE

Before, Sandy felt like she wasn't in control of her health, weight, or aging. "Now," she said, "I feel at least 10 years younger!"

Beauty styling: Makeup, Colleen Kobrick; Hair, Missy Kovato; Wardrobe styling: Pamela Simpson

LOOK AT ME

- Lowered total cholesterol **10 points**

- More than tripled her energy level

- No more skin flaws

- Weight lost: **3.8 pounds**

- Inches lost: **7**

Tip **EATING HEALTHY DOESN'T HAVE TO BE DIFFICULT.** I thought eating healthy would be too costly and time consuming. My husband and I started eating tons of fish like trout and haddock, which I didn't know about before. Plus, I noticed my taste buds change after a few weeks of eating the fresh, clean foods on the plan.

ENGAGE

Connect with Your Best Self— And the World around You

Think of the excitement and energy with which you plan a vacation: those bucket lists of activities and new-slate visions of how you'll feel once you can finally calm down and lose yourself in a book or a landscape. Or the deep gratification that comes from finding the time to think about launching that dream business or reconnecting with family and friends. You can channel these intentions as you plan this next phase of your life—and all of those to come.

So consider the next 8 weeks a permission slip to prioritize your personal and professional happiness and fulfillment at this important crossroad in your life. This chapter offers many ways to get there.

On your travels, you'll search for *duende*. A term from Spanish folklore that loosely translates as "inspiration," *duende* is the fire in your soul—and with the tips in this chapter, you'll be on your way to rekindling it. Week after week, our test panelists excitedly reported doing things they haven't done in years—dragging out their oil paints, reconnecting with singing partners to let loose, leaving the familiarity of a long-time job for the challenge of a new position. They were describing *duende*, and you can get it, too.

What's missing from your life? What consumes you with curiosity? What long-held dreams can you resurrect and what regrets can you finally own so you can move beyond them to what's next? In other words, who are you now, and who do you want to be in your Second Act?

This chapter zeroes in on your attitude and spirit—the inner you. You'll find strategies, many of them designed by our advising psychologist Suzanne Segerstrom, PhD, that can help you release stress and find peace, cultivate curiosity or a more positive mind-set, hold on to hope or let go of past hurts, take a step toward the career you always wanted or the dream you dismissed years ago. Some strategies will be familiar; others, new. But each invites you to reconsider the way you view the world and interact with others and challenges you to reach for your best self.

As you read through these strategies, pay attention to which ones resonate with you, and note those you want to try. (Be aware, too, of strategies that elicit an I-could-never-do-*that* reaction—a sign that they might actually teach you something.) Once you begin the 8-week plan, we'll help you incorporate a new strategy each week. For now, let their transformative power inspire you.

Get Enough Sleep

The first step in finding *duende*? A good night's rest.

Like a healthy diet and regular exercise, adequate sleep—7 or 8 solid hours a night—is a key pillar of health. Remove it, and well-being comes crashing down. Studies link chronic lack of sleep to high blood pressure, diabetes, weight gain, and possibly even cellular aging, according to one study. Subjects whose quality of sleep was poor or who slept less than 7 hours per night had significantly shorter telomeres. And older participants who did get enough sleep had telomere lengths that looked years younger. Too little shut-eye may also age the brain. One 15,000-person study found that those who averaged less than 5 hours of sleep per night for several years experienced a decline in memory performance equivalent to 2 years of brain aging. Yikes!

If you skimp on sleep, you're aging unnecessarily. It's time to reclaim its rejuvenating power. Not only will you awaken refreshed and alert, you'll be more likely to stay on plan. Here are four ways sleep helps you turn back the clock and find inner strength.

It helps keep weight on track. Sleep helps maintain a healthy balance of the hormones that make you feel hungry (ghrelin) or full (leptin). When you don't get enough, ghrelin rises and leptin falls. The result: You feel hungrier than when you're well rested. In one study, those who slept less and stayed up later consumed significantly more calories than those who went to bed at 10 p.m. and got a full night's sleep. If you habitually munch along to your favorite late-night talk show, getting to bed earlier may make a significant difference in your weight.

Sleep also affects how your body reacts to insulin, the hormone that controls blood sugar. Sleep deficiency results in a higher than normal blood sugar level, but improving your sleep habits can help turn that around. In a group of normal sleepers, researchers found that even 3 nights of catch-up sleep improved insulin sensitivity by 31 percent, compared to those who continued to have poor sleep schedules.

It revs your immune system. Sleep boosts immunity; sleep deficiency impairs it. People who get less than 7 hours per night are three times more likely to catch a cold, one study found. And if you get a yearly flu shot, consider this: Compared with those who were well rested, sleep-deprived subjects had only half as many disease-fighting antibodies 10 days after the vaccination.

It sharpens your decisions and keeps you in control. After several nights of lost sleep, your ability to function suffers as if you haven't slept at all for a day or two. Lack of sleep affects your ability to make sound decisions (there's a reason for the expression "let me sleep on it"). The lack of impulse control induced by sleep deficiency may also trigger a meltdown. Sleep deficiency weakens the connection between the part of the brain that regulates emotions (the amygdala) and the part that makes high-level decisions (the prefrontal cortex). When you run on no sleep, you say or do things you wouldn't have had you gotten the rest you needed.

It may even make you lustier. There's little that helps you feel younger than a toss in the sheets, and sleep may make a difference in your sexual desire. In women, just 1 extra hour of sleep accounted for a 14 percent increase in the likeliness of having sex the next day, a study found. Those "extra hour" women also reported being better able to climax compared to women who didn't get the additional sleep. It may be that hormonal changes due to sleep loss translate to poorer sexual function.

In Week 1 of our plan, your better-sleep campaign kicks off with two specific tips (see page 191). Start adding the strategies below, and before long, you'll sail through your days and sleep soundly all night.

Turn in and get up at the same time. Do this even on weekends, within

Renew Right Now

FALL ASLEEP FAST WITH THIS BREATHING TECHNIQUE

Too keyed up to sleep? Long, slow abdominal breathing can make that hamster in your head get off its wheel and relax. In a small Harvard study using yoga breathing techniques to treat insomnia, all volunteers reported that the quality and quantity of their sleep improved.

To sleep better tonight, try a breathing technique called the 4-7-8 breath exercise.

1. With your tongue resting on the roof of your mouth, just behind your upper teeth, exhale completely.

2. Close your mouth and inhale through your nose for four counts.

3. Hold your breath for seven counts.

4. Then exhale (with your tongue in the same position) for eight counts.

Repeat this cycle three more times.

---

an hour of your weekday rise and sleep times. Staying up late and sleeping in late on weekends can disrupt your internal body clock's sleep-wake rhythm. Turn in at around the same time every night and wake up at the same time in the morning, and you'll begin to find it easier to drop off and get up energetically.

Get some morning light. Spend time outside, even on a cloudy day. It will tune up your body's internal clock and help you maintain a healthy sleep-wake cycle. At the very least, try to expose yourself to natural light for at least 20 minutes first thing in the morning—so throw open the curtains, sit by a window, and lap up those gentle rays. (Bonus: extra time for you.)

Move each day. As you have already read, exercise helps you drop off faster and sleep more soundly for longer periods. Just end your sweat session 4 hours before bedtime (so if you turn in at 10 p.m., hit the shower at 6 p.m.). That's because 30 minutes of vigorous aerobic exercise elevates your body temperature for about 4 hours, which can make it hard to fall asleep. Give your body time to cool down, and you'll enter dreamland just fine.

Quit caffeine by 2 p.m. Or earlier—the effects of caffeine can last as long as 8 hours. If you're really sensitive to caffeine, consider limiting chocolate and tea, as well (they contain smaller amounts of caffeine).

Nap smart, not long. If you find it hard to fall or stay asleep at night, a daytime nap will likely disturb your nighttime sleep patterns even more. But if you do decide to nap (and studies show myriad benefits, including increased productivity and reduced production of the stress hormone cortisol), finish it by midafternoon and limit your snooze to no more than 20 minutes.

Avoid large meals close to bedtime. Heavy meals take longer to digest, so if you turn in too quickly afterward, acid reflux can keep you uncomfortably awake. Also, avoid spicy, acidic, and fried foods, which in some people can lead to indigestion and GERD. A light snack before bed is fine. Just remember to pair proteins with carbs (for snack ideas, see page 174).

Have an early nightcap. A glass of wine or a cocktail before bed may help you *fall* asleep, but once it wears off, you won't *stay* asleep; alcohol can cause arousal and sleep disruption later in the night. After Week 3, if you opt for a daily libation, stick to just one at least 3 hours before you turn in.

Create a pre-bed chill-out ritual. Physically and emotionally stressful activities trigger the release of cortisol in your body, which increases alertness and arousal. Take a warm bath, read a calming book, or sip a cup of herbal tea before bed.

Make your bedroom a sleep sanctuary. Keep your room cool (65°F is

Turn-Back-the-Clock Breakthrough
SLEEP TO TAKE OUT YOUR BRAIN'S TRASH

Here's another reason to get more sleep: It purges your brain of gunk that ages it.

When scientists at the University of Rochester used special microscopes to observe the brains of sleeping mice, they discovered a kind of plumbing system that rids the brain of unwanted waste. This cellular trash includes a number of proteins, such as beta-amyloids, the buildup of which is associated with cognitive problems, including Alzheimer's. The researchers coined the term *glymphatic system* (a mash-up of glial brain cells and lymphatic system) to describe a brain-cleansing mechanism akin to the lymphatic fluid that clears toxins from the body.

This system becomes twice as active during restful sleep, the researchers found, which allows the brain to vastly increase its removal of potentially harmful gunk. Conversely, sleep too little and your brain might get overrun with destructive neurological trash. This could explain the demonstrated loss of gray matter in Alzheimer's and aging, the study said. ▪

optimal). If you're menopausal and prone to night sweats, dress lightly (or not at all). Above all, keep your laptop, smartphone, or tablet in another room. The glow from this gadgetry may pass through your closed eyes into the region of the brain that controls sleep—the hypothalamus—delaying your brain's release of the hormone melatonin, which promotes sleep.

"Do" Optimism

You probably have that friend who has a knack for bringing down any mood. At a holiday gathering, she'll mention some new viral epidemic going around. At an outdoor picnic, she'll belabor the bad weather and mention the possibility of lightning storms. This buzzkill attitude was hilariously captured a few years ago in a *Saturday Night Live* character named Debbie Downer, who continually deflated her friends' positive vibe with a string of negative one-liners punctuated by a close-up of her dour face and the *wah-wahhh* sound of a sad trombone.

Debbie sees only dark clouds, never silver linings. And while her negativity makes for good comedy, the tendency to be a wet blanket in just about any situation—a trait experts call dispositional pessimism—doesn't merely ruin a good time. It can affect your health.

First, though, it's worth clarifying that optimism and pessimism aren't just a matter of feelings. They're about what you believe about the future. In broad strokes, optimists believe that the future holds more good than bad. Pessimists expect the opposite—a dark or uncertain future, rather than a hopeful one.

And so research has found that optimists do better in most avenues of life, whether it's work, school, or relationships. They get depressed less often than pessimists, make more money, and have happier marriages. There's even evidence that they live longer, healthier lives, with less chance of developing heart disease, high cholesterol, or diabetes, which suggests that optimistic people may take better care of their health.

All of this is awesome news—if you're a born optimist. But what if, like Debbie, you tend to see the glass as half empty? Actually, there are techniques you can learn to flip the switch and "do" optimism so you reap the same health benefits as optimists, says Dr. Segerstrom (whose book, incidentally, is called *Breaking Murphy's Law: How Optimists Get What They Want from Life—And Pessimists Can Too*).

To do optimism and find *duende*, you don't need a personality makeover. (Besides, some pessimists—and even their loved ones—may value their cynical or darkly funny outlooks.) To benefit from optimism's boon to health and productivity, you just have to think and behave a bit differently in certain situations. The following tips can give you a head start.

Don't force it. Pushing yourself into an upbeat mood can backfire. In one of Dr. Segerstrom's favorite studies, researchers asked one group of people to use classical music to raise their moods, and they had other volunteers simply listen to the symphony with no forced outcome. The result: The concert was no help for those who were trying to lift their spirits—but the other group felt much better.

In other words, if you want to be happy, stop trying so hard. Don't even monitor yourself (*Do I feel better yet? How about now?*). Instead, aim to be *engaged*.

When you're fully immersed in something, it can distract you from a pessimist's favorite pastime—rumination. (That's shrink talk for when you obsess endlessly over problems or concerns.) When you ruminate, it's not just a bad day—it's *always* a bad day, on top of which you have a lousy life, because you're a bad person. With that kind of bleak perspective, it's really impossible to see a solution.

When you're mired in negative thoughts, turn to an activity that demands your full attention. Going for a jog or other type of workout fits the bill (you'll fall on your face if you don't focus on what your body is doing). If you're at the office, you might check in on a colleague you know who could use a boost herself (helping someone else takes the focus off you). Or go out and buy a "just because" card, write an encouraging message, and mail it.

Go for the (realistic) goal. Optimists and pessimists don't differ in the number of goals they set, nor in how important they think their goals are. But optimists have higher expectations for meeting their goals and put more effort into achieving them.

Pause to consider what your personal goals might be. Big, long-term goals—a 50-pound weight loss, a more exciting or challenging job, a wider social circle—take time and effort to achieve. Aiming for lofty goals can set you up for failure because they just feel unattainable. Instead, begin with one or two simple, short-term goals—say, to walk at least 30 minutes, 4 days a week for a month, or to learn to make soup from scratch, or to start a blog. When you achieve that small goal, set another.

If you don't manage to knock out even a small goal, don't beat yourself up. Instead, refocus on the big goal that the small goal was leading to (lose 15 pounds, cook more dinners, start a blog), and find another small goal to take its place, Dr. Segerstrom suggests. Or consider three new ways to try to achieve the original goal and commit to trying them all in the next week. (Hold yourself to it by putting those steps in your daily calendar.)

Over time, start to make your goals bolder. Slowly increase the amount of time and effort they'll take to achieve. Commit yourself and keep moving forward. Dare to care, strive, and even endure a setback or two. It's a sneaky way to build toward that big-picture goal while enjoying the ride.

Dig deep and lean in. Why do optimists seem to have all the luck? Long after pessimists have given up and gone home, optimists continue to try to solve problems. In one study, optimists continued to work on unscrambling an impossible-to-solve anagram 50 to 100 percent longer than pessimists.

"Whether the glass is half empty or half full, it needs to be washed, dried, and put away in the cupboard, and optimism affects whether or not you are motivated to get that done," Dr. Segerstrom says. In other words, optimists' positive expectations increase their motivation and effort; pessimists' negative expectations decrease their motivation and effort.

So about that goal. Even if you don't fully believe you'll achieve it, you have to *act as if you will*. That means you keep hammering away at it. That's "doing" optimism. And think about it—when you never give up on a goal, you increase the likelihood that your persistence will pay off, and you'll get what you want out of life now and in the future.

Don't let failure faze you. When good things happen, pessimists tend to dismiss these events as flukes, while optimists typically take the credit. When bad things happen, pessimists blame themselves and expect to suffer a long time; conversely, optimists see bad events as having little to do with them and as problems that will pass quickly. In other words, optimists view success and failure quite differently than pessimists do.

Setbacks are a part of life. It's nothing personal. To help ensure that they don't sap your positivity, use this trick: As setbacks occur, write out what happened, along with how you interpret both the causes and their impact on your life. Then make a conscious effort to explain the situations differently, and focus on nonpersonal, changeable causes and outcomes.

For example, if you were let go from your job, don't tell yourself that you are talentless and will wind up living under a bridge. Instead, tell yourself that this particular job wasn't the perfect fit for you—and look for some positive takeaway from the negative experience (like you realize now that you don't love managing others, or you need to work for someone who communicates more clearly, or it's the sign you've been waiting for that you're burned out and ready to search out a new field). See this setback as an opportunity to find a better situation.

Indulge your doom-and-gloom. That work deadline you missed? It's pink-slip city, permanent unemployment, and a box under the highway. Is that just a headache—or could it be brain cancer? This mental process of making an event worse than it actually is—what therapists call *catastrophizing*—is an example of irrational thinking. And while the worst-case scenarios above may sound absurd, play them out in your head enough, and they can seem not only logical but inevitable. And as any optimist will tell you, they're not.

To snap yourself out of it, exaggerate those doomsday scenarios in your

Renew Right Now

TRY THESE SNAP-OUT-OF-IT MOVES

You don't have to spend years in therapy to become more upbeat about life. In a landmark study, a team of researchers, led by positive psychology pioneer Martin Seligman, turned to volunteers to test five strategies that were purported to increase happiness and reduce symptoms of depression. Their findings were, well, super positive: Three of those strategies really did boost happiness—and it took just a week to make a dent. Here's what you need to do.

WRITE DOWN THE GOOD. Every day for a week, participants wrote down three things that had gone well for them and why they thought these things had happened. Not only did the exercise have an immediate mood boost, the participants reported feeling happier for 6 months afterward.

USE YOUR STRENGTHS IN A NEW WAY. Volunteers were asked to think about their top five strengths—generosity, say, or creativity—and then were told to use one of these strengths in a new and different way every day for a week. The result? They measurably increased their happiness for—again—a full 6 months.

PAY A GRATITUDE VISIT. People were given 1 week to write a letter of gratitude and deliver it in person to someone who'd been especially kind to them, but whom they had never properly thanked. The happiness boost from this experiment lingered about a month.

mind to the point of hilarity. For example, say to yourself, "Oh, come on. Will I *really* end up in a box under the highway because I'm a day late on this project?" Don't stop there. In your mind, trap squirrels for dinner. Then paint the opposite scenario. Your project makes your company a bazillion dollars—and you're promoted to CEO!

Finally, write down the most likely outcome. Chances are, it won't include the executive suite—or the underpass. The beauty of this goofing around is that you feel a bit of power over your thoughts and the situation. That sense of control is the antidote to pessimism.

Get a Handle on Stress

Asked in his later years to define *stress*, Hans Selye, the scientist who coined the term in 1936, answered, "Everyone knows what stress is, but nobody really knows." What he meant was that because none of us respond to stress in quite the same ways, stress can be difficult to define. Some of us get headaches and backaches; others rant, drive like maniacs, and eat all the doughnuts; still others become anxious and irritable. Moreover, the same experiences that stress you out may roll off someone else's back.

Stress isn't always a bad thing, either. If you're at zero stress, you've probably got no pulse. In fact, some stress can save your life. *Acute stress* is the reaction to an immediate threat, commonly known as fight-or-flight mode. The threat can be real (a near-collision on the highway) or perceived (a jackhammer under your window). Acute stress triggers the release of chemicals and hormones, like cortisol and adrenaline, that prepare your body to face a threat or to flee it. Your pulse quickens, you breathe faster, your muscles tense, your focus narrows while your brain activity increases—all of which were immensely useful survivalist reflexes when early humans needed to kill or outrun predators.

But with fewer real enemies in sight, our stress response is triggered more frequently, and often chronically, by situations like job pressure, financial worries, relationship issues, caring for aging parents, and even loneliness. *Chronic stress* (versus acute stress), left unmanaged, can mess with your mind and body in serious ways. With chronic stress, those same chemicals that in short bursts can save your life now suppress functions you don't need for immediate survival. Here are just a few of the ways chronic stress can wreak havoc on your health.

Stress steals your sleep. Chronic stress can cause hyperarousal, a physiological state that upsets the balance between sleep and wakefulness and makes it hard to fall and stay asleep.

It makes you scatterbrained. You may be unable to focus or think straight, either at work or home. You also may find it harder to learn and retain new information; studies have linked long-term exposure to high cortisol with a shrinking of the hippocampus, the brain's memory center.

It makes you crave crap food. Along with insulin, cortisol and other glucocorticoid hormones appear to be responsible for stress-related cravings for sugar, salt, and fat.

It messes with blood sugar. People with type 2 diabetes may find that their blood sugar is higher when they're stressed out. (Physical stresses, such as illness or injury, can raise blood sugar levels, as well.)

It causes or worsens back pain. When you feel like you're under siege, every muscle in your body clenches up, including those in your neck and back. If you're stressed all the time and those muscles stay tight, it can eventually cause major pain.

It expands your waistline. One study linked high-fat, high-sugar foods to more fat storage in the trunk region and insulin resistance, but *only* among women who were chronically stressed.

It puts your heart at risk. Under stress, the body releases inflammatory substances into the bloodstream, which can aggravate heart disease or increase the risk of heart attack or stroke. Also, under chronic stress, you may smoke, overeat, and stop working out—unhealthy behaviors that jack up the risk for high blood pressure, high cholesterol levels, and heart disease.

It may shorten your telomeres. In one study of 647 women, researchers measured subjects' telomere length (from a blood sample) and stress hormone levels (from their urine). The women also filled out a questionnaire to gauge perceived stress, or how stressed out they felt. Those who were found to have above-average stress levels had slightly shorter telomeres (or DNA "youth caps") compared to their low-stress sisters. But the difference in telomere length was most dramatic when researchers also looked at the women's levels of perceived stress; in this group, telomere length was impacted similarly to the effects of obesity, smoking, or 10 years of aging!

The bottom line: Stress will suck you dry if you let it. Instead, learn to control your response to stress, so it doesn't control you. How to do it?

This, once again, is a matter of body chemistry. Just as the body reacts to acute stress with a cascade of arousing chemicals and hormones, when the immediate threat passes, stress hormone levels return to normal. The *relaxation response,* which can be triggered by activities like deep breathing exercises and muscle relaxation (more on those in a minute), can help accelerate this return to normal, Dr. Segerstrom says.

It's tough to rekindle your *duende* when anxiety continually threatens to suffocate it. But, the first step to managing stress is to become consciously aware of when you feel it and to identify your specific stress triggers.

The exercise below can help you identify those triggers. Take a moment to think about your responses, and then write them down (use the journal you may have started for tracking your progress or just scribble in the margins here). Try to be as detailed as possible.

IDENTIFY YOUR STRESS TRIGGERS

1. How do you know when you are stressed? What are your personal stress signals?
   - List the symptoms of stress that you feel in your body (headaches, digestive issues, muscle tension, low energy).

   - Jot down any ways that stress affects your mental or emotional states (you feel anxious, angry, irritable, or out of control; you can't concentrate or make decisions).

   - List the ways in which stress affects your behavior (you snap at people, hoover up sweets, reach for a cigarette when you quit years ago, and so on).

2. Mentally review your typical day and week and jot down the events or situations that trigger stress for you. Are they related to your children, family, health, finances, work, relationships?
3. Review the stress-relieving tips and techniques in this chapter, from sleep to work strategies. Select a few that you're willing to try and write them down.

When Stress Hits, Breathe It Out

Breathe out stress. One key to mastering stress is to have a focused exercise in your pocket for tough situations, and this simple breathing technique, called *circle breathing,* can melt stress fast.

1. Inhale and stretch your arms over your head, giving a sigh of relief and lowering your arms as you exhale. Relax and keep your arms lowered for the rest of the exercise.
2. Now imagine that you're inhaling a stream of peaceful energy into a spot a few inches below your navel.
3. Inhale the warm stream into the base of your spine, and then imagine it traveling up your back to the top of your head.
4. Exhale and mentally follow your out breath back down the front of your body to the point below your navel where you'll begin the next in breath. Your breath has now come full circle.
5. Continue this breathing pattern for five to 10 circle breaths. You can also use circle breath for a longer period as a relaxing form of meditation.

Four Pleasure-Packed Ways to Cut Cortisol

PRODUCED BY YOUR ADRENAL GLANDS, the stress hormone cortisol helps regulate blood pressure and the immune system in a sudden crisis, whether from a physical attack or an emotional setback. Though it means well, cortisol just doesn't know when to quit.

Fortunately, the body has evolved an antidote to its fight-or-flight mode: the relaxation response. Here are four ways to boost your Zen and dampen stress—and in some cases, cut your cortisol levels nearly in half. (No, doing them all at once probably won't erase every last bit of anxiety, but try them individually to defuse stress sessions.)

TO CUT CORTISOL 66 PERCENT—GRAB YOUR HEADPHONES. Music can help calm your brain, especially if you're coping with a super-stressful event. When doctors at Japan's Osaka Medical Center played tunes for a group of patients undergoing colonoscopies, the patients' cortisol levels rose less than those of others who underwent the same procedure in a quiet room.

To forestall cortisol spikes in other anxiety-producing situations—when you're working on a tight deadline, paying your bills, or hosting dinner for your in-laws—pipe in some background music. To wind down faster at bedtime, switch off the TV and listen to soothing music instead.

TO CUT CORTISOL 50 PERCENT—TURN IN EARLY OR TAKE A NAP. What's the difference between getting 6 hours of sleep and getting the suggested 8? Fifty percent more cortisol in the bloodstream, experts say. When a group of pilots slept 6 hours or less for 7 nights while on

Guide Yourself to Calm

With a technique called guided imagery, you focus on a specific image that helps you return to tranquility. You can use audiotapes or books to guide you. The Academy for Guided Imagery (acadgi.com) offers a dozen simple guided imagery techniques to ease stress, which you can download instantly.

Escape into Sensuality

We mean any action that involves your senses—touch, smell, taste. When you're at the height of stress, endorphins released into the brain relieve pain and begin a recovery period. You can mimic this stress-busting process by doing things that feel good physically, such as taking a warm bath or shower,

duty, their cortisol levels jumped and stayed elevated for 2 days, according to a study from Germany's Institute of Aerospace Medicine. The recommended 8 hours of nightly shut-eye allows your body enough time to recover from the day's stress. When you fall short of the 8-hour mark, take a nap the next day. Pennsylvania State University researchers found that a midday snooze cut cortisol levels in subjects who were sleep-deprived the previous night.

TO CUT CORTISOL 47 PERCENT—SIP THE "CUP THAT CHEERS." Tea has deep associations with comfort and calm (think of how the English revere their late-afternoon teatime). And science confirms the connection. When volunteers at University College London were given a stressful task, the cortisol levels of regular black-tea drinkers fell by 47 percent within an hour of completing the assignment, while others who drank some kind of fake tea experienced only a 27 percent drop. The researchers suspect that natural chemicals such as polyphenols and flavonoids may have calming effects.

TO CUT CORTISOL 25 PERCENT—SEEK THE SPIRITUAL. Religious ritual fortifies many people against everyday stresses, and it can also lower cortisol secretion, according to University of Mississippi researchers. Churchgoing study subjects had lower levels of the stress hormone, on average, than those who did not attend services at all. If organized religion isn't your bag, head for "nature's cathedral" and de-stress in the woods, a meadow, or a stretch of water.

going outdoors and taking a deep whiff of the roses or lilac trees in your yard, or preparing a fragrant cup of herbal tea and steeping yourself in its scent and flavor.

Connect with Others

Whether you cook a big meal with friends or family, volunteer with religious or community groups, or go for a hike with your kids or a colleague, you're bonding with others. As you catch up, share intimacies, vent frustration, and get or give a sympathetic ear, you feel connected and energized. But there's more to it than good vibes. Social relationships—both in quantity and quality—affect our immediate and future physical health and mental well-being, and they even influence how long we live.

Researchers who investigate the link between health and social ties have turned up some fascinating findings. For example, having fewer and flimsier social ties has been associated with inflammation and lowered immune function. Other research has linked strong social bonds with longevity. In one survey, researchers looked at data from a whopping 148 previous studies, comparing people's social habits with their health records over more than 7 years. What they found: Strong social connections boosted odds of survival by 50 percent compared to those with weak social ties. In fact, lack of social connection was a stronger risk factor for death than even lack of exercise and obesity.

One reason for this effect is that when you're connected to a group and feel responsibility for others, the sense of purpose you feel spurs you to take better care of yourself. Other studies have found that social connection acts like a shield against stress, which, as you know, can hammer the heart, immune and digestive systems, and insulin regulation. It could even be that when we care for others, our bodies release a protective hit of stress-quenching hormones.

You don't need to be a social butterfly to benefit. If you feel loved and content within a small social circle—partner, dog, a casual work buddy, one BFF with whom you can share all—that's great, too. It's feeling lonely that's unhealthy. In fact, one study found that feelings of loneliness were associated with higher mortality, and it didn't matter whether subjects were married, had friends or relatives close by, or had some kind of unhealthy habit, like smoking. In other words, whether you feel connected—not the number of connections you have—is what matters.

"Social networks are not something you *have* so much as something you *do*. They are the reflections of your actions to build, maintain, or even prune back your social relationships," says Dr. Segerstrom. Just as you can "do" optimism without being an optimist, you can broaden your support network without having to doggedly work your Rolodex. These suggestions can get you started.

Do for others. Get involved in a cause or volunteer project that's important to you (see page 103 for more tips on how to do this). You're likely to meet others who share similar interests and values.

Pop up, pop in. Ever get a positive, potential-pal vibe from someone you see frequently at work, the gym, or your favorite coffee shop and wish you could get to know that person? Stick to a routine that puts you where you know she will be, and strike up small talk each time. In one experiment, strangers of the same gender had several face-to-face conversations, and then rated how much they liked one another. Turned out that each encounter upped the positive feeling between the two people. (If you can't get out on a certain day, it's useful to know that repeated online chatting had the same positive effect.)

Forget yourself and focus on others. Loneliness can set in when you spend too much time in your head. Ruminate too much and you can create "back off" vibes, leading others to think you're aloof or not interested in connecting. If you can muzzle those negative thoughts, it'll be easier to let others in. According to one review of loneliness-reducing techniques, the most effective strategies teach people to break the cycle of bleak thoughts about their self-worth and being judged. Go back to the "'Do' Optimism" section on page 89 and focus on the exercises that aim to reverse negative-thought spirals. Or if rumination has been a lifelong pattern, consider counseling to help you learn new strategies.

Be yourself. If you sincerely want to expand your social network, these tips are a great start. But if you're content with the connections you have, don't force it. Going against your nature is likely to stress you out. Be who you are, as long as you have at least a few rock-solid connections to cheer you on—and up.

Build Resilience

When challenges, setbacks, or even tragedy hits—family conflicts, a financial reversal or health scare, even divorce or death—some people crumble, while others adapt and bounce back relatively quickly. Why? Psychologists credit *resilience*, the ability to adapt well in the face of adversity. There's evidence that this take-a-licking-and-keep-on-ticking quality may help you stay happy and healthy as you age.

Greater resilience to stress is consistently linked to happiness and other positive emotions. Research on these bounce-back personalities, conducted on the oldest old to young soldiers in battle zones, suggests that these individuals:

- Tend to be optimistic, persistent, and determined

- Have realistic and attainable expectations and goals

- Show good judgment and problem-solving skills

- Care about how others around them feel

- Feel like they are in control of their lives

While genetics may play a role in resilience, it's also possible to develop it. Then its effect snowballs; once you begin to manage life's challenges and setbacks without falling apart, you'll feel stronger and more positive in general. That positivity can have a protective effect on your health, particularly on the immune system. (Studies have linked contentment and joy with robust immune system function.)

Resilience also opens your eyes to your inner strength and resources. While resilience won't protect you from grief (even the most resilient people bear emotional scars), it will carry you through the bad times until the good ones return. And when you're resilient, you actually believe that they will.

Strengthen your resilience muscles using the tips below.

Take care of yourself. As you face the headwinds of a tough situation, immerse yourself in an activity that relaxes you and gives you pleasure. Meet a friend for coffee, paint your toenails, putter in the garden. Get enough sleep, eat a healthy diet, and exercise regularly. Good self-care primes your mind and body to deal with difficult circumstances.

Lean on others. In times of stress or adversity, friends, family, and others typically offer a sympathetic ear and a shoulder to cry on. Accept their offers of support with a grateful heart; help from those who care and are willing to listen strengthens resilience. You may find that involvement in civic groups, faith-based organizations, or volunteer work gives you the social support you need to make it through.

Cut back on TV, Internet, and radio news. In a crisis, the last thing you need is more bad news—and you certainly don't have to watch it unfold on cable. Research led by psychologist Turhan Canli, PhD, has demonstrated that emotionally intense images get deeply etched in memory because they activate the amygdala, the part of the brain that processes threats to our survival. Why program it with anxiety-producing images that stay with you? To avoid becoming emotionally and physiologically overwhelmed, ration your consumption of news media. Place inspiring images where you'll see them often, because you'll remember them just as vividly as distressing ones.

Explore faith and spirituality. While you don't need to be religious to be resilient, it can be helpful to have a sense that life has purpose. Even exploring different religious and philosophical traditions can deepen your sense of why you're here and what the purpose of your life might be. Attend a religious service, read a good book of philosophy—or spend a quiet moment reading a poem or two.

Make Time to Meditate

Meditation isn't just for the hippie fringe. Today, 18 million Americans say they maintain some kind of meditation practice. Although the word might conjure a yogi sitting cross-legged for hours, chanting and channeling life's sacred truths, in fact, there are many ways to meditate, many of them simple and requiring just a few minutes to reap benefits. Do it regularly to calm your mind, reduce blood pressure, boost immune function, keep stress in check, or get relief from insomnia, compulsive eating, or depression.

Much of the research on meditation has focused on a specific type, called mindfulness meditation. To be mindful is to tune in to the moment and observe, rather than react to, both your inner sensations and the world around you. You just focus your attention on your breath and body sensations, rather than the jumble of thoughts and feelings that can crowd your mind and lead to stress. It's simple but powerful medicine for our distracted, gerbil-on-a-wheel way of life. There's evidence that a regular meditation practice can:

- Lower blood pressure
- Reduce anxiety
- Reduce pain
- Boost gray matter
- Heighten creativity
- Boost immunity

And meditation may even lengthen your telomeres, extending life span. In one study, researchers investigated the effects of a 3-month meditation retreat on telomerase activity, or the production of telomere-protecting hormones. They found the meditators had on average about 30 percent more telomerase activity than nonmeditators—evidence that the mind really does influence the body.

Maybe you're ready to give meditation a try. But how to begin? These guidelines for a basic mindfulness meditation exercise from the New York Insight Meditation Center can help you nail down the basics.

Pick a place . . . If you can, devote a space exclusively to meditation. It doesn't have to be big, just relatively quiet and large enough for a chair or cushion. Feel free to add candles or photos to inspire a meditative mood.

. . . And a time. Ideally, you'd meditate in the morning, before the demands of the day crash down on you. If you can't, don't let that stop you. As with exercise, the best time to meditate is the time you can fit it in. For you, that might be during your lunch break, when you get home from work, or your evening quiet time.

Start short, go longer. Ten minutes might seem like an eternity at first, but stick with it. The practice gets easier and more rewarding over time, and before long, you'll find that you can meditate for longer periods.

Set your intention before each session. Are you meditating to become calmer and more open? To reduce stress? To explore your inner depths? Whatever your intention, state it silently to yourself before you begin. It will help you remember what you stand to gain.

Perfect your posture. Sit on a chair or cushion, straight and tall. (If you're a meditation newbie, try sitting against a wall so you know what a straight back feels like.) Rest your hands in your lap and close your eyes, focusing your attention inward.

Relax and let go. Don't skip this—consciously releasing the tension in your body helps you stay open to thoughts and feelings that arise during your session. Keeping your back straight and breathing through your nose, relax and soften each part of your body. Start with your face and move slowly downward—neck, shoulders, back, and so on. When you breathe, inhale and exhale as naturally as you can, filling your lungs with air and gradually expelling it.

Choose a focus. Holding an alert, open posture, decide where to fix your attention as you meditate. You can focus on your breath (each inhale and exhale through your nose), the rise and fall of your chest or belly, or body sensations as they come up.

Ignore inner chatter. Count on it: Your mind will wander, or you'll find yourself immersed in inner dialogue. When this happens, gently lead your attention back to your focus.

No time or inclination for long bouts of meditation? Even 5 minutes can reduce anger and cause positive changes in mind and mood, research suggests.

Turn-Back-the-Clock Breakthrough
MEDITATION TAMES MONKEY MIND

Monkey mind is a Buddhist term, stemming from the Buddha's observation that, left untrained, our minds tend to be distracted and unsettled, swinging and hopping from one thought to another.

Meditation is the antidote to that chattering chimp in our heads. In a Yale study, several minutes a day of mindfulness meditation reduced activity in the brain's default mode network (DMN)—the part involved in distraction and rumination. Since research has linked a wandering mind with unhappiness, meditation's gentle "pipe down!" message to the DMN may help you develop the calm, alert, aware mind that Buddha praised— that of a forest deer. ∎

Lend a Helping Hand

Pick up a ladle, grab a hammer, or stuff envelopes for a cause. When you do unto others, those you help aren't the only ones who benefit. A few hours of volunteer work each week confer an array of health perks. One giant study of more than 70,000 adults found that mortality rates fell 24 percent among those who volunteered regularly. When you help strangers in need, the researchers surmised, the feelings of usefulness and altruism you experience may cause your brain to produce more oxytocin and progesterone—good-vibe chemicals that curb stress and reduce harmful inflammation. Here are a few more volunteering perks.

You'll find balance. If life is a blur of deadlines at work and demands at home, and assuming you long ago let go of the "I'll sleep when I'm dead" philosophy, you may feel that you can't squeeze even one more thing into your schedule. You might want to rethink that, though: Carving out time for volunteer work may actually gift you with that elusive work-life balance you seek, a recent study found.

Swiss researchers had 746 workers take an online survey designed to measure their levels of stress and burnout and how they viewed their work-life balance; 35 percent of the group reported volunteering at least once a week. Compared to nonvolunteers, those who gave their time reported having a better work-life balance and feeling less stressed and exhausted by the demands of their jobs.

In their paper, the researchers referenced a previous study that found that although time famine—i.e., the "there aren't enough hours in the day" phenom—is pervasive in our hard-driving culture, study subjects who gave away precious hours through volunteering felt like they had more time than they actually did. That kind of makes sense—the social boost you get from volunteering may give you the energy to do other things you thought you didn't have time for.

You'll improve your health. Older adults who volunteered in elementary school classrooms at least 15 hours a week for a year doubled the number of calories they burned, a Johns Hopkins University study found, reducing their risk of weight gain and obesity-related conditions. In another study, people over 50 who volunteered for roughly 4 hours a week were less likely to develop high blood pressure than nonvolunteers.

You'll be happier. After 8 years, adults who volunteered had a significantly lower risk of depression compared with those who never lent a hand, a study from the University of Texas at Austin and Duke University found. Other studies have linked volunteering with greater life satisfaction. Volunteering increases empathy, which makes you appreciate all the good stuff in your own life. Particularly relevant to those going through a career downshift, volunteering may also give you a greater sense of purpose and accomplishment.

But there's a catch: To derive health benefits from volunteering, your motives have to be pure. In one study, participants who volunteered with some regularity lived longer, but only if their intentions were truly altruistic (as opposed to doing it because someone made them pitch in).

Even if you don't have time on your hands to volunteer, it's worth finding ways to squeeze in a little pro bono action. Here's how to start the process.

Match pitching in with passion. What do you truly love or want to learn more about—history, plants, working with numbers? Who, or what, do you have a soft spot for—teens, animals, babies? Follow that desire, and it's likely that you'll zero in on the organization that best matches both your gifts and your passions. Think of volunteer work as a chance to pursue interests you sidelined for years. You don't always need to be an expert. Organizations don't necessarily need those; they need people who really want to help.

Go surfing. Many Web sites match organizations with volunteers. For example, you can log on to VolunteerMatch, plug in your zip code, and choose from 29 categories, such as crisis support and politics. Another Web site, Senior Corps, is for people 55 and older who want to become foster grandparents, help homebound seniors, or share their skills through community service, such as beautifying their neighborhood. You can also contact local organizations directly, or call your city or county volunteer center.

Give for a day. If your schedule's too packed to pitch in regularly for a cause in your community, you can still make a difference. Got a free Saturday? Sign up for a charity walk, park cleanup, or soup kitchen. If you're game, you might even arrange to become an organ donor.

Find Your Second Act

This period in your life is like an amazing novel you're halfway through: Anything can happen, and you're dying to see what comes next. The best part? You're the main character. So plunge into your Second Act with that same I-gotta-know excitement. The Second Act is a regret-free zone where you let go of disappointments and do what you've always wanted to do, personally and professionally. "Compared with people in their twenties, people in midlife and older actually have more psychological resources, such as happiness, optimism, and self-control, that can help them go after dreams and goals," says Dr. Segerstrom. "So it's a perfect time of life to do that."

The influential 20th-century psychoanalyst Erik Erikson knew how pivotal midlife was (you can credit him with developing the concept of the identity crisis). His best-known work theorized that there are eight stages of life, each associated with a particular psychological struggle that shapes our personalities. At midlife, which Erikson defined as ages 40 to 65, our major developmental struggle is *generativity* versus *stagnation*. In other words, right now, we face a choice. We can cease to grow or generate something worthwhile, usually through helping future generations.

In young adulthood, our major "task" is love. We form relationships and identities that shape us. At midlife, the task is parenting—not just to our children, according to Erikson, but to the next generations. This makes sense—today, we have more opportunity to engage with the world and step up not just as mentors and leaders but as creators. This is an amazing moment to use our experience, skills, and energy to transcend regret—to release our disappointments over the person we didn't become or the dreams we didn't fulfill. In the Second Act, we get to transform those regrets into pursuits that give our lives meaning and purpose.

While that purpose can be found in hobbies or leisure pursuits, work can fire up that *duende*, too—if your job or career engages you. If it doesn't, you are so not alone. A 2014 Gallup survey revealed that over half of American workers—51 percent—are not engaged in their jobs, defined as involved in, enthusiastic about, or committed to their work. More than 17 percent are "actively disengaged." In your Second Act, you have the opportunity to change that, whether by making a career switch, striking out on your own, or even finding a new and more gratifying role in your current workplace.

Take a moment to consider where you are in your career. Are you fulfilled and looking forward to many good years doing what you love? Or are you burned out and craving a change? Do you have lists of plans and goals for postretirement life, or is that future hazy? The suggestions below can help bring that future into focus.

Try some DIY counseling. Career coaches often use tests or comprehensive questionnaires to assess someone's skills, interests, values, and personality traits. Typing "career assessment test" into your search engine will bring up those you can take for free. While they won't provide all the answers, they can jumpstart your thinking about what you really want and need from work and which careers fit your values and personality.

Consider a career coach. A coach who specializes in the career you want to transition into, with a proven track record of success, can help you define and achieve your career goals faster and with minimal bumps along the way. Be aware, though, that anyone can call themselves a career coach. So check out candidates carefully, both as you search and during your initial interview (often by phone). One way to search: Type "career coach" and your area of interest into your search engine. For example, "teaching" and "career coach" results in a listing of coaches with that specialty. Review their Web sites, do separate Web searches to get a sense of their reputations, and arrange interviews with those you like best. And definitely ask about fees; they typically start at $75 an hour.

Test-drive your Second Act. Internships, volunteer work, college courses, or apprenticeships allow you to gain hands-on experience and see if your dream career is a good fit. Want to teach? Try substitute teaching, and work with different age groups to see what feels right. Thinking about nursing school? Volunteer at a hospital first. Dreaming of making your living as a gardener? Take a low-paying job at a plant nursery before you sign up for a degree in horticulture.

You might also consider joining a movement that combines making a living with making a difference. An organization named Encore.org helps harness midlife talent and skills to create a better future for young people and future generations. People in the program move from accounting to helping low-income people do their taxes for free, from teaching children to mentoring them, from selling insurance to working with disadvantaged teens. To take a first step into your Second Act, log on to encore.org.

Take the first step to a start-up. Always wanted to run your own show? You're not alone; 39 percent of Americans ages 50 to 70 share the same dream, a 2014 survey by Encore.org found, and a growing number are turning interests, hobbies, or skills into a small business. The US Small Business Administration offers free or low-cost help to wannabe entrepreneurs, including free online webinars and courses for those over age 50. Poke around on sba .gov/content/50-entrepreneurs.

Try Out a New Hobby (Or Pick Up an Old One)

Whether you love to paint, craft, or play games, participating in such brain-stimulating hobbies throughout your life can help keep your mind functioning smoothly as you get older. In a study published in *Neurology*, adults who practiced arts and crafts (like drawing, pottery, or sewing) or who regularly socialized with friends were less likely to suffer from age-related memory or thinking problems later on.

Learning new skills that challenge your brain, like picking up a musical instrument or focusing on a complicated craft, can sharpen your cognitive ability at any age. And it's never too late to start: In a University of Texas study, one group of adults over 60 was assigned to learn a new skill (such as digital photography) for 15 hours a week; a second group engaged in familiar activities (like listening to classical music); and a third group simply upped

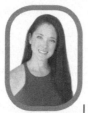

Dr. Vonda Wright says . . .
PUSH PAST YOUR COMFORT ZONE

As I approach 50, I find myself in continual reflection about my whirlwind of a life since the age of 18, when I left the Kansas farm I grew up on. As I think about who I am and who I still want to be, I also consider what I've learned in Act One so I can apply it to my Second Act. I'm the kind of person who likes to make lists, and I've started a list of everything I've done this decade, from having a child to beginning my second career as an orthopedic surgeon. It's an amazing exercise in remembering, engaging, and thinking about what I've done and learned and what the next decade could hold.

One key lesson from this exercise: Take risks. I always said that I wanted to climb to great heights and that if I fell, I'd want to fall from high enough to feel the wind in my hair. I certainly have climbed high and fallen far, only to rise and climb again.

To me, to engage is to push yourself—to purposefully choose to do something that doesn't come naturally. If you spend most of your days using your brain and not your body, you might train to run your first marathon (which I did to prove to myself that I was strong enough). If you're shy, you might join a group. If you have a tight-knit circle of friends you've hung out with for years, you might get to know someone completely unlike you.

That's the direction in which I've pushed myself lately. While I can speak in front of thousands of people comfortably, I'm what you'd call an extroverted introvert. While I draw energy from others, I need time alone to regenerate. In the last 3 years, I've come from behind the shield of my professional self to engage in the lives of women in my home city of Pittsburgh in a more personal way. At first, this wasn't entirely comfortable. Now, it's amazing. I organize an annual conference in Pittsburgh called Women's Health Conversations. This year, for the first time, I invited the 14 savvy, dynamic women who support this effort to my house for lunch—not to talk about our plans for empowering women, but to cook for them, engage in conversations about their amazing lives, and just give thanks for the bounty of good in their hearts.

No matter what your age while you are reading this, there's still plenty of time for an epic Second Act. In what ways might you push yourself? What joys might that push bring into your life? Notice who you are, think about who you want to be, and then engage like you never have before.

their activities that required social interactions, like field trips or going to the movies. At the end of the 3-month study, the new-skills group showed more improvements in memory compared to the other two groups.

What is it about hobbies that keep the brain young? New, stimulating experiences challenge the mind, most likely protecting brain cells from death and encouraging the growth of new ones, the study said.

Hobbies feed the soul as well as the brain. In addition to your usual hobbies, think about trying something new. The mental challenge of the new skills—not just using the same skills that you've had for a while—will stimulate your brain.

Don't have a hobby? Look to your childhood or young adulthood to pinpoint contenders. Did you always want to learn sign language, grow orchids, braid rugs, write short stories? Now's the time! The more complex and intricate the hobby, the better it is for you. The only "must" is that you enjoy it enough to do it at least a couple times a week.

Take a Quick "Nature Dip"

Some scientists think we evolved to enjoy places rich in natural resources because they represented good things to come. Studies that focus on the health benefits of nature suggest that whether we're in green meadows or pine forests, nature affects our moods and even our bodies. We care more and are more generous. We're more tranquil. One study found that long walks through forests over 2 days lowered stress-hormone levels, pulse rate, and blood pressure. We have more energy after just 20 minutes a day in nature, research shows. We may even feel ecstatic. Neuroscientists say viewing natural settings increases interactions in the brain's pleasure receptors. We're also less likely to feel blue. A 30-minute walk in a green scene reduced depression in 71 percent of study participants.

Nature heals us like nothing else can, so soak it up at every opportunity, big or small. Even if you live in a city or the suburbs, it's usually not hard to find a place to nature bathe, as the Japanese call it—and a quick dip is all you need. The nearest local or state park is fine, and if you spend time under trees, rather than in open fields, you'll take in more phytoncides— airborne antifungal and antibacterial compounds that, when inhaled, appear to boost a type of white blood cell that attacks tumors and viruses.

Reconsider Retirement

DO YOU DREAM OF RETIREMENT, or do you dread it? Do you picture it as a time to revive youthful dreams or goals and to live *your* way, or do you see it as a stressful time marked by boredom or even an identity crisis? Well, you might want to stay at a fulfilling job, or go full Second Act. Several studies suggest that postponing retirement may confer perks more valuable than a gold watch.

For one: cardiovascular health. In a study published in the journal *Social Science & Medicine*, Harvard researchers examined rates of heart attack and stroke in the ongoing US Health and Retirement Study. Those who'd said sayonara to their jobs were 40 percent more likely to have suffered a heart attack or stroke compared to those who still worked.

People who continue to work rather than retire feel healthier, too. In one study, researchers found that retirement reduced the likelihood of enjoying "very good" or "excellent" health (as reported by the participants) by 40 percent. It also raised the probability of developing at least one health problem, and taking medication to treat it, by 60 percent.

If you absolutely can't stand your job, however, retirement may actually improve your health and well-being. A study of workers found exactly that, linking retirement with improved self-perceived health for those in poor work environments, as well as those with health complaints before they retired. In other words, if you're a take-this-job-and-shove-it type, retirement may actually boost your health. But it's vital to have a plan for active retirement, because a cross-country trip only takes so long.

Leave your phone in the car so that all of your senses can get their fill. The effects are enhanced if you pay close attention to nature, immersed in its beauty. And if you're so inclined, it's okay to roll in leaves, jump in puddles, or, yes, hug a tree.

Make Love Tonight (Or This Morning)

While you focus on eating fruit and veggies at every meal, using sunscreen daily, and working out religiously, take a look-younger shortcut that will curl your toes: Have sex. A study conducted in Scotland suggests that an active love life can make people look up to 12 years younger than they actually are. Seriously! Over 10 years, a panel of judges periodically watched 3,500 men and women through a one-way mirror. (Not having sex!—Just interacting.) Their mission: to guess the age of each. One bunch of participants, nicknamed the "Superyoungs," were consistently estimated to be 7 to 12 years younger than they actually were. Among this group, an active sex life was one of the strongest correlates of a youthful appearance. On average, Superyoungs reported that they had sex three times a week, compared to a control group's average of twice a week. One notable detail: Researchers observed that the faces of sexually active couples were less lined and wrinkled, and their skin was smoother and suppler. The researchers credited oxytocin, a chemical released during sex that reduces stress. As a bonus, they reported that they felt "comfortable and confident" with their sexuality. Great skin and body confidence, too! Rock on, Superyoungs.

There are so many convenient reasons *not* to have sex: You're too tired; you're fuming at your partner over some slight; sex actually has been hurting down there. If the fire down below is more like a smolder, one or more of the tips below may lend a spark.

Read to yourself—or each other. For many women, erotic literature can help jumpstart arousal. If you're truly inspired, invite your partner into bed (wine and clothes optional) and take turns reading to each other from an erotic book. You might try the *Herotica* series, written by women. Or delve into the erotica of Anaïs Nin, the Paris-born writer, diarist, and sexual adventuress who set the gold standard for female-penned erotica. (Nin's *Delta of Venus* is a classic.) Spicy books help take the pressure off you and your partner to initiate sex—and will likely inspire a few new ideas to try out.

Get competitive. A little healthy competition can do wonders for your sex drive. That's because competition boosts dopamine—also released during sex—which tricks your body into arousal. Challenge him to a game of cards, basketball, or even a board game. Then up the stakes: Whoever wins gets whatever he or she wants in the bedroom when the game is done.

Easy does it. In menopause, hormonal changes cause vaginal walls to become thinner, dryer, and less elastic—and that means sex can hurt. Don't let pain rob you of pleasure. Once the reason for the pain is identified, it can be treated. A simple over-the-counter lubricant may help ease the discomfort of drier, thinner tissues. If the pain continues, see your health-care provider or gynecologist. Two possible treatments: topical estrogen applied inside the vagina, to help thicken vaginal tissues and increase moisture and sensitivity, or an oral estrogen treatment.

Find a Furry Ally

It's amazing how easy it is to fall down a clickhole of watching cats jump out of boxes or dogs wear their "guilty" face. But pets can heal hearts as well as steal them. Study after study has shown that people who own and care for a companion animal reap big health benefits, both physical and emotional.

Owning a pet—a dog, especially—may help reduce the risk of cardiovascular disease, according to the American Heart Association. Pet owners are more likely to have lower blood pressure and a better cholesterol profile, to be less vulnerable to the negative health effects of stress, and to survive a heart attack. Dog owners are also more likely to exercise, thanks to all that walking.

Pets may also calm the body's reaction to mental stress, as plenty of post-traumatic stress disorder patients and military veterans have discovered. (A few schools and universities are even using pet therapy to calm students before exams.) Pets have a measurable effect on the body's physiological reactions to stress, as one study published in the journal *Hypertension* clearly showed. Researchers treated subjects with high blood pressure and high-pressure jobs either with blood pressure medication alone or medication and the instructions to adopt a pet. Although both groups saw a drop in resting blood pressure, only the pet adopters saw a drop in blood pressure while under mental stress, and the effects were even greater 6 months later.

The emotional bond between you and your pet also seems to account for some of a companion animal's power to heal; pet owners feel less lonely and like they have constant social support. Playing with or snuggling with a pet releases hormones like oxytocin and dopamine, which boost feelings of closeness and happiness. Here are a few more ways to get a pet boost.

Bond. If you already have a dog or kitty, spend extra time exchanging deep, loving gazes or leaning in close to listen to your pet's purrs or grunts of pleasure. And, of course, give lots of strokes, hugs, and caresses.

Play. Engage in purposeful play. Hide kitty treats around the house, or teach your dog a new trick or enroll him in an agility class.

Walk. Take a long ramble with your dog. It's a treat for your pet and a stress buster for you. Do it daily, and it'll help keep you at a healthy weight. If your pet is overweight, the walks will benefit his health, as well.

Screen Your Screen Time

If there was a binge-watching Olympics, some of us would surely bring home a medal. The average American spends 35.5 hours a week in front of screens watching and streaming media (and in a recent Netflix survey of 1,500 online respondents, 61 percent said they binge-watch regularly).

But there's good reason to go dark more often. As you surely know, a ton of research links a sedentary lifestyle in general (and prolonged TV watching in particular) with a shortened life span and an increased risk of heart disease, type 2 diabetes, and obesity.

One study published in the *British Journal of Sports Medicine* put TV's health impact into grim perspective. You've heard of FOMO, or fear of missing out? This study looked at what we literally miss out on by spending so much of our time plugged in. Crunching data from a huge Australian epidemiological health study (and folding in mortality statistics, too), researchers calculated that in 1 year Australians ages 25 and over watched 9.8 billion (*billion!*) hours of TV, the equivalent of 286,000 lost years of life. Moreover, every hour of TV watched after age 25 was associated with a 22-minute reduction in life expectancy. (Those who averaged 6 hours of TV a day lived an average of 4.8 years less than those who didn't watch any.) If you're thinking, "That sucks—*for the people of Australia*," the study noted that the effects do apply to other industrialized countries, too.

Another reason to give binge-watching the boot, especially if you monitor your blood sugar: Every extra hour a person with prediabetes spends watching the tube each day raises type-2-diabetes risk by 3.4 percent, according to research.

You know you're not giving up TV. But it *is* possible to convert your Netflix or Hulu habit into a not-so-guilty pleasure.

Watch for fun, not for stress management. Watchers who tuned in to de-stress were more likely to have insomnia, one study showed.

Be picky. You've given up crap food. The next step: giving up crap TV—and you'll feel just as good. It may even help you lose weight. In another study, women snacked 52 percent more during yawn-worthy shows. So make a new TV rule: Watch only what engages you. Your favorite drama series or a documentary on a topic that interests you? Enjoy. Another rerun of a '90s sitcom or reality show? Ditch it. Instead, dig into a book, write in your journal, or take any other action, no matter how small, that expands rather than numbs your mind.

Embrace the cliff-hanger. Avoid the temptation to blow through an entire season in a weekend, no matter how the plot thickens. Stop at a 1-hour episode (or less) per day and you're golden. Suspense never killed anyone, after all.

Cultivate the Ability to Be Awestruck

The word *awesome* has been cheapened by overuse. "That pizza was awesome!" you might crow, or "What an awesome haircut!" But the ability to experience awe—real, jaw-dropping reverence in the face of something powerful or beautiful (art, nature, music)—has enormous health benefits, such as lowering stress and boosting immunity. One study suggested that feelings of awe may lower levels of proinflammatory cytokines, proteins that tell the immune system to work harder. (Cytokines help fight illness and infection, but when they cruise around the body without an ailment to fight, they can be harmful, leading to disorders such as arthritis, clinical depression, type 2 diabetes, heart disease, and Alzheimer's.)

No need to watch the sun rise over the Grand Canyon or cry at the opera to reap this benefit. Some researchers have observed that people can be awestruck even by small occurrences. Try to build minimoments into each day that have the power to make you sigh, cry, or stare in wonder. Here are some ideas to get you started.

- Pause when you see an anthill, and watch the ants at work. (Yes, get right down on the ground; ants put on quite a show.) Or pick out one honeybee and observe its path from flower to flower.

- When a thunderstorm hits, take in the flashes and mighty rumbles from the safety of your porch.

- Visit the largest church or other house of worship in your town and sit in silence.

- Go outside and watch a meteor shower predicted in your area. Or gaze at a full, silvery moon.

- Listen to a piece of music that has always moved you.

Feeling the first stirrings of *duende*? Ready to take your Second Act on the road? That's an amazing place to be as you launch your rejuvenated self. You've learned the important steps to take to renew yourself from the inside. Now let's look at how you can turn back the clock on the outside, too.

LOOK AT ME Annie Raines, 58

- Reduced high LDL cholesterol **20 points**
- Reduced high blood glucose level **12 points**
- Boosted confidence **3 points (or 33 percent)**
- Improved back pain
- Weight lost: **16.8 pounds**
- Inches lost: **6.5**

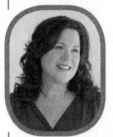

MY STORY: The Younger in 8 Weeks program gave Ann a chance to take her get-healthy goals to the next level. She shaped up her diet by cutting out sugar and refined carbs and eating more vegetables. For exercise, she added variety to her workouts, including strength training, extra stretching, and more walking throughout the day. "My mom lives a block and a half away, and now I usually walk there instead of driving," she said.

But it wasn't easy. "The second day, I felt like I had the flu. The next day, I had a bad headache and low energy," she said, attributing her symptoms to detoxing from sugar, refined carbs, and coffee. But thanks to the support of the group, she stuck it out. Within a few days, her acid reflux had started to subside (and now she no longer needs medication), she was sleeping better, and she had more energy.

By the third week, the pounds started to come off and her arthritis pain began to ease. The morning foot pain that Ann had suffered with for years was gone, and stairs were no longer a problem. "I can walk down the stairs one foot per step now," she said. "I've regained my mobility and my dignity."

SUCCESS!

Sandy Franklin, 55

MY STORY Sandy Franklin is a new grandmother, but lately people have been mistaking her and her daughter for sisters. Five years ago, this wouldn't have been such a surprise. "At 50, people told me I looked 35, but at 55, I look 55," she said before starting the program. After eating her way through menopause and gaining 50 pounds, Sandy threw in the towel. "Once you see the wrinkles and weight gain, you realize you're not going to look like you did when you were 50 or 40, and it's easy to say, 'Why bother?'" But it wasn't just looks that were making her feel old. This former avid runner and skier could no longer enjoy those activities because of chronic knee pain. "I had let myself go," she admitted.

But with her first grandchild on the way, she was inspired to become a role model for her daughters. "I can only do that by taking care of myself," she said.

First, she got back into the kitchen and started to enjoy cooking healthy foods, like beans and quinoa. And she gets more protein from foods like tofu and tempeh instead of meat. "I'm now eating to live long, rather than living to eat long!" she said. The pounds were melting off, and Sandy's energy level soared.

The extra energy came in handy when she hopped back on her bike, an activity she could do without knee pain. She started with 30 minutes three times a week. "I forgot how good those endorphins feel! It's like a happy drug, but it's free and has no side effects." Sandy even uses her time on the bike to pray and meditate. "It sets the tone for my day," she said. She increased her riding to 5 days a week, logging up to 20 miles some days. When the weather turned cold, she took spin classes or rode her bike in her basement.

Now she was feeding her body, but Sandy knew she needed to feed her soul. "I got back into a Bible study with some dear friends I had lost touch with," she said. She also pulled out her paintbrushes, needlepoint, and crochet needle: "I realized that it is important to take care of myself by doing things I enjoy."

And she enjoys shopping again, now that she's dropped nearly three sizes. But the changes that no one else sees are also important. Her blood glucose level is no longer prediabetic, and she lowered her high cholesterol and high blood pressure to healthier levels.

"Now I feel like someone my three grown daughters and my new granddaughter can look up to," she said. "I want to stay healthy so they don't have to take care of me, and I can help them instead."

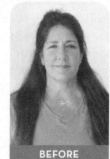

BEFORE

Beauty styling: Eva Scrivo; Wardrobe styling: Erin Turon

LOOK AT ME

- **No more joint pain**

- **Thicker hair**

- **Fewer and less noticeable crow's-feet**

- **Sharper memory**

- **Weight lost: 25.2 pounds**

- **Inches lost: 16**

Tip **DIVIDE AND CONQUER. To** make the skin-care routine easier, I stored my morning products in one little basket and the evening ones in another basket. I stocked both with cotton pads and kept them next to my sink. It saved time, and I didn't have to remember what to use when.

GLOW

Look as Good as You Feel

Yes, beauty comes from within. But it's equally true that self-esteem and appearance create their own virtuous cycle—when you look your best, you tend to feel that way. And while age-related changes to skin and hair can't be stopped, our experts have tons of simple, smart, and downright sneaky ways to slow them down.

Crucial to more youthful skin is a strong prevention plan—plenty of sleep, a daily sunscreen, a healthful diet packed with free-radical-chasing plant foods—and 10 products that both protect and repair skin. Hair changes with age, too (as you surely know all too well), and the right cut, color, and care can make yours softer and shinier and give it the volume and bounce you remember.

Our skin-care routine—created by Jeannette Graf, MD, assistant clinical professor of dermatology at the Icahn School of Medicine at Mount Sinai in New York City—creates clearer, more luminous skin and, as a few of our panelists found, even lightens brown spots.

The hair and makeup sections are courtesy of Eva Scrivo, owner of the Eva Scrivo Salons in New York City and the artist behind our panelists' remarkable "after" looks (at the end of Week 8, page 276). Her strategies can help you transform your appearance and camouflage common age-related beauty challenges, from wrinkles to dull and thinning hair.

Our panelists followed the experts' lead, and even strangers noticed their glow. At the end of a long day, panelist Lisa Boland, checking off the last item on her to-do list, picked up her eyeglasses at a local vision center. "I felt exhausted, but the optician actually commented on my 'beautiful complexion,'" Boland says. "It was a nice way to end my day."

The Skin Solution:
Fuss Less, Glow More

We begin life with smooth, rosy, unblemished skin containing ample amounts of collagen and elastin, the stuff that gives skin its youthful firmness and springiness. We take that perfect skin for granted during decades of sunbathing, eating an imperfect diet, and pulling all-nighters. Somewhere in our midthirties, though, our skin begins to morph. What infernal process triggers the crinkles, dullness, slackness, and spots?

It's a combination of the normal aging process, called *intrinsic* aging, and damage from outside influences (*extrinsic* aging). Controlled mostly by genes, intrinsic aging is behind the visible lines (often from decades of smiling or squinting), the loss of youthful fullness, and the emergence of thinner, drier skin. Extrinsic aging shows up as a thickening of the skin's outer layer; a premature loss of collagen, elastin, and skin-hydrating glycosaminoglycans; age spots; and wrinkles. These changes make the skin appear rough, saggy, uneven in tone, and adorned with creases and spots.

Ultraviolet (UV) light—which we soak up from the sun and man-made sources like tanning beds—is the biggest cause of extrinsic aging, so damaging to skin it even has a name: photoaging, directly linked to wrinkling and skin cancer. Another extrinsic skin ager: invisible airborne particles of crud, including smog, soot, and cigarette smoke. Chemicals called polycyclic aromatic hydrocarbons cling to these particles and are converted to quinones—highly reactive molecules that can age skin in the same ways that chronic exposure to UV light can, a study published in the *Journal of Investigative Dermatology* found.

But even if you already have visible signs of premature aging, positive lifestyle changes can turn your skin around. So can a healthy diet, adequate sleep, and simple morning and evening skin-care routines that emphasize both protection and rejuvenation. What follows is Dr. Graf's fast, least-you-can-do skin-care routine that can make a significant difference in as little as 4 weeks. Flip to the Product Guide on page 407 for a list of recommended brands.

Note: If you follow the skin-care routine and develop burning, stinging, itching, or redness—even if it's minor—discontinue the routine immediately and consult a dermatologist, says Dr. Graf.

The Morning Routine: Protect

When you're in a hurry in the morning, it's easy to shortchange your skin. But it's important to safeguard it from harm. "During the day, skin is busy fending off environmental aggressors like sun, wind, and pollution," says Dr. Graf. "So morning skin care focuses on protection." Our a.m. routine consists of four simple steps.

STEP 1: CLEANSE

Even if you cleanse your skin at night (which you will on our plan), you have to cleanse it again in the morning, says Dr. Graf, because as skin renews itself overnight, impurities come to the surface and need to be whisked away. But if you're cleansing with soap and water, stop right there. "Many women splash their faces with water in the morning, but water alone on your skin is not a great thing," says Dr. Graf. Prolonged water exposure wears away the skin's lipid barrier to the point that it can't defend itself against damaging irritants and UV light. And bar soap can leave skin tight and dry because it removes oils that help keep skin supple. (That squeaky-clean feeling? That's a sign of overdrying—and your skin compensates for the lack of oil by producing extra oil.)

Dr. Graf recommends using cleansers that are wiped off instead of rinsed off with water. One such product is micellar water cleanser—purified water with tiny oil droplets dispersed throughout. These work well for all skin types, she says, and are ideal for women who want a one-step process. Just apply to your face and neck, and then wipe it off with a cloth or cotton ball. The oil particles will break down any residual makeup and oil on your face, while the water whisks them away.

If your skin is on the oily side, you may want to consider a cleansing oil instead. While cleaning your face with oil may sound like a recipe for break-outs, surprise: Cleansing oils are actually *best* for skin that's prone to clog-ging, like oily or acne-prone skin. The reason: Water-soluble cleansers won't penetrate to your oil glands because water repels oil, whereas an oil-based cleanser can cut through the oil on your skin and unclog dirt in your pores. Rinsing with water whisks away all the excess oil and leaves your skin soft and clean, rather than taut and dry, as it is when it's been stripped of its natural oils by regular soap. To use a cleansing oil, massage it into your skin and then splash your face with water.

STEP 2: APPLY A PROTECTIVE ANTIOXIDANT SERUM

Free radicals are rogue molecules in the body generated in part by pollution and sun exposure, and they're like kryptonite to your skin's metabolism. "Free radicals damage DNA—and it's our DNA that dictates how our cells function," says Dr. Graf.

To the rescue: antioxidants. Not the ones you eat (although a higher veggie intake is good both for health and glowing skin), but the ones you apply to your skin. Serums are liquids—typically water based—with a high concentration of active ingredients. Because they're made of very small molecules, the skin absorbs them quickly and deeply. Serums that contain antioxidants,

---

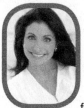

Dr. Jeannette Graf says ...
SIP A GREEN JUICE FOR GLOWING SKIN

For extra radiance, pack your blender with carrots, cantaloupe, and other carotenoid-rich produce. One study found that, within weeks, the skin of people who consumed a daily equivalent of 15 milligrams of beta-carotene supplements took on a golden tone that others perceived as attractive.

But why pop a supplement when you can sip the delicious real deal? This 2-serving smoothie packs more than 6 milligrams of beta-carotene into less than 100 calories. (Save your second serving in the fridge for up to a day.)

1 cup chopped kale

2 large kiwifruit, peeled and chopped

1/2 cup fresh orange juice or tangerine juice

1/2 cup cilantro sprigs, chopped

1 rib celery, chopped

1/4 cup ice cubes

Blend all the ingredients.

PER SERVING: 92 calories, 3 g protein, 21 g carbohydrates, 3 g fiber, 12 g total sugar, 1 g fat, 0.5 g saturated fat, 36 mg sodium)

---

such as vitamins C or E, help shield the skin from environmental threats, reduce inflammation, and even out skin tone, keeping your skin bright and youthful. Smooth one on your skin immediately after cleansing.

STEP 3: MOISTURIZE

As we age, oil-producing glands in the skin become less active, which means that skin dries out. Moisturizers trap water in the skin, helping to reduce the appearance of lines and give you a brighter, more youthful complexion. Dr. Graf recommends selecting a product that contains at least one of the ingredients below (look especially for the first two), which help skin retain moisture and temporarily plump it.

Hyaluronic acid. Produced naturally by skin, "hyaluronic acid is a moisture magnet—it pulls moisture into the skin," says Dr. Graf. But hyaluronic acid levels decrease with age, leaving skin less plump and with deeper wrinkles. If your skin is very dry, a moisturizer with hyaluronic acid is a good option.

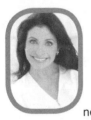

Dr. Jeannette Graf says . . .
THERE'S A RIGHT WAY TO APPLY SUNSCREEN

When choosing a sunscreen for your body, use the same principles for choosing one for skin below the neck (broad-spectrum protection; SPF of around 30). Here's how to apply it correctly.

- Cover all exposed skin. That'll take about 1 ounce of sunscreen, the amount that would fill a shot glass.
- Apply to dry skin 30 minutes before you head outdoors. If you use topical medications, apply them first, let them dry, and then apply sunscreen.
- Choose a water-resistant sunscreen if you know you'll be active, swimming, or sweating.
- Reapply sunscreen either every 2 hours or immediately after you swim or towel off.
- On days when the sun is blazing, slip on a shirt or other cover-up, slap on a hat, and don wraparound sunglasses. The shades help protect not just the delicate skin around your eyes but also the eyes themselves.

Glycerin. Another moisture magnet, glycerin draws moisture into the skin and is good for parched skin.

Ceramides. These lipids mimic the natural fatty acids in skin that seal in moisture.

Peptides. The building blocks of proteins, peptides signal cells to produce more collagen and help facial muscles relax, which helps make lines appear less prominent.

Dr. Graf's p.m. routine includes a line- and wrinkle-smoothing retinoid (see page 124), so your moisturizer doesn't need to include one. However, there is one last ingredient you can look for in a moisturizer: a broad-spectrum sunscreen, your complexion's first line of defense against photoaging.

Whatever type you choose, use a gumdrop-size dollop of moisturizer, and make sure to cover your entire face (be careful around your eyes). Apply also to your neck and chest. If you select a moisturizer with a broad-spectrum sunscreen, skip Step 4 (though read more about what "broad spectrum" means, below).

STEP 4: SHIELD

Only 30 percent of women (and 14 percent of men) report using sunscreen regularly, according to recent research. But to avoid a leathery face and décolletage and protect against skin cancer, everyday use—not just during beach season—is a must.

Choose broad-spectrum protection. A broad-spectrum sunscreen is the cornerstone of any youthful skin strategy. To understand what the term *broad spectrum* means, you need to know that the sun emits two kinds of ultraviolet (UV) rays—UVA and UVB. All sunscreens protect against UVB, the main cause of sunburn. But UVA rays need to be screened out, too; they penetrate the skin more deeply than UVB and contribute to both premature skin aging and skin cancer. A broad-spectrum product protects against both kinds of rays. (Unlike UVB rays, which are highest during the summer, UVA is the same level all year round, which is why you really should wear sunscreen in winter.)

To ensure you've got a broad-spectrum product, check the packaging for one of the following active ingredients, all of which filter out UVA rays: Avobenzone (Parsol 1789), ecamsule, titanium dioxide, or zinc oxide (which is especially suited to sensitive skin).

Go with an SPF of around 30. A product's SPF, or sun protection factor,

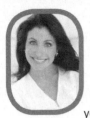

Dr. Jeannette Graf says ...

HERE'S ALL YOU NEED FOR DAILY SKIN CARE

Now that you know the right way to apply your skin-care products, here's a recap of all you'll need for younger, dewier skin. See the Product Guide on page 407 for my brand recommendations.

A.M. ROUTINE

Micellar water cleanser or cleansing oil

Antioxidant serum

Moisturizer

Broad-spectrum sunscreen

P.M. ROUTINE

Retinoid cream

Night cream (optional)

Eye cream

---

is the level of protection it provides against sunburn-causing UVB rays only. While you can find sunscreens with SPFs of 50 or even 100, beyond SPF 30, the difference in protection is negligible.

Apply the sunscreen to all exposed areas of your face and neck. What about the rest of you? See the box on the previous page.

The Evening Routine: Repair

"At night, your skin does the bulk of its repair work, such as creating new cells and mending or shedding old, damaged ones," says Dr. Graf. Your nighttime regimen can be just as streamlined as your morning routine, requiring only two additional products (or just one, if you prefer).

STEP 1: WIPE AWAY THE DAY'S DIRT AND DEBRIS

Cleanse your face and neck exactly as you do in the morning, says Dr. Graf, especially if you wear makeup (for the correct way to remove it, see page 217 in Week 3). "At the end of the day, there are bacteria, parasites, and broken-down skin particles on your face, and you need to clean them off," she says.

STEP 2: APPLY A SKIN-BRIGHTENING RETINOID

There's no all-around age reverser as powerful as this derivative of vitamin A, says Dr. Graf, thanks to its ability to increase collagen production and cell turnover. According to a study published in the *Archives of Dermatology*, retinoids accelerate skin's natural sloughing process, which slows down considerably as we age. Using a retinoid can help make skin brighter and smoother—and less likely to break out, too.

If you're a retinol newbie, start with over-the-counter retinoid products, which contain varying amounts of retinol, says Dr. Graf. If you have sensitive skin, she suggests using a product formulated with retinaldehyde, which can be less irritating.

If you use an over-the-counter retinol for a while and notice a plateau in your skin's improvement, it may be time to consider a prescription retinoid, says Dr. Graf. There are many prescription-strength formulations, and a dermatologist can recommend the best formulation for you. For the best results—and less chance of flaking or irritation—follow these guidelines.

Over-the-counter retinoid: Cleanse your face and neck, apply the product, and then wait a few minutes to apply moisturizer.

Prescription-strength retinoid: Cleanse. Next, making sure that your skin is totally dry, dot a tiny amount of prescription-strength product on each part of your face and blend. Apply moisturizer immediately. "Prescription-strength retinoids penetrate the skin so rapidly, you don't have to wait," says Dr. Graf.

STEP 3: MOISTURIZE

If you're happy with the moisturizer you applied in the morning, there's no need to buy a special night cream, says Dr. Graf. However, if your skin is extra parched, consider using a thicker moisturizer. Ingredients to look for: fatty acids such as ceramides to repair skin's natural moisture barrier; hyaluronic acid and glycerin to attract water to the skin; and petrolatum, mineral oil, and dimethicone to seal in moisture. Stick with balms or creams; most lotions aren't hydrating enough for dry skin. Whether you use your daytime moisturizer or a heavier night cream, apply it *over* your retinoid, says Dr. Graf.

STEP 4: DAB ON AN EYE CREAM

Why not just use your moisturizer? "Because many contain water, which can puff up the eye area," says Dr. Graf. She recommends eye creams formulated with retinol, peptides, and vitamin C, which are ideal for the thin skin around the eyes, providing wrinkle relief without irritation, while hyaluronic acid and peptides hydrate and repair collagen. There are also eye creams that lighten dark circles with licorice, niacinamide (a form of vitamin B), and green tea, all of which target uneven tone and pigmentation.

When you apply eye cream, use your ring finger to gently tap in the product. Also, apply it not just to crow's-feet but to the entire eye area (the skin on the brow bone, too). Start your application on the inner brow, next to your nose, and then go around the upper brow, outer crow's-feet, and under the eye.

Healthier Hair: Styling Secrets for a Lusher, More Youthful Look

In times of change, hair is often the first thing we want to overhaul—not just to look more polished, but to send a different message or explore a new identity, says our beauty expert, salon owner Eva Scrivo. "Today's you is different from the 20- or 30-something you, often in amazing ways. You've evolved. You've grown. And a new style or color can reflect those positive changes," wrote Scrivo in her book, *Eva Scrivo on Beauty*.

Maybe you're panicked by the prospect of changing your hair. No doubt about it—it's a gutsy move, especially if you've worn the same style for years. To cut your signature waist-length hair shorter; to play with different, more flattering color; to settle in the stylist's chair and hold your breath, half-terrified, half-exhilarated—it's an act of faith, a kind of private coming-out party for the wiser, more mature self you're now exploring. A more youthful style or color takes years off, and that perk is often accompanied by an emotional sense of freedom and release. You feel more alive, more energetic, and ready to take on this next phase of your life. "Accepting your age does not mean giving up," Scrivo says. "It means doing things differently than you did them 20 years ago."

Your hair should reflect the woman you are today—and to find that style requires embracing and working with your physical changes. When it comes to aging and hair, Scrivo preaches the three Cs:

- **Cut:** Your hair should have lift and movement, and the style should complement the shape of your face.

- **Color:** The right color adds depth and fullness to the cut and complements your skin tone.

- **Care:** In your twenties, your hair may have been stronger and fuller. After 40, hair care changes. "You need to take a more strategic approach," says Scrivo. That means using products that strengthen and fortify the hair and nourish the scalp. "A healthy scalp equals healthy hair," she notes.

What follows is a breakdown of the three Cs. This will be the next best thing to sitting in Scrivo's chair. Once again, if you want specific brand recommendations, see the Product Guide on page 407.

The Best Cut for You

"A great haircut is your most powerful accessory to make you feel more confident and beautiful," says Scrivo. That's why it's important to give this decision the deliberation it deserves. Discuss the questions below with your stylist before getting a new style so you're both on the same page.

What do you want to keep—and what are you looking to change? Maybe you're fond of your wavy hair but not the way it frizzes. You may want to keep your hair long but hate that it gets flat on top. Conversely, you may prefer a shorter style but fear that it looks matronly or unfeminine. Or you might be looking for a style that plays up your best features (your eyes or cheekbones) or camouflages challenges (a receding hairline). "A good haircut is a problem solver," says Scrivo.

What's your hair texture? Hair's texture and density (whether curly, frizzy, coarse, straight, or fine), and especially the cut, affect how hair falls

Renew Right Now

A SIMPLE BUT SMASHING CHANGE: BANGS

A change as basic as bangs can transform your entire look, says Scrivo—and there are so many ways to wear them. They can be blunt, textured, and side swept, and they can conceal fine lines and cover a short or high forehead. "Bangs can make you look younger because they soften your face and play up eyes and lift cheekbones," she says. And they can be the perfect answer if you're seeking a change but don't want to cut your hair short.

and moves. For example, if you have curly hair and it feels too puffy, you may want to wear it longer, as length weighs hair down, helping it to behave better. Alternatively, if your hair is long and you want to bring out the curl, cutting it shorter will help to add bounce and definition. The latter would also be true if your hair is fine, as a shorter style can add volume.

What's your face and body type? Is your face long and narrow, heart-shaped, round, or square? Do you want to create a stronger jaw line or a longer or shorter neck or play down jowls? A talented stylist can see where the lines of a haircut should hit to create a flattering optical illusion.

If you're larger framed, consider growing out your hair to your collarbone or longer to slim and elongate your face and body. "The right length and lines in your hair can make you appear thinner and taller," says Scrivo. So will adding height at the crown (the top of your head). "With the right style, you'll naturally have volume at the top of the head by virtue of how the hair is cut," she adds. And you won't have to rely on teasing or too many products.

How much maintenance are you up for? Do you have 5 minutes to style your hair in the morning, or 20? If the style you want requires a blow-out, will you do it, or would you prefer a less care-intensive, wash-and-go style?

What's your personal style? The image you project to the world is the X factor that allows you to carry off an unexpected length, style, or color. "With the right balance and sound execution, rules can be broken," Scrivo says. "One of my regular clients is 75 and wears her brunette (colored) hair flat-ironed below her shoulders. She can carry this look because she takes good care of herself, is slim, has beautiful skin as well as a refined sense of style."

ANTIAGING CUT #1: LONG LAYERS

Why it works: Serious hair loss is determined by a genetic lottery, but hair thins for nearly all of us after 40. Long layers make up for lost density by adding volume at the crown and sides of your head, says Scrivo.

Best for you if: Your below-the-shoulder hair is dragging you down and making you look older, but you don't want to lose length. Face-framing layers strengthen your bone structure, says Scrivo.

Ask for: Long layers throughout the hair, with shorter layers around the face that graze the lower cheekbone and end at the jaw, midneck, and clavicle. A few pieces snipped at eye level will draw attention there, Scrivo explains.

ANTIAGING CUT #2: MODERN SHAG

Why it works: The shag's layers keep your hair from being weighed down by extra length and add volume at the root—and make hair look thicker, too.

Best for you if: You are too rushed to blow it dry or are just bored with your midlength style.

Ask for: A midlength cut with gradual, choppy layers around the face and slightly longer layers in the back. Antiaging bonus: Bangs disguise prominent forehead wrinkles. Blunt, straight-across bangs work best on narrower face shapes, while sideswept fringe suits women with rounder faces.

ANTIAGING CUT #3: LONG BOB

Why it works: Your hair's outer layer becomes more fragile after 40, and a drop in keratin protein makes hair weaker and less elastic, so it will break rather than snap back when pulled or stressed. The long bob creates more bounce because hair is blunt and full at the bottom, creating a nice swing

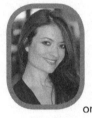

Eva Scrivo says ...

THESE HAIRCUTS WILL *ADD* YEARS

Just as the right hairstyle can roll back the years, the wrong one can add them, says Scrivo. If you're wearing one of the styles below, consider updating your look.

THE HELMET. "With this style, hair is set and heavily sprayed and has an equal length around its entirety—typically 3 to 4 inches from the scalp on the top, sides, and back," says Scrivo. "It's a style similar to that of our grandmothers after their weekly 'wash-and-set' at the beauty parlor."

THE MOM-LET. This is what Scrivo calls a variation of the dreaded mullet. "In an attempt to gain height while leaving the hair long, short layers are cut at the top of the head and the back and sides are left too long, creating yet another unflattering version of this 1980s trend," says Scrivo.

THE WITCH. Overly long, unstyled, wild hair that has been neglected and allowed to go completely gray can add years to a woman's appearance, says Scrivo. But there's no need to go super-short. "Whether you're an ex-hippie or a bohemian at heart, you can remain true to your soul by cutting your hair 3 to 4 inches below your shoulders, including face-framing layers, and blowing out a few sections, especially at the front, for added polish," she says.

when you walk and making it look healthier, Scrivo says.

Best for you if: You want to go short but not really short. This longer-in-front cut is also ideal if your idea of styling is running your hands through your hair before you head out the door; this style will still look good even if your air-dried hair waves and bends at will.

Ask for: A long bob that sits just above or below the clavicle (no longer), with some layering at the nape of the neck and minimal layering in front.

ANTIAGING CUT #4: PIXIE

Why it works: A natural loss of fatty acids and keratin protein makes hair more vulnerable to damage, so things you've always done (color, heat style, etc.) now rough up the hair's surface and damage its outer cuticle layer. The pixie enhances shine and amplifies texture by lopping off hair that's been damaged by chemical, thermal, and environmental stresses.

Best for you if: You're a wash-and-go type; most of the work this cut requires is simply washing, air-drying, and adding a little pomade to finish it off.

Ask for: A pixie, but specify that you'd like it to be soft, not severe, around the edges of the cut, and be clear about how long you'd like it to be, especially on top. Usually, a pixie is no longer than 3 inches, but you can request 4 or 5 inches (a good option for broader faces, says Scrivo). You can also pair it with soft, sideswept bangs for a more feminine feel. Ask your stylist to leave the hair an inch longer around the perimeter for a softer, less severe result (this can always be adjusted when the hair is dry).

Do Color Right

If you already color your hair, you know how good it looks and feels afterward— softer, smoother, less frizzy. Scrivo notes that because color fills in the cuticle of each strand, hair feels silkier and reflects more light, while the extra layer of pigment adds volume and density to strands, giving your locks that lush, youthful appearance.

If you don't color, it's time to give it serious consideration. Because whatever your hair woe—frizz, lack of volume, the fading of your natural color, or coarse and wiry gray hair—coloring can improve it. "Hair color acts as a permanent cosmetic," says Scrivo. "The right hue can brighten your complexion, make you look more refreshed and rested, and give the impression of thicker hair."

The caveat: It's vital to use the right color formulation for your hair type *and* your skin tone. Because coloring your hair can make your appearance or break it, Scrivo recommends that you get your hair professionally colored—and not because she owns a salon. "Most salon-grade hair color is made with finer and more expensive colorants and conditioning ingredients, which prevents the hair from becoming dehydrated and gives it greater shine," Scrivo says. Also, a salon colorist creates a color formula just for you, which means it's customized and the result is more multidimensional. "A good colorist is part chemist, part artist and considers your complexion, eye color, percentage of gray, and shape of the cut," she adds. Finally, it's difficult to apply one's own color well—even professionals have others do it for them, since it's hard to see the top and back of your head.

The DIY option has become increasingly popular as at-home formulations have improved, but there are a couple of things to keep in mind. First, you want to avoid flat, one-dimensional hair. You can do that by not always pulling the color all the way to the ends of your hair from the roots or by leaving it on for less time (the ends absorb color more quickly). Look for at-home kits that have built-in highlights and color gray hairs differently from the rest of the hair. Also, many women make the mistake of going too dark, which can look ghoulish, because older skin tends to be sallow. Pick a lighter hue, but for best results, don't stray too much from your natural hair color.

If you go the at-home route, think about having your hair professionally colored every second or third time, Scrivo advises. This helps ensure that your color is evenly applied, as good hair color is half formulation and half application. And a colorist can correct any gaffes that you make on your own, even out any spots you missed, and prevent dark ends.

CHOOSING THE RIGHT FORMULATION

Hair color comes in different formulations, from temporary color—which sits on top of the hair strand and washes out after one shampoo—to semi-permanent, which lasts 8 to 10 shampoos. There's also demi-permanent color, which contains peroxide and lasts up to 24 shampoos, and permanent formulations that contain a bit of ammonia to completely penetrate the strand. (In other words, permanent color doesn't wash out; it grows out.) When selecting a formulation, ask yourself these questions:

How gray are you? If your hair is less than 50 percent gray, consider a demi-permanent formula, which blends the grays instead of covering them, says Scrivo. If your hair is more than half gray, a permanent formulation, which covers gray 100 percent, may be the better option. "Gray hair needs a more potent formula to open the cuticle and get the pigment into the hair strand," Scrivo explains.

What color are you going for? If you want to go two or more shades lighter than your current color (whether it's natural or colored), opt for permanent color, with or without highlights, says Scrivo. Looking for a less dramatic change? Go with a demi-permanent formulation, which is also a good choice if you have only a few grays, she says.

What condition is your hair in? If it's dry, damaged, or *porous*—meaning that it sucks up water and moisture like a sponge—it's likely to suck up hair color, too. So be aware that if your hair is porous, using a semi- or demi-permanent formulation may give you a darker-than-expected result.

What kind of upkeep are you ready for? Once you start to color, you'll have to do it regularly to keep that fresh, glossy look. Just as you considered how much time you're willing to spend on styling your hair, you'll have to decide how often you're willing to go to the salon for upkeep. Usually, semi- and demi-permanent formulations require the least amount of upkeep and the fewest trips to the salon, says Scrivo. Depending on how fast your hair grows, root touch-ups usually are needed every 3 to 4 weeks.

PICKING YOUR PERFECT HUE

Choosing the right hair color for your skin tone may be the most painless way to look decades younger, Scrivo says. As we get older, our complexions become duller and paler, and having the wrong hair color can worsen the effect by washing you out.

"Older women often tell me that no matter how much rest they get, they look tired," says Scrivo. "That's because their hair color is off. When you get hair color right, it frames the face and illuminates the skin."

Finding the right color for your skin tone can be tricky. Women often go too light, says Scrivo, and their hair color ends up almost matching their skin tone. At the other extreme, women also go too dark in an attempt to color gray hair, which draws attention to wrinkles, sallow skin, and thinning.

Scrivo's recommendation: Stay within one to two shades of your natural color (or, if you're gray, what your color once was), and add a few highlights. Golden colors make hair and facial features softer and younger on those with pale or yellow undertones, she says. Choose shades that are ashen color when you have pink or blue undertones. Those with olive-toned skin would do best to add red-toned highlights instead, since red balances green in the law of color theory.

One of the fastest ways to take years off your face: adding highlights around the hairline, says Scrivo. They help catch the light, illuminating the face for a more youthful appearance. Highlights also camouflage emerging grays around the hairline. Because the success of highlights depends on their subtlety and nuances of tone, Scrivo recommends getting them done at a salon, where a stylist can help you choose the right color and technique.

Caring for Your Hair

If you invest in a great cut and professional color, it makes sense to use superior products, too. Generally speaking, salon-grade shampoos and conditioners contain higher-quality ingredients. Drugstore shampoos tend to have higher levels of detergent, or sulfates, to produce immediate lather, which can strip hair of its natural oils (and the salon color you just invested in). Mass-market conditioners usually contain silicone, which mimics moisture, making hair feel slippery, and can build up a barrier that prevents healthy conditioning ingredients from permeating it, says Scrivo. If you're going to buy drugstore brands, look for shampoos and conditioners that don't contain sulfates, parabens (a preservative), or mineral oil, Scrivo says.

The bottom line is that you should buy the products that make your hair look and feel best. "If a product works well for you, then it's a good value. If it dries out your hair or strips your color, then you're paying much more for it than you realize," Scrivo says.

SHAMPOO ON YOUR HAIR'S SCHEDULE

While many women wash their hair every day, that's usually not necessary—and can even backfire. Just as overcleansing your skin can cause it to produce more oil to compensate, stripping the scalp can also lead to an overproduction of oil. Scrivo's guideline for shampooing: Wash when your hair feels dirty or your scalp itches. That might be every day if your hair's on the oily side or two or three times a week if your hair is dry or curly. The less you wash, the more natural oils stay in your hair, helping to tame any frizziness. And you don't have to wash your hair every time you go to the gym; perspiration is mostly water, not dirt.

Whether you want to add volume, bust frizz, or protect hair color, you'll find a shampoo that's made for the job. If the vast amount of choices confuses you, ask your stylist for a recommendation. The person cutting, coloring, and styling your hair is the one who knows it best.

CONDITION FROM THE BOTTOM UP

"Conditioner does for the scalp what moisturizer does for the face after makeup removal; it replaces the moisture removed during cleansing," says Scrivo. Again, let your hair type and style be your guide. Some products offer volume, while others tame frizz, quench dry or damaged hair, or protect color. Whichever you use, apply it to the ends first. Then, work your way up your hair, applying more as you move up your head. If your hair is oily, there's no need to condition your roots, says Scrivo. Your scalp's natural oils act as a built-in moisturizer.

USE A CLARIFYING SHAMPOO

Styling products can leave a buildup on your scalp that many shampoos can't penetrate. "This buildup of gels, mousses, and sprays can cause scalp irritation, flakiness, and inhibit the hair's natural shine," Scrivo says. "It also can be a barrier when using conditioning masks and treatments."

Removing product buildup will make your hair look and feel invigorated. There are a bunch of clarifying shampoos on the market. Or make your own, Scrivo says: Just add 1 tablespoon of apple cider vinegar to the dollop of shampoo you'll be using to wash your hair. Let it sit on your hair for a few minutes, rinse, and then shampoo and condition as usual. Because clarifying treatments can remove hair dye, it's best to use one the night before you head to the salon for your color appointment.

BRUSH 100 STROKES

That "100 strokes a day" advice is no beauty myth, says Scrivo. Brush for 2 minutes each night before bed, and in 6 weeks your hair will be shinier, softer, and more manageable, she says. Nightly brushing distributes the oils from your scalp to the ends of your hair, removes dead skin cells that can clog hair follicles and inhibit new hair growth, and also stimulates circulation. Don't use a brush with plastic bristles, though; they don't do a good job of redistributing oil through hair. Invest in a natural-bristle brush instead.

COMBAT FLAKES AND ITCHINESS

If your scalp itches, or you're dealing with flakes or dandruff, treat your scalp with essential oils. Rosemary oil can help with dandruff, neem oil can treat light flakiness, and tea tree oil can soothe an itchy scalp, says Scrivo. (Just be aware that tea tree oil can fade hair color.) If your scalp is oily, lavender oil can help balance oil production.

Essential oils can be powerful stuff, so use them sparingly. Add one dropper full to an ounce of seed or vegetable oil (sunflower oil or quick-absorbing jojoba oil works well). Right before bed, massage the mixture onto your scalp for several minutes, and wash it out in the morning when you shower. Don't worry about your pillowcase; natural oils absorb easily into the scalp and hair and won't stain it (but you can cover the case with a towel if you like).

GET THICKER-LOOKING HAIR

As estrogen levels decline over time, hair naturally thins out. Stress or sudden trauma can also be the culprit behind a dwindling hairline or small bald patches. If these are issues for you, flip ahead to the "Reverse Hair Loss" section on page 239, which we'll cover in Week 5 of the plan.

To disguise or mitigate gradually thinning hair, the tips below are tried-and-true techniques to help.

Brush, brush, brush. Another reason for those nightly strokes: It helps stimulate circulation to the scalp and exfoliate the skin to unclog hair follicles and promote growth, says Scrivo. You don't have to brush hard. Lightly set a soft, natural-bristle brush on your head, and gently press down while moving it in tiny circles (be careful not to tangle your hair). Or give yourself a nightly scalp massage with your fingertips.

Go shorter. Cutting even a couple of inches can help your hair look thicker and bouncier. Layers add volume, too; ask that layers be concentrated near your face while the back is left full to create the illusion of body and thickness. "A side part or side-swept bang also helps to mask a thinning hairline," says Scrivo.

Have your hair professionally colored. The color swells your hair's cuticle, increasing its diameter and lending extra volume. (Scrivo particularly likes Goldwell hair color, which is low in ammonia and high on shine.) To avoid overprocessing delicate hair, touch up roots no more than every 3 weeks and highlights every 2 to 3 months.

Use a volumizing shampoo. Choose one without sulfates (detergents that are harsh on hair but not necessary for a cleansed scalp). This formula removes excess oils that make hair look limp but is gentle enough to support a healthy shine.

Achieve liftoff. After a shower, when your hair is damp, work a volumizing mousse or spray into hair near the root. Make sure to use smaller amounts if using more than one product.

Back off on the blow-dryer. "One sure way to fry your hair is to smash the nozzle of the blow-dryer right up against it," says Scrivo. Hold the dryer about an inch away from the brush, which also helps hair keep more shine, since direct heat removes the top layer of moisture and makes hair look dull, Scrivo says. To protect hair from the heat of a blow-dryer or curling iron, use a shielding serum with heat-buffering dimethicones, which will help prevent split ends.

To give your hair a break from the blow-dryer now and again, sop up water from hair with a T-shirt (cotton is softer on the cuticle and doesn't rough it up like a typical towel, which could result in frizz), and then finger comb it with a smoothing lotion so it won't frizz. Be sure to use a styling product made specifically for fine hair that will not weigh it down.

Shake off thinning spots. Hair fibers are amazing. Shake the pigmented cellulose fibers over a wide part or a thin bald patch, and it disappears. These are like false lashes for your hair; the fibers (which come in different shades) cling to your hair and appear to thicken it. You'll find hair fibers in most large drugstores.

Consider hair extensions. Hair extensions can add fullness and density to thinning hair of any length, says Scrivo. The key: Choose quality extensions and have a professional stylist cut and blend them into your hair.

Scrivo recommends the Invisi-Tab line of extensions, made of human hair (visit invisitab.com for a salon locator). "They're very natural looking. The hair is soft, doesn't tangle, and, if necessary, can be colored or highlighted to blend perfectly with your natural hair," she says. You can opt for Invisi-Tab's tape-in extensions, which attach to your existing hair with a special double-sided tape and can be left in for several months. For fullness with convenience, the clip-on variety can add volume where you need it in minutes. The stylist will attach them or show you how to clip them in. "Clipping in two or three pieces on each side of the head, just below the parietal ridge (the bone that protrudes a bit on either side of the skull), will give your hair added fullness," she says. Used this way, the extensions cost $200 to $600.

Change Your Makeup: Put Your Best Face Forward

Learning to apply cosmetics more artfully can take years off your appearance and enhance what nature gave you. "When it comes to makeup, details make all the difference," Scrivo says. For brand recommendations of the products she suggests using in this section, see the Product Guide on page 407. (Going out for the evening? See page 215 in Week 3 for Scrivo's tips on how to transition makeup from a natural day look to a more dramatic evening look.) Here are a few guidelines to help you get the best and most natural results.

Apply your makeup in the right order. Follow the sequence in these pages and you'll glow for hours without streaks, smears, or midday makeup fade-outs. Do you have to use every product listed? Of course not. If you want to skip particular products, simply move on to the next cosmetic.

Invest in good tools. A flawless face begins with the right application tools, says Scrivo, and they don't include the puffs and brushes that come with makeup. The right tools can help you apply makeup flawlessly—no more raccoon eyes, clown cheeks, or lipstick-smeared teeth. Here's a primer:

- **Makeup sponges** for foundation. If you use an inexpensive brand, use a fresh one each time and then toss it. More expensive, higher-quality alternatives can be washed after each use and last 2 to 3 weeks. Scrivo recommends sponges by Alcone, which will last for months if washed after each use.

- A **powder puff** made of velour or down. Handwash it every couple of weeks.

- Separate **brushes** for concealer, loose powder, brow powder, eyeliner, eye shadow, lip color, and blush. Buy brushes as a set (they're less expensive), and buy the best set you can afford. "If you take care of them, they can last more than 10 years," says Scrivo. Choose brushes with rounded bristles rather than blunt edges.

    To extend the life of your brushes, store them bristles-up in a cup and wash them every 2 weeks. Washing them is simple: Just swirl the bristles in a bowl of warm water to which you've added a small amount of shampoo. Swirl for a minute or two and rinse under the tap in the direction of the bristles. Squeeze the water from the bristles (be gentle!), reshape the bristles, and let them air-dry on a clean tea towel.

    Armed with the right set of brushes, you'll be able to use less makeup to better effect, says Scrivo. If you've always applied lipstick straight from the tube or used the cheap brushes that come with eye shadow or blush, you'll be amazed at the soft, natural effect good brushes deliver.

Start with less, add more. As counterintuitive as it may seem, a flawless look is achieved not by using more product but by using less. (This is especially true of foundation, which is supposed to enhance your skin rather than conceal it.) Scrivo's advice: Use very small amounts of product and build up the color if you need to. It's so much easier to add more rather than have to remove it. Also, when you dip your brush or sponge into a product, do not apply it directly to your face, she says. Rather, pause for a moment to tap or wipe your brush or sponge on the back of your hand to remove excess product. *Then* apply it.

Take your time—and a seat. "I recommend sitting at a vanity to do your makeup," she says. When you stand at the bathroom mirror (as so many of us do), it's easy to rush through the process, which can result in crooked lines or too-heavy application. "If you sit down, you'll do a much better job," she says. If possible, consider making a dedicated space for applying makeup, with a good-sized mirror and natural lighting. Your makeup will look more polished, and you'll be gifting yourself with a small oasis of time dedicated totally to you.

PRIMER: SMOOTH FINE LINES AND LARGE PORES

Good painters sand and prime the walls before painting. It's just as important to prime your skin for foundation. "It allows foundation to sit more evenly on skin, which makes for a smoother surface, so it reflects more light," Scrivo says. Also, primer prevents your skin from soaking up your foundation and cheek color, so your makeup stays put.

Many primers contain silicone, which fills in pores and fine lines. Silicone-based primers are great for dry skin. If your skin is on the oily side, though, a brand with silicone may plug your pores, so opt for a water-based primer instead. Match your primer formulation to your makeup formulation: If your foundation is water-based, use a water-based primer; if it's silicone-based, use a silicone primer. Can't tell? Ingredients that end in -cone, -methicone, or -siloxane signal a silicone formula.

If you prefer, you can wear primer alone, over sunscreen, to blur fine lines and large pores. "You get a bit of coverage without a lot of weight, especially with a drop of concealer under your eyes," Scrivo says.

Apply with light strokes, feathering with your fingertips over your entire face.

FOUNDATION: LIGHT COVERAGE, LUMINOUS SKIN

There are tons of foundations on the market. So which one is right for you? It depends on your skin type, Scrivo says.

IF YOU HAVE . . .	CHOOSE A . . .
Dry skin	Cream or hydrating liquid foundation
Oily skin	Powder or mineral-powder foundation
Combination skin	Oil-free, water-based foundation
Sensitive skin	Fragrance-free liquid foundation or tinted moisturizer

Next, decide what color suits you best. Scrivo has two rules of thumb for choosing a foundation color.

Select a hue that matches your skin. No matter what your skin tone, you want foundation to be invisible on your skin, says Scrivo. "It should disappear when you apply it. Your foundation and skin should be one." Don't overdo it; just one drop of foundation can deliver even, radiant skin with undetectable coverage.

Ideally, you should buy foundation at a department-store cosmetics counter so you can actually test out a few. Don't wear foundation, and take a small hand mirror with you. The salesperson will help you select several hues and give you samples on a cotton swab. Take the swabs to the nearest window and swipe them on your jaw in natural light (fluorescent bulbs alter the color's appearance). "If you can see it on your jaw, then it's the wrong color," says Scrivo.

If you buy foundation that you can't test, shop for it bare-faced so you get the truest sense of your natural skin tone. To find a match, hold three shades up to your face—one that looks just right, one that's darker, and one that's lighter. Check the colors near a window with natural light.

Start with moist skin. You've already applied moisturizer, sunblock, and primer, but if your skin doesn't feel moist, apply one more drop of moisturizer. "Moisture is the secret to a flawless finish," says Scrivo.

For smooth, even, glaze-thin coverage, place one drop of foundation, about the size of a pea, onto the back of your hand and apply to your face with a makeup sponge. "Really wiggle the sponge and work the foundation into your skin," Scrivo says. Then follow with light, feathery strokes of the sponge to further blend. (If you wear eye shadow, also apply foundation to your lids to neutralize darkness or redness.) If you need more, apply it in small amounts and blend. Then, place a tissue over your face and blot to remove any excess foundation.

CONCEALER: CAMOUFLAGE FOR IMPERFECTIONS

Concealers come in different formulations and offer varying amounts of coverage, so pick the best type for the job. Stick concealers deliver the most coverage and are best for blemishes or hyperpigmentation. Liquid concealers are best for dark circles under the eyes because they're light, creamy, and easy to blend. And when you have a blemish or purplish under-eye circles, you'll want a special type of concealer, called a color corrector. Applied before regular concealer, green and yellow correctors neutralize redness; salmon correctors neutralize dark spots and bluish under-eye circles.

Concealer should always be applied with a brush rather than a finger; imagine "erasing" broken capillaries, dark circles, and spots with just the tips of the bristles, says Scrivo. Place a tiny amount on the back of your hand, and dab the tips of the bristles into it. Remove the excess and then apply, brushing and blending carefully.

To conceal spots and broken capillaries: With a clean brush, dot the blemish with a green concealer. (Just the blemish, not the skin around it.) Use a cotton swab to dot on a liquid concealer that matches your foundation or skin tone exactly. Blend into the skin around the blemish, and then set with loose powder.

To hide dark circles: Pick a concealer one shade lighter than your foundation. Apply it in two layers, Scrivo says. Apply one layer with a brush and tap it with your ring finger to blend. Apply a second layer, and tap again.

LOOSE POWDER: OUTSMART MAKEUP FADE-OUTS

Loose powder has two important functions: It absorbs moisture from other products you've applied, such as moisturizer and foundation, and sets makeup so it lasts longer without streaking. The traditional light, medium, and dark color choices work for most women, says Scrivo. If you are having trouble choosing between two colors, you can mix them or use a colorless, translucent powder.

Many women apply loose powder over the entire face, which can make them look like they've been dusted with flour. This application method, which requires both a powder puff and a powder brush and applies powder only in certain areas, avoids that chalky look.

1. Place a small amount of powder into your hand, and then press your puff into the powder.
2. Press the puff into your skin. Apply *only* between your eyebrows, around the corners of your nose, just under your lips, at the cheekbones, and just below the cheekbones (where you would apply blush). Don't use too much loose powder around your eyes, as it can collect in wrinkles, making your skin look crepey. (If you wear eye shadow, powder your lids, too, so your shadow won't crease.)
3. Remove excess powder with a clean powder brush.

EYEBROWS: MAKE THEM REAPPEAR

"Full brows are a sign of youth," Scrivo says. They frame the eyes, flatter eye shape, and balance out facial features. Unfortunately, they are often ignored in a makeup routine. (To identify and create a brow shape that complements your face, and to follow Scrivo's grooming tips, see page 227 in Week 4.) An eyebrow pencil is the easiest way to add more definition or (if you need it) more length. Brow pencils are typically light, medium, and dark brown. You'll need a wax-based eyebrow pencil that's a shade lighter than your natural hair color. If your brows are very sparse, add a stiff-angled brush and eyebrow powder.

1. With a very sharp pencil, use light, feathery strokes to draw in brows. Make sure there's no makeup or lotion on your brows. If there is, your feathery strokes may slide off and not hold.
2. Run your eyebrow brush over your brows to soften the pencil strokes.
3. Press a trace of loose powder into your brows to set the pencil with a puff.
4. If your brows are very sparse, apply eyebrow powder after the pencil with your stiff-angled brush to fill in and shade any empty patches. The powder clings to the pencil's waxy base and creates a "furrier" look.

EYE SHADOW: OPT FOR SUBTLE, BRIGHTENING COLOR

You've already primed your lids with foundation and loose powder—now comes the fun part. To brighten your eyes during the day without piling on the color, choose warm tones, which make you look well rested. If you're fair-skinned, opt for peach, or a very light pink. Taupe and light to deep chocolates work well for darker skin tones.

If you want only a dusting of color, stop after Step 1.

1. Apply the shadow over your entire lid, from lashes to crease.
2. To add an accent color or contour, use a small amount of shimmer at the top of the lid or the brow bone.
3. For contour, apply a darker shade (dark taupe, chocolate, gray, navy, or black) to the outer corners of the eyes, blending into the crease. For a more dramatic effect, apply it close to the lash line.

EYELINER: RECLAIM YOUR LASH LINE

If your lashes have gotten sparser with age, you probably want to use eyeliner—but women often make the mistake of drawing a dark, heavy line to re-create their lash line. The solutions: a very sharp eye pencil and a feather-light touch. Scrivo recommends lining your upper lids with a fine line. "A heavy line under the eyes typically makes a woman look older, and the product tends to fall and collect in wrinkles," she says.

Most women find an eye pencil easiest to use. But because its waxy texture can smear or fade after a few hours, Scrivo recommends a two-step process for the upper lash line. You'll need two types of eyeliner—a very sharp pencil and a liquid liner.

To find the right color, match the color of your lashes, not your hair color. (If you're a blonde or a redhead, opt for dark taupe, navy, gray, or warm brown.) Tip: To correct a wobbly line or other mistake, erase it with a tiny bit of foundation on a cotton swab.

1. Starting at the middle of the lid, dot on pencil eyeliner between each lash. (Now you know why your pencil needs to be sharp!) Stop when you get to the outer corner of the lid, then return to the middle where you started. Next, "connect the dots" from the inner corner of the eye to the middle. Voilà—you've just subtly enhanced your lash line with no

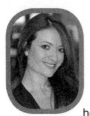

Eva Scrivo says ...

TAKE THE MYSTERY OUT OF MAKEUP: GO PRO

Worn cosmetics for years but want to update your look? Or are you a makeup newbie who never really learned how to apply it? Either way, consider educating yourself with a private lesson with a professional makeup artist.

How it works: You bring all of your makeup (or just yourself). The makeup artist assesses your products, separating those that suit your skin type and coloring from those that miss the mark. You'll also be shown how to get the most from the cosmetics you have and learn about products you may want to try.

Why not just head to a department store for a free makeover? Because at cosmetics counters, most recommendations are driven by sales, says Scrivo. A professional can be more objective about brands, and the lesson itself is more technique-based and less product-focused. While a session can typically cost anywhere from $75 to $200 depending on where you live and whom you see, "it's smart spending because you can learn how to properly use the makeup you've already purchased," says Scrivo.

thick, heavy lines. "You'll use less liner this way, and it will look more natural," says Scrivo.

2. On to your liquid liner. Remove the excess from the brush on a tissue. Then begin at the center of the top lash line and gently trace your pencil line to the outer corner of the eye. Stay as close to the lashes as possible. The line should be barely visible at the inner corners of your eyes and more prominent at the outer corners.

LINING YOUR LOWER LIDS

If you do choose this option (which you might if you can't bear not to line the lower lashes), you can either select a shade lighter than your natural lashes or get creative with color, Scrivo says. Green eyeliner flatters redheads, a plum hue works for brunettes, and a soft gray looks great on blondes. Whatever your coloring, a touch of silver, gold, or bronze pencil liner along your lower lids, around the lash line, will brighten your eyes.

If you're unsure of using a bold accent color on its own, try mixing a bit of it with your brown or black eyeliner, right on top of it. "It blends together nicely and adds a bit of softness to a dark color," says Scrivo. If used sparingly, a bold accent color can be used on the lower lash line on its own, she says.

1. With your (very sharp) eye pencil, place a small dot in between each lash, as you did on the top lash line. Alternately, with liquid liner, trace the faintest thin line across your lower lash line. "There should be almost no liner on the brush, and just tickle the brush between the lower lashes," says Scrivo.

2. With a clean brush, soften that delicate line by smudging and blending with the tip of your brush.

MASCARA: A MUST FOR EYES OVER 40

On their own, thickening and volumizing mascaras fall short. As a team, they give you the full, long lashes you remember. This application technique can help you reclaim (okay, fake) the lashes you've lost to time. Work on one eye at a time, because the moment mascara dries, it becomes hard to adjust. Here's what you need.

- An old-school metal eyelash curler, such as the one made by Shu Uemura ($20). Curling your eyelashes opens and brightens your eyes and gives you a wide-awake look.

- A thickening mascara

- A volumizing mascara

If you've always worn black mascara, you may want to try brown/black, which gives a lot of definition and looks less harsh, Scrivo says. But there are many shades of brown, and it's important to choose the right hue. Brown/black is best for dark hair. If you're blonde, opt for ash brown. If you're a redhead, select a brown with an undertone of red.

One last tip: For those of you wondering about waterproof mascara, it is a necessary evil for emotional events, such as weddings. It also can be a last resort for women who feel that no matter what brand of mascara they use, it always collects under their eyes. Using this type of formulation is safe as long as you remove it correctly. Scrivo recommends a warm washcloth with a mineral oil–based remover. For all other formulations, Cetaphil wipes remove all eye makeup beautifully. (To remove makeup correctly, see page 217.)

1. Warm your eyelash curler with hot water from the tap, dry it off, and press your lashes. The heat from the water helps curl them. (Never heat a metal curler with your blow-dryer!)
2. Apply one coat of thickening mascara. Start at the base of your top lashes and wiggle very gently to the left and right, back and forth. That wiggle distributes a little bit more product to the base of your lashes, which helps lift them. Then move the brush up and outward toward the mirror. Apply whatever is left on the wand to the bottom lashes in the same manner, so the coating is lighter.
3. While the thickening mascara is still wet, apply one coat of volumizing mascara and repeat the wiggle-and-lift technique.

LIP LINER/COLOR: SIMPLE STEPS TO PLUMPNESS

If you typically apply lipstick throughout the day, straight from the tube, there's a better way that has more staying power: Use a lip pencil.

Lip pencils not only increase the staying power of lip color, but they also can add definition, making lips that have thinned look fuller, Scrivo says. She likes a thinner lip pencil over the "chubby" types (they replace lipstick rather than a liner) because it delivers a more precise line. For daytime, choose a color that matches your natural lip color—typically, pale pink, rose, plum, or natural brown.

Lip color comes in many formulations—tinted balms, glosses, stains, satins, matte formulas. For day wear, Scrivo recommends a lip pencil on your lips, with a slick of transparent (but colored) lipstick over it. This combo wears well and has a more polished look than gloss, she says. If you love the staying power and glamour of matte lipstick, start with natural lip balm and apply a thin layer of color with a brush. (Keep your balm with you and reapply as needed.)

While lip color is a personal choice, there are a few guidelines for better results. For example, if your lips have lost fullness, avoid dark lip colors and choose cream-based lipsticks with a satin finish, which can make lips look fuller. Also, be cautious with shades that have a frosty finish, especially lighter hues like pinks and peaches, which can look dated and emphasize aging around the mouth. If you have frosted lipsticks in your makeup collection, apply the lipstick, and then add a slick of gloss on top, which tones down some of the frostiness, says Scrivo.

While red lips are classic, it's important to choose the right shade, says Scrivo. Be guided by your skin's undertone. A blue-based red complements porcelain skin. If you have reddish or pink skin, try a brown-based red or a dark, blue-based cherry (think black cherry rather than a bright Maraschino). Olive or yellowish skin tones brighten with warmer lip colors, such as reds with a blue or orange base. A knowledgeable salesperson at a beauty counter can help you with the right selection.

1. With your fingers, coat the lips with a thin layer of natural lip balm to create a smooth base for lip color and help color stay true. Blot.
2. Using light, feathery strokes and a very sharp pencil, draw a thin line around your lips. Don't try to redraw the shape of your mouth; that line will be there when your lipstick wears off. Blot the liner with a tissue.
3. Apply your lip color with a brush, which will help you apply a sheer layer of pigment evenly and precisely, Scrivo says. Can't use a brush all day? At least use one in the morning.

BLUSH: BRING SKIN FROM DULL TO RADIANT

Still look pale and tired after a full 8 hours of sleep? Blush can help you look younger and healthier. If you like a dewy complexion, choose a cream or stick blush. For a matte finish, opt for a powder/compact blush.

Blush is intended to capture a natural, rosy glow, so think of the color your skin would naturally blush, and match it. For lighter skin, opt for a pink-rose, while a deeper rose-brown works for darker skin, Scrivo advises. If your skin has reddish or pinkish undertones, or if you suffer from rosacea, go with a soft apricot or brown. You may also try using a bronzer, which can give a nice glow without adding more pink to your skin. For darker skin tones, good options include deep berry, plum, or wine.

Dewy finish: Apply translucent powder just on your T-zone (forehead, nose, and chin). Apply cream or gel blush to the fingertips of your dominant hand—Scrivo recommends using your middle and ring fingers. Then, gently press the pads of your fingers to your cheeks. Concentrate on the apples and feather the color toward your hairline, says Scrivo (but not into your hairline, of course). Pat and blend the color up to your cheekbones.

Matte finish: Using a powder compact blush and a large powder brush, make soft, sweeping strokes, starting under the cheekbone. Use many strokes to blend—15 to 20 for each cheek. "With each stroke you blend the makeup better, making it look seamless with your skin," says Scrivo. "Only use a small amount of product and concentrate on the blending rather than applying more color. Artists use many brushstrokes when creating their work, so blend, blend, blend," she says.

The End of the Beginning

To end with our experts' strategies for ageless beauty seems fitting. We hope it's clear that while any woman can learn the routines and skills in this section, beauty transcends external appearance. To feel beautiful is a choice. So is pursuing beauty; the simple act of applying mascara can be good for the soul. The moment you reach for beauty, you become beautiful, and everyone can see it.

That's an amazing place to be as you launch your rejuvenated self. For the next 8 weeks, you'll use all that you've learned so far to renew every part of you, inside and out. If you feel a bit nervous, that's normal—but don't worry, we'll be journeying with you. Get ready to EAT, MOVE, ENGAGE, and GLOW, for real.

SUCCESS!

Lisa Boland, 50

MY STORY Lisa Boland is lucky to be alive. In January 2012, she faced not just one but two life-threatening health crises—a heart attack and a perforated colon—within 9 days of each other. During the long recovery, she gained 40 pounds. That may seem like a small price to pay, but this mom of a 12-year-old boy was feeling the effects of the excess weight—fatigue, joint pain, trouble sleeping—and she knew that things would only get worse. "The clock is ticking, and I need to make changes now," she said before starting the Younger in 8 Weeks Plan.

During the first week, Lisa had an epiphany that set the stage for her success. "It occurred to me that one of the biggest reasons I didn't make better choices for my health in the past was my own belief that I wasn't strong enough to resist temptation or make myself exercise," she said. "Well, yesterday proved to me that I *am* strong enough. I *can* do this!"

Lisa's biggest change was taking control of her stress eating. "I'd reach for sweets or salty snacks whenever my stress level was high," said Lisa, who works full time as an administrative assistant and has a jewelry design business on the side. "The junk food would make me feel better briefly, but then I'd feel guilty for eating it and end up feeling even worse than before."

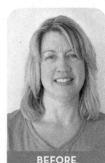

BEFORE

To her surprise, the antidote was exercise. "I used to dread working out," she said. "But now, she discovered that it relieved her tension. "Instead of eating when I'm feeling overwhelmed or have had a rough day, I exercise. Sometimes it's a brisk walk, sometimes strength training, or even yoga. Afterward, my head is clear and I'm reenergized to tackle the problem at hand."

Each good choice that Lisa made increased her confidence (an 80 percent bump over the 8 weeks) to make more good choices—even during crunch times before jewelry shows. She also lowered her blood pressure from borderline high to healthier levels.

Now she's ready for new adventures. When her son suggested they go geocaching (a high-tech scavenger hunt), she was game. "I discovered how much I missed being out in nature. Now I love hiking. And more importantly, I have the energy to do it."

Another secret to her success: "For the first time ever, I'm doing this for *me*. Not for an event, not to please someone else, not to fit into a bathing suit. I'm taking care of me because I want to be healthier and enjoy every bit of my life. I have no intention of stopping this journey."

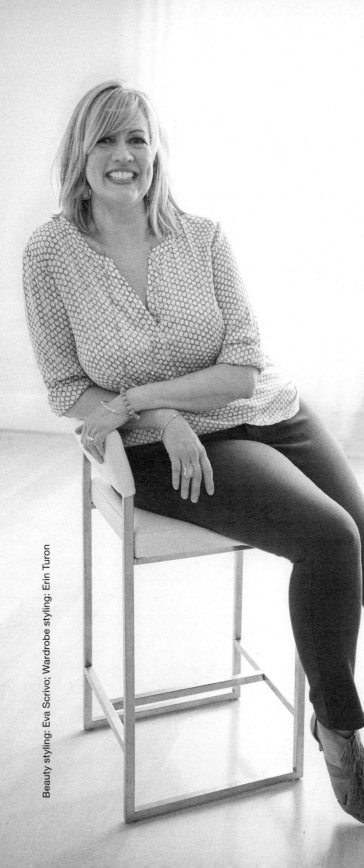

Beauty styling: Eva Scrivo; Wardrobe styling: Erin Turon

LOOK AT ME

- Joints no longer hurt

- Lowered borderline high blood pressure **15 points**

- Sleeping better

- Reduced skin blemishes and fine lines

- Weight lost: **11 pounds**

- Inches lost: **6.75**

Tip BE KIND TO YOURSELF.
When I stopped the negative self-talk, I quickly learned that one slipup or less-than-perfect choice wouldn't derail my entire day if I didn't let it. My next choice could easily get me right back on track.

PART

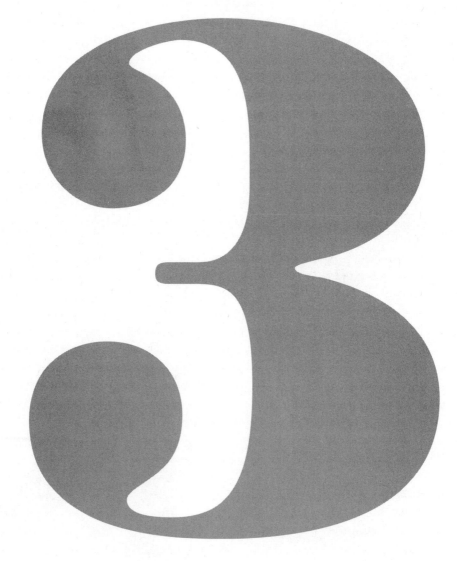

THE YOUNGER IN 8 WEEKS PLAN

8 Weeks to a Younger You

Now that you've read through the science and strategies that make up our Younger in 8 Weeks Plan, it's time to put them to work and grow younger every day. Think of this plan as a menu. This is how to "order" each week.

Set Your Daily Intention

Success begins with a vision. Where do you want to be in 8 weeks in terms of your health, your energy, and your appearance, and what small step can you take today to edge closer to it?

To stimulate that process, each morning for the next 8 weeks you'll set an *intention*—a personal goal for the day. (We'll explain how when we get to Week 1.) It takes just 2 minutes, and it will set you up for success each day, helping you stay on plan and shape your vision of what might come next for you. Don't blow this off. It's scheming and dreaming about tomorrow that keeps you young.

Hit Your Weekly Goals

Each week of the plan introduces different goals along with a to-do list to help you achieve them. Week by week, you'll systematically topple common issues that stand in the way of a more youthful and healthy you. For the first 4 weeks, you'll strive to eat clean, get quality sleep, begin the exercise plan, embrace a new skin-care regimen, and learn strategies to shrug off the stress that ages you. Later on, you'll tackle more specific goals—banish bothersome aches and age-related annoyances, manage blood pressure naturally, protect your hearing and vision, sharpen your memory.

As the goals progress from week to week, you'll delve ever-deeper into the constants of the plan: EAT, MOVE, ENGAGE, and GLOW. Here's an overview.

EAT

Yes, it's a challenge to change the way you eat. But we've made it a *tasty* challenge. First, you'll follow our 4-day Jumpstart to shed bloat. You'll score a nice (if temporary) weight loss and a welcome burst of energy. Next up: our Clean & Green plan, which includes selections from 76 delicious recipes designed by dietitian Andie Bernard Schwartz, RD. In Week 3, you graduate to dining out and planning your own meals and snacks. Just plug your favorite healthy foods into the Meal Builder on page 173. No need to count calories, either (they are accounted for through food choices and portion sizes), but you'll consume around 1,400 each day. From the Zesty Pork Tenderloin Wrap (page 359) to the Double Chocolate Pudding (page 402), we're sure you'll find your meals to be delicious—and the furthest thing from abstemious.

MOVE

You've no doubt started and stopped many exercise programs in the past. This is the one that will stick. That's because it's well rounded (so you won't burn out on any one aspect of it) and designed to ramp up gradually, so you feel solid gains each week. Endurance, strength, flexibility, balance—our workout routine helps improve them all, and, like our panelists, you'll be blown away by how good it feels to be active again (or to turn your activity up a notch if you've already got a routine). In Week 1, you'll start with an invigorating daily stretch to center body and mind. In Weeks 2 and 3, the spotlight's on cardio—steady paced at first, followed by interval training. You'll pick up weights or resistance bands for the strength routine in Week 4. After that, you'll keep on nudging up the speed and intensity. You can go at your own pace, and soon enough, you'll feel so energized by the results you won't want to quit.

Safety and injury prevention are accounted for in every move, even if you have never followed a formal workout routine or haven't exercised in years. You'll do dynamic stretching before cardio and strength workouts to prepare your body for exercise. We offer an optional balance routine starting in Week 5. When you're done, a short flexibility routine will increase your range of motion and further protect against injury. If you're often sore and achy, consider a foam roller (borrow one if you're not ready to commit). As a number of our panelists can attest, that dense log of foam can feel amazing on shoulders, hamstrings, or other sore spots.

ENGAGE

It's time to unleash the powerful, positive you that's been under wraps, perhaps for far too long. Week by week, you'll step further outside your comfort zone in search of age-defying *duende* (for a sense of purpose) and the activities that make you amazingly, passionately happy. You might reach out to old friends or endeavor to make new ones, learn to meditate for real this time, dust off your piano, pivot to a new and soul-satisfying career, or decide to go back to school. Whatever your passion, get off the couch, turn off the tube, and make it happen! Each week, challenge yourself to audition different ENGAGE strategies to see which ones resonate most.

GLOW

In this part of the plan, changes arrive both gradually and right away (instant gratification is the greatest). In Week 1, you'll start the morning and evening skin-care routine. By Week 3, you're likely to see visible changes in your skin, and the makeup makeovers you'll find that week will be outright transformative. Because we know you want to feel better—and look younger—right now, keep an eye out for the "Instant Glow" and "Slimmer in a Minute" tips each week.

Splurge!

Every other week (Weeks 2, 4, 6, and 8) features a splurge—that is, a goodie that isn't strictly necessary but adds fun and a bit of decadence to your program. While splurges are optional, these periodic rewards will help keep you motivated. And feel free to swap one splurge for another or treat yourself to a splurge that's not "on the menu."

Journal Your Journey

Some of our panelists kept a journal to document their transformations. We invite you to do the same. It's a place to set your ongoing goals; record your workout progress; do the thought exercises and check-ins throughout the book; and learn which foods, recipes, and antiaging strategies work for you (and which don't). Keeping a record of this time, chronicling how you change on the inside and on the outside, can help ensure your goals are drawn the way you want.

Our test panelists used their private Facebook page as a safe, welcoming place to share triumphs and setbacks, receive support, and even have an occasional meltdown. So think about asking others to join you on this journey, and then set up a Facebook page or WhatsApp group so you can check in regularly. Whether your fellow "travelers" are local or far away, you'll be able to get and give support whenever it's needed—support that can help keep you on the path to a lifetime of health and happiness.

How to Eat Clean & Green

Okay, you're *almost* ready to start the plan.

First, though, you need a little more information about the powerful antiaging foods you'll be eating more of and the youth-stealing foods you'll be eating less of on the Clean & Green plan. (Happily, no food is entirely off the table. Wine and other alcoholic beverages come back in Week 3 after the Jumpstart, and sugar—in moderation—shows up in Week 4.) We even include beverages and foods that are proven to stop cravings cold. "I designed this plan to keep your taste buds happy and your belly satisfied," our nutritional advisor, Andie Bernard Schwartz, RD, says. "It's amazing how intensely flavorful healthy foods can be."

The "At a Glance" table on the next page gives you an idea of how you'll be filling your plate. Later in the chapter, you'll find our Meal Builder, which you can use to create meals from your favorite healthy foods. Don't forget, too, that we've got 76 Clean & Green Recipes, starting on page 334, designed to work with the plan. And if you want to know the brands that get a thumbs-up from Schwartz, see the Food Shopping Guide on page 403.

Finally, we encourage you to take a chance on a vegetable or whole grain you've never tried. Become a regular at local farmers' markets and natural foods stores. Study the organic section of your supermarket. You'll readily find everything you need. More important, you'll be actively engaged in improving your health, making smart food choices, and discovering flavors that are just as satisfying—and arguably even more so—than the age-accelerating diet you may be accustomed to.

At a Glance: What You'll Be Eating

MORE OF THESE	LESS OF THESE	BEVERAGES	CRAVINGS CRUSHERS
Vegetables and fruits	Added sugar	Water	Avocados
Whole grains	Animal proteins	Plant-based milks	Dark chocolate
Meatless proteins (such as beans, nuts, and seeds)	Dairy (except yogurt)	*Optional:* Coffee, green tea, red wine	Nuts
Fish	Processed whole grains		
Prebiotics and probiotics (especially yogurt)			

Eat More of These

We call our plan Clean & Green because it's high in plant foods (with an emphasis on ones with cell-nourishing, deep colors) and as free as possible from health-compromising chemicals used on produce and in food processing. Each day, you'll eat 7 to 9 servings of fruits and veggies, plus multiple servings of whole grains, beans, and nuts and seeds. (In most cases, 1 serving fits in your hand.) This dietary mix is high in antiaging powerhouses, like meatless proteins (plus fish!), healthy fats, and telomere-lengthening antioxidants, which will help turn back the clock from the inside out.

How many servings you consume depends on your age, gender, and activity level. Eat the minimum if you're small and sedentary, the maximum if you're tall and active.

Veggies

AIM FOR: AT LEAST 6 TO 7 SERVINGS PER DAY.

What's a serving? ½ cup cooked or 1 cup raw.

Biggest nutritional payoff: Focus on leafy greens and brightly colored veggies (pumpkin, eggplant, tomatoes), as well as cruciferous versions (broccoli, cabbage, cauliflower). Remember: Deeper hues mean more antioxidants. Seek out organic to avoid pesticide residue; if you have to go conventional, scrub your veggies clean with water, even if you're peeling them.

Tip: Have veggies at breakfast. It sets the tone for the day. Think spinach and mushrooms in your eggs, kale in your smoothie, a tall glass of green juice. If you hate veggies, try baby versions, which tend to be less bitter, with just as many health benefits.

Fruits
AIM FOR: 1 TO 2 SERVINGS PER DAY (AFTER THE JUMPSTART).

What's a serving? ½ cup sliced fresh, frozen, or canned (fruit only—no syrup!); 1 whole small fruit; or 2 tablespoons dried.

Biggest nutritional payoff: Again, the brighter (or deeper) the hue, the better. And berries pack more fiber and youth-extending antioxidants than most fruits.

Tip: Pass on fruit juice, which is high in both natural and added sugars. To control your appetite, dig into an avocado (yep, it's a fruit). For more on avocado's hunger-crushing power, see page 171. Fresh fruit is better than dried, which is more calorie-dense.

Whole Grains
AIM FOR: UP TO 5 SERVINGS PER DAY.

What's a serving? 1 slice whole grain bread, 1 cup whole grain cereal, ½ cup cooked whole grains or whole grain pasta.

Biggest nutritional payoff: Get down with brown! Brown rice is an inexpensive source of trace minerals, such as selenium, magnesium, and niacin. And unprocessed whole grains—like barley, farro, millet, quinoa, wheat berries, and wild rice—are super-high in fiber and more nutritious than white rice or white-flour pastas because the nutrients (primarily fiber and B vitamins) are concentrated in the husks, which are removed when grains are refined. Whole grains are generally chewier than the refined types and have a nuttier flavor. (White rice will start to taste downright bland!) When you're buying bread, look for nutrient-packed sprouted-grain kinds over traditional whole wheat breads (for recommendations, see the Food Shopping Guide, page 403).

Tip: To cook grains quickly, let them sit in water for a few hours before cooking. Just before dinner, add extra water if necessary, and then cook. Grains keep 3 to 4 days in the fridge and take just minutes to warm up with a little added water or broth. Use the leftovers for cold salads; just toss them with chopped veggies and a healthy olive oil and vinegar dressing.

Up Your Fruit and Veg Intake with Green Juices and Smoothies

AS OFTEN AS POSSIBLE, OPT FOR whole foods over liquid versions. However, green juices and smoothies are a quick and easy way to down part of your daily quota of phytonutrients. Since you're going to get friendly with your blender over the next 8 weeks, here are a few things to keep in mind.

GREEN JUICES: A GREAT MEAL SUPPLEMENT. Green juices are made with leafy greens, like spinach and kale; other green veggies, like parsley, celery, and cucumber; and the occasional fruit (kiwifruit, banana) for taste. You'll find our Green Juice Blend recipe in Day 2 of the Jumpstart and our Super Green Smoothie (a hybrid beverage) in Day 4. You'll also find hundreds of variations on the Web if you plug "green juice" into your browser. Just steer clear of recipes that contain more than 1 serving of fruit or are sweetened with juice. Because all of the health-boosting fiber has been strained out of juice, it makes a great supplement to a meal but should not be considered a meal replacement.

Green juice blends, which can taste grassy and a little bitter, are not to everyone's liking, although they were a hit with some of our panelists. Give them a shot if you have a juicer (or consider investing in one).

SMOOTHIES: A NUTRITIOUS MEAL REPLACEMENT. Whole-food smoothies are a nutritionist's dream. When smoothies blend healthy carbs, like veggies and fruits, along with protein and fat from milk, nuts, avocado, and/or unsweetened protein powder, they're nutrient-dense, bona fide meals.

To build the perfect smoothie, use this blueprint.

CHOOSE A BASE. Keys to a perfect smoothie: texture and consistency.

Beans (and Other Legumes, Including Peas, Lentils, and Soy)

AIM FOR: 1 TO 3 SERVINGS PER DAY.

What's a serving? ½ cup cooked beans, peas, or lentils; ½ cup tofu.

Biggest nutritional payoff: All legumes (beans and peas are varieties) are great sources of fiber and protein (whole or mashed) as well as disease-fighting phytochemicals. Eat them every day if you can. They'll help you hit the recommended 25 to 30 grams of daily fiber.

Half a frozen banana delivers both, but for a low-sugar shot of healthy, satisfying fats, try avocado. Avocado is high in fiber, too. Use 2 to 3 ounces of avocado per 8-ounce serving.

OPT FOR A LOW-SUGAR LIQUID. Skip the juice and add ½ cup of an unsweetened plant-based milk, such as almond or coconut. Check the list of ingredients to avoid sweeteners before you buy. Add another 2 to 4 ounces of water if you're adding greens

ADD SOME GREENS. Use a handful of spinach, kale, or similar leafy greens. You'll get less sugar by default and more antioxidants and fiber.

SWEETEN WITH BERRIES. Berries are tiny treasure chests of nutrition. (For instance, blueberries get their deep-blue hue from anthocyanins, anti-oxidants that fight inflammation and oxidative stress.) So satisfy your sweet tooth with ½ cup of fresh or frozen blueberries, strawberries, raspberries, or blackberries rather than higher-sugar fruits, like mango and pineapple. Bonus: Berries are high in vitamin C, so they boost plant-based iron absorption while mellowing the taste of the greens.

PUMP UP PROTEIN. Toss in ½ to 1 cup 2% plain Greek yogurt, 2 tablespoons chia seeds, 2 tablespoons natural almond or peanut but-ter, or 1 scoop protein powder. If you use powder, skip the kinds with added sugar or artificial sweeteners. See the Food Shopping Guide for Schwartz's protein-powder picks.

MAKE ADD-INS COUNT. For an extra dash of flavor and antioxidants, try sprinkling in a bit of carob or cocoa powder or matcha (a green tea powder loaded with disease-fighting power).

Tip: Cooking your own legumes is easy. Rinse and soak them overnight in the fridge, and then cook them in water for the time suggested on the pack-age. (They keep in the fridge for up to 2 days, too.) Also consider stocking up on canned beans—black, white, kidney, and instant bean soups—so you'll always have the core of a clean and tasty meal. Just rinse them first, since many varieties are packed in a high-sodium liquid. Frozen edamame (raw, whole soybeans) is easy to prepare in the microwave; pop the beans on salads or sprinkle with a little salt as a snack.

(Mostly) Meatless Protein Powerhouses

IN THE UNITED STATES, THE RECOMMENDED Dietary Allowance for protein—which boosts muscle mass and keeps hunger at bay—is 46 grams for women and 56 for men. Even if you get enough protein each day, you probably do it unevenly—consuming most of it at dinner, while breakfast is typically carb-rich and protein-poor. But a study published in the *Journal of Nutrition* found that people who paced out their protein intake over the course of a day saw a 25 percent boost in muscle mass compared with those who ate the same amount of protein at night.

PROTEIN POWERHOUSE	AMOUNT	PROTEIN (GRAMS)	EAT IT LIKE A PRO
Chia seeds	2 tablespoons	6	Add these tiny black-and-white seeds to smoothies, yogurt, or oatmeal.
Chickpeas	½ cup	7	Toss them whole onto salads, roast them with spices, whip them into hummus. Chickpeas (aka garbanzo beans) assume the flavor of whatever they're in. Plus, chickpea flour is a tasty gluten-free alternative.
Edamame	1 cup (shelled)	16	Steam these soybean pods whole to preserve the nutrients (boiling can release them into the water). Eat whole, toss on salads, or mash and spread on toast.
Eggs	1 large	6	Like they say: incredible, edible—and versatile. Hard- or soft-cooked, scrambled or baked into a frittata, eggs will be your new best friends. Choose the cage-free variety; it's more humane for the chickens, and it's nutritionally better for you, with two and a half times more omega-3s and twice the vitamin E of regular eggs.
Greek yogurt	1 cup	29	A little more protein-rich than regular yogurt. Enjoy it for breakfast, but use it as a tasty substitute for sour cream and mayo, too. Before you buy, check the label to avoid added sugar.

Nuts and Seeds (Including Nut Butters)
AIM FOR: 1 TO 3 SERVINGS PER DAY.

What's a serving? 1 ounce nuts or seeds; 1 to 2 tablespoons nut butter.

Biggest nutritional payoff: All nuts are good sources of protein, healthy fats, vitamin E, magnesium, and phytochemicals. Walnuts have the

Looking for more healthy ways to get your protein quota? The following chart contains the top plant-protein powerhouses. If you eat a variety throughout the day, you'll easily meet your daily protein needs. You'll also get more fiber and/or beneficial plant chemicals and less sodium and saturated fat than if you ate meat. (Yeah, we've included eggs and yogurt in here; since these are so nutritious, they've got a spot on the table in our plan.)

PROTEIN POWERHOUSE	AMOUNT	PROTEIN (GRAMS)	EAT IT LIKE A PRO
Lentils	½ cup	9	Great in soups and salads, they cook up quickly. To keep lentils crunchy, don't add salt until the beans are cooked completely.
Peanut butter	2 tablespoons	8	Your childhood sandwich spread grows up when stirred into hot oatmeal or eaten on a sliced pear. Opt for natural brands with peanuts, maybe a little salt, and nothing else.
Quinoa	½ cup	4	Cook one big batch of quinoa and use it for days—as a hot cereal, as a binder in homemade bean burgers or salmon cakes, or as the base for a grain salad. To get that ideal fluffiness, drain quinoa in a fine-mesh strainer after it's cooked.
Seitan	⅓ cup	21	Made with the gluten from wheat, seitan is firm and chewy and a perfect substitute for meat in stir-fries or casseroles. Go easy on the salt, as some packages have nearly 13 percent of your daily sodium intake.
Tempeh	½ cup	15	This nutty-tasting kin of tofu tastes great in stir-fries and as a meat replacement in burgers. Like its cousin tofu, tempeh loves a good marinade (just a quick brush of soy sauce can do wonders).

highest content of brain-boosting omega-3s of any nut, and they are also rich in vitamin E. As for nut butters, Schwartz recommends venturing beyond peanut butter to try almond or sunflower butter. "These nuts contain even more healthy omega-3s and higher amounts of iron, magnesium, and vitamin E," she says. But natural (no sugar added!) peanut butter is fine, too.

Meanwhile, chia seeds and flaxseed have significant amounts of omega-3 fatty acids, and chia in particular can fill you up because it absorbs water. Sunflower seeds, which are unusually high in vitamin E and iron, are great to pop as snacks or sprinkle on salads.

Tip: While a handful of nuts and seeds make a good snack, it's easy to sprinkle them on foods like salads, veggies, yogurt, and even oatmeal.

Fish

AIM FOR: AT LEAST 1 SERVING TWO TO THREE TIMES A WEEK (OPTIONAL, OF COURSE, IF YOU'RE GOING VEGETARIAN).

What's a serving? 3 to 4 ounces cooked or ¾ cup flaked (like tuna).

Biggest nutritional payoff: Fish is high in protein (about 7 grams per ounce), contains brain-boosting omega-3 fatty acids (and less saturated fat and cholesterol than red meat), and has a higher water content than most meats, so you can satisfy your hunger on fewer ounces.

Tip: Bake, grill, broil, or poach—just don't fry your fish. And opt for low-mercury choices, including trout, salmon, cod, and tilapia fillets and canned anchovies and light tuna, which are super-high in omega-3s. Avoid shark, swordfish, king mackerel, and tilefish, the fish highest in mercury. Review our basic guidelines for choosing fish on page 55.

Prebiotics and Probiotics

AIM FOR: AT LEAST 1 SERVING PER DAY.

What's a serving? Depends on the food. If you can do veggies and yogurt every day, you're definitely good to go.

Biggest nutritional payoff: This plan features plenty of prebiotic (high fiber) and probiotic (high in the good-for-you bacteria) foods, both of which are key to balancing your gut health and boosting your immune system. Most of these are foods you're very familiar with. Prebiotic powerhouses include almonds, apples, artichokes, asparagus, bananas, bran, garlic, leeks, onions, plums, and tomatoes.

The queen of probiotic power foods is yogurt, and because it's such a key player in our longevity plan, it merits its own section (on the next page). Other potent probiotic foods include kefir, fermented soybeans (tempeh), miso, and fermented vegetables, such as kimchi, sauerkraut, and cured Greek olives.

Cook with Healthy Fats

THE DAYS OF NONFAT FAD DIETS are gone, and although saturated fats aren't as categorically heart-unhealthy as once thought, unsaturated fats keep your blood vessels flexible, lower total cholesterol levels, and fight inflammation. Unsaturated (you may have heard of "mono" and "poly" unsaturated) fats are primarily found in plant foods (nuts, grains, olives, and avocados), while omega-3 fatty acids are most prevalent in seafood.

When cooking, opt for healthy cooking oils, such as **extra virgin olive oil**. Schwartz particularly likes **extra virgin coconut oil**, which contains a type of saturated fat that is more easily metabolized by the body than other saturated fats.

If you love the rich flavor of cooking with butter, look for **grass-fed butter** or **ghee** (a clarified butter used in Southeast Asian cuisine), which you can find in many specialty stores and high-end supermarkets. It contains omega-3 fatty acids (from the grass the cows ingest) as well as hard-to-find vitamin K, which keeps calcium from lodging in the arteries, Schwartz says.

Tip: Try kimchi or sauerkraut in small amounts as a flavoring on a grain bowl or with a rice dish. Drink kefir or pop cured olives as a snack. And miso is a wonderful flavor that adds a meaty taste to bean dishes and soups.

Yogurt

AIM FOR: AT LEAST 1 SERVING EVERY COUPLE OF DAYS.

What's a serving? 1 cup (8 ounces).

Biggest nutritional payoff: Schwartz recommends either 2% plain Greek or 2% plain grass-fed yogurt (if weight loss isn't an issue for you, whole is more satisfying—and both should ideally be organic). Grass-fed yogurt is from cows that graze in pasture year-round, which makes the yogurt richer in omega-3 fats and CLA (conjugated linoleic acid), a beneficial fatty acid. Meanwhile, with its hint of sweetness and creamy texture, 2% plain Greek yogurt tastes downright decadent. It's also significantly higher in protein than regular yogurt—just 1 serving delivers 38 percent of your daily protein needs—and lower in carbohydrates.

To get the greatest probiotic benefit, pick a brand that goes beyond "live active cultures" and choose one containing additional potent bacteria. The label will say *Lactobacillus (L. acidophilus)* and/or *Bifidobacterium (B. bifidum)*.

Tip: Always check the ingredients for added sugar. Yogurt naturally contains 6 to 12 grams of sugar in a 6-ounce serving, the size of most individual yogurts. Pass up brands with more than that. (Heads-up: Nondairy yogurts—often made from soy, coconut, or almond milks—may contain added sweeteners and stabilizers to mimic the taste and consistency of dairy yogurt.)

Eat Less of These

Added Sugar
LIMIT YOURSELF TO: NO MORE THAN 6 TEASPOONS (9 FOR MEN) A DAY (STARTING WEEK 4).

What's a serving? Remember: 4 grams = 1 teaspoon.

Nutritional drawback: Sugar is associated with so many negative health outcomes, from inflammation to diabetes and brain fog. For the first 3 weeks, our plan eliminates added sugar, the kind that flavors processed foods or that you sprinkle onto food or stir into beverages. (And artificial sweeteners are also a no-no because they can trigger cravings.) Thereafter, the plan allows 6 teaspoons (or 24 grams) a day for women, which means you can splurge on the sweet treats in the Food Shopping Guide (page 403). Or choose your own desserts starting in Week 4 as long as you stay within the 24-gram limit.

Animal Protein
LIMIT YOURSELF TO: 1 SERVING OF RED MEAT ONCE A WEEK; 1 SERVING OF CHICKEN/POULTRY TWO OR THREE TIMES A WEEK.

What's a serving? 3 to 4 ounces cooked.

Nutritional drawback: This plan doesn't contain much red meat (beef, pork, and lamb), given that it's highly caloric and a steady consumption of it has been linked to diseases like cancer, Schwartz says. If you miss red meat, it's okay (but hardly necessary) to have it once a week. Chicken is lower in saturated fat, so you can have it a bit more often.

When shopping, look for organic or grass-fed beef or lamb, which has more omega-3 fatty acids, and "pasture-raised" pork. (How to know for sure? Look for third-party certification, such as the American Grassfed Association, Certified Humane Raised and Handled, Animal Welfare Approved, or USDA Organic.) For poultry, opt for organic or pasture-raised.

Tip: Use meat as a condiment. Think of spicy sriracha sauce—a little goes a long way. Build your meals around beans, veggies, and whole grains, and add an ounce or two of red meat for flavor.

Dairy
LIMIT YOURSELF TO: AS INFREQUENTLY AS POSSIBLE.

Nutritional drawback: Dairy products, like milk and cheese, are good sources of protein and calcium, which we need to build muscle and bone. However, they're calorie-dense and high in saturated fat and cholesterol—so minimize them in favor of the protein and calcium you can get from whole plant foods (yogurt, as you know, is exceptional). Of course, use milk in recipes that call for it (though plant milks can often work, too). And our snack plan allows for a limited amount of cheese combined with a fruit and/or whole grain, a cravings-killing combo.

Tip: If you're interested in trying some nondairy cheese options while on the 8-week plan, see the Food Shopping Guide on page 403 for Schwartz's recommendations.

Processed Whole Grains
LIMIT YOURSELF TO: AS INFREQUENTLY AS POSSIBLE.

Nutritional drawback: Ideally, all of your grain intake would come from whole, unprocessed grains. Once whole grains are pulverized into flour and restructured into bread, cereal, or pasta, your body digests them nearly as quickly as it does sugar. But in the real world, a bowl of cold cereal makes for a simple breakfast, sandwiches are quick and convenient, and pasta does sometime whisper our names.

Fortunately, Schwartz has recommended specific brands of processed whole grain products that—while not healthier than unprocessed grains—are healthy enough (and delicious). Check the lists in the Food Shopping Guide on page 403 for these options.

Delicious No-Grain Pasta

IF YOU'RE A DIEHARD PASTA LOVER, consider investing in a spiral slicer, says Schwartz. These nifty gadgets turn fresh veggies into the pasta you crave. For example, you could make "zoodles"—that's noodles made from zucchini—which are a tasty fiber-filled pasta substitute. Squash makes for a tasty "pasta," too.

You can find spiral slicers in the kitchen department of most big-box stores. "I just got one recently and love it!" says panelist Kathy McCarthy. "I have so much zucchini from our garden, and zoodles have become a family favorite."

Beverages

Water

AIM FOR: AT LEAST 1 GLASS PER MEAL, AND SIP WHEN YOU EXERCISE.

What's a serving? 8-ounce glass.

Biggest nutritional payoff: It's not inherently nutritious, of course, but water is the ultimate longevity drink. Adequate hydration supports cellular and organ function and keeps your digestion trucking along, particularly with all that good fiber you'll be eating. How much water you need daily depends on a bunch of factors, including outside temperature and activity level. The Institute of Medicine has set "adequate intake" levels of 125 ounces (about 15 cups) for men and 91 ounces for women (about 11 cups), but most of us can get about 20 percent of that from food. Schwartz's "Aim for" recommendation will keep you on target.

Tip: If you don't care for its taste, try our flavored waters, on page 170. Mix up a batch in Week 1, and enjoy them throughout the plan.

Plant-Based Milks

AIM FOR: AS A SUBSTITUTE FOR REGULAR MILK—IN COFFEE, SMOOTHIES, AND HOT OR COLD CEREAL.

Biggest nutritional payoff: From smoothies to cold cereals, plant-based milks are rich in disease-fighting flavanols and low in (or devoid of) saturated fat or cholesterol. There are many varieties, made from unsweetened nuts (almond, cashew), coconut (a great nut-free option), grains (quinoa, oat, rice), or seeds (flax, chia, hemp), which generally taste a bit like the foods they're made from. While soy milk is rich in female–friendly B vitamins, potassium, and magnesium, it tends to be more processed than the other plant milks, Schwartz says. If you're looking to limit your intake of soy overall (some studies have linked its plant estrogens to increased breast cancer risk), it's better to get your soy from whole or minimally processed sources like edamame and tofu.

Tip: Always opt for unsweetened plant milks; some brands pack more than 20 grams of sugar per glass. And avoid brands that contain carrageenan, a type of seaweed used as a thickener and emulsifier; research has shown a link to gastrointestinal inflammation and colon cancer in animals.

Unsweetened nut milks tend to be thicker but low in protein (surprise: even almond!), though you can buy many plant milks with added protein. You'll find Schwartz's favorite brands on page 405.

Optional: Coffee
AIM FOR: NO MORE THAN 2 TO 3 CUPS A DAY (1 PER DAY ON THE JUMPSTART).

What's a serving? 8 ounces.

Biggest nutritional payoff: Researchers are always uncovering new reasons to drink coffee; its high antioxidant content is associated with longevity, sharper memory, and weight loss. But don't go overboard. The FDA's 3-to-5-cup-a-day recommendation equals about 400 milligrams of caffeine, which is a lot. Too much can decrease the body's ability to absorb calcium and reduce water intake. That's why Schwartz likes 2 to 3 cups.

Tip: For healthier add-ins, swap cream for lower-fat dairy milk or unsweetened nut milks. For sweetness, add a splash of vanilla or a sprinkle of cinnamon.

Optional: Green Tea
AIM FOR: AS OFTEN AS YOU LIKE (AND AS A COFFEE SUBSTITUTE).

Biggest nutritional payoff: Green tea is majorly high in antioxidant polyphenols, and drinking it regularly has been found to do everything from lower cancer risk to sharpen memory. Three 8-ounce cups a day, served hot or iced, will net you a healthy 300 milligrams of polyphenols. Bottled teas contain significantly less of the good age-defying stuff than home-steeped, and many contain added sugar, so brew your own. Note that

Four Refreshing Soda Swaps

NOT SO KEEN ON PLAIN WATER? Give these naturally flavored waters a try. Place the ingredients in a 2-quart jar, crush them with a wooden spoon, and cover with 6 cups of ice. Fill the jar with water, stir, and chill in the refrigerator for several hours to let the flavors infuse. Strain before you drink. These concoctions will keep in the refrigerator for 2 or 3 days.

SPICY CITRUS BLAST

1 slice (3") of fresh ginger, peeled and grated

1 cucumber, peeled and thinly sliced

1 lemon, peeled and thinly sliced

Fresh mint to taste

CUCUMBER-JALAPEÑO QUENCHER

2 cucumbers, peeled and thinly sliced

2 jalapeno peppers, seeded and sliced (wear plastic gloves!)

MINTY MOJITO

6 mint sprigs

2 limes, peeled and thinly sliced

VANILLA LATTE

2 whole vanilla beans

2 cups whole coffee beans

green tea does contain caffeine (about 40 milligrams per tea bag), though far less than coffee.

Tip: Be sure to choose a high-quality tea, such as The Republic of Tea or Tazo. If you opt for loose leaves, use 1 teaspoon leaves to 6 ounces water. Let the tea steep for 2 to 3 minutes to extract the most health-boosting phytonutrients.

Optional: Red Wine

AIM FOR: NO MORE THAN 1 GLASS A DAY, THOUGH SCHWARTZ RECOMMENDS LIMITING IT TO TWICE A WEEK AND IDEALLY NOT AT ALL DURING THE PLAN.

What's a serving? A 5-ounce glass

Biggest nutritional payoff: The plant compound resveratrol found in red wine has been shown to boost telomere length, and its antioxidant content has heart-protective effects. These benefits have been found in moderate drinkers; go beyond 5 ounces a day, and the benefits are negated. Not to mention the unwanted calorie punch, if you're counting (one glass of red wine is 125 calories). Which is why Schwartz recommends skipping it entirely for the next 8 weeks.

Tip: If you like drinking red wine, consider opting for pinot noirs grown in cool, rainy climates; they have the most resveratrol, according to one study. Also, opt for a dry red—the sweeter the wine, the lower its flavonoid levels.

Cravings Crushers

Avocados

AIM FOR: HALF A MEDIUM AVOCADO A DAY (OR 2 TABLESPOONS GUACAMOLE).

Biggest nutritional payoff: You may already know that these buttery green orbs get their creamy goodness from healthy unsaturated fats. What you may not know: Adding avocado to your lunch can cut hunger nearly in half. In one study, volunteers who ate half an avocado at lunchtime stayed satisfied for up to 5 hours. Just as impressive, their appetites were reduced by as much as 40 percent, which meant less late-afternoon snacking. Its nutritional pedigree also includes soluble fiber, vitamin E, folate, and potassium.

Tip: A medium avocado packs around 320 calories and 30 grams of fat, so it would be tough to fit a whole one into your daily diet. But half is definitely, deliciously doable. Here are a few ideas.

Make an avocado "margarita." Drizzle an avocado half with lime juic, sprinkle with sea salt, and dig in.

Revamp a sandwich. Turkey sandwich for lunch? Swap the mayo for mashed avocado flavored with your favorite spice (like ground red pepper or curry). Or replace the mayo in tuna salad with mashed avocado.

Get your guac on. To make a fast dip, stir store-bought salsa and finely chopped red onion into mashed avocado.

Whip up a smoothie. In a blender, combine ½ ripe avocado, ½ cup stemmed and torn kale leaves, ½ banana, ½ cup ice cubes, and ¼ cup orange juice. Blend until smooth. Serves 1.

Make a next-level salad. In a bowl, combine ½ diced ripe avocado, 1 tablespoon plain yogurt (Greek or regular), ½ teaspoon fresh tarragon, ½ tablespoon lemon juice, ¾ cup shredded chicken, and 1 tablespoon diced shallots. Serve over greens.

Dark Chocolate
AIM FOR: 1 SERVING PER DAY STARTING IN WEEK 4.

What's a serving? 1 ounce.

Biggest nutritional payoff: Dark chocolate is packed with flavonoids—natural compounds that relax blood vessels, thereby lowering blood pressure. To reap cardiovascular benefits, you have to get 200 milligrams of cocoa flavanols daily. You'll find Schwartz's chocolate recommendations on page 406.

Tip: Plagued by cravings for chocolate or other sweets? Try this tip from Will Clower, PhD, neuroscientist and author of *Eat Chocolate, Lose Weight*. Twenty or 30 minutes before your meal, pop a piece of dark chocolate as big as the top joint of your thumb. Let it melt on your tongue. Repeat immediately after your meal. This simple tip works because the cocoa butter in those small amounts triggers the hormones in your brain that say "I'm full," according to Dr. Clower.

Nuts
AIM FOR: ONE 1-OUNCE SERVING PER DAY.

What's a serving? Depends. It's roughly 35 peanuts, 24 almonds, 18 medium cashews, 15 pecan halves, and 14 walnut halves.

Biggest nutritional payoff: You've already read about how nuts are high in protein, heart-healthy fats, vitamin E, and magnesium. Keep an eye on portions; as tasty as they are, nuts are calorie-dense. You can sprinkle them on salads, swirl them into yogurt, or enjoy them straight or with some dried fruit as a snack. You won't overdo it if you count them out and zip them into single-serving snack bags.

The Meal Builder

Now that you have a clearer picture of what you'll be eating more (and less) of, we want to give you the tools to start crafting your own meals, which you'll do starting in Week 2. Plug your favorite foods into the Meal Builder and you'll know that virtually every meal will be plant-based, healthy, and insanely good. Here's your template.

1. EAT THREE MEALS PER DAY—TWO OF THEM PLANT-BASED, THE THIRD WITH ANIMAL PROTEIN (IF YOU WISH).

Here's the shorthand version: Envision your empty dinner plate. Devote one-quarter of the plate to protein and one-quarter to whole grains. The other half of your plate? Pile it high with veggies, cooked or raw. Here's how it breaks down.

EACH MEAL SHOULD CONTAIN THE FOLLOWING:

Veggies: 1 to 2 servings. One serving is ½ cup cooked or 1 cup raw.

Whole grains: 1 serving (optional). One serving is ½ cup cooked.

Protein: 1 serving. One serving is 3 to 4 ounces, regardless of whether you choose plant or animal protein. Again, opt for plant protein more often than not. You can also choose fish twice a week, red meat once a week, and chicken two or three times a week.

AIM TO INCLUDE THESE INGREDIENTS SOMEWHERE ON YOUR PLATE, TOO:

Healthy fats: 1 serving at meals and snack time. A serving is one of the following: 1 teaspoon oil (healthy ones such as olive or coconut) or grass-fed butter, 1 ounce nuts or seeds, 1 to 2 tablespoons nut butter, or 2 tablespoons guacamole. (As you've noticed, many of the healthy-fat-containing plant foods are also healthy proteins—win!)

Prebiotic or probiotic foods: Try to add one to meals or snacks (like a sprinkling of chopped almonds in your oatmeal or sauerkraut as a side). See page 48 for a list of prebiotic and probiotic powerhouses.

Fruit: 1 to 2 servings a day *after* the 4-day Jumpstart. One serving is ½ cup sliced fruit, 1 small whole fruit, or 2 tablespoons dried fruit.

2. EAT TWO SNACKS PER DAY.

Snacks should ideally consist of a protein (and/or a healthy fat, which typically are found together in the same food), and a whole food (a fruit, veggie, or whole grain). Portions are smaller than at meals, of course.

HERE'S WHAT A SNACK SHOULD LOOK LIKE:

½ **serving protein** (ideally containing a healthy fat, for example, 4 ounces Greek yogurt, 1 tablespoon chia seeds, ¾ cup cooked edamame, ¼ whole avocado)

with

1 fruit/vegetable serving (for example, 1 small apple, 1 cup sliced carrot sticks, 1 cup steamed broccoli, ½ medium-size banana)

or

1 serving whole grains (for example, 1 rice cake, 1 serving healthy crackers [serving sizes vary based on cracker size; my recommendations can be found in the Food Shopping Guide, page 403], 1 slice bread [for peanut butter or hummus], ¼ cup healthy granola)

Once or twice a week, feel free to have a packaged snack from the Food Shopping Guide (page 403). Pair it with 1.5 to 2 ounces vegetable- or animal-based protein.

3. HAVE DESSERT AFTER DINNER!

You can enjoy it every night following the 4-day Jumpstart, but stick to no added sugar (have naturally sweetened foods, like fruit) for the first 3 weeks.

Whatever your indulgence, don't exceed 6 teaspoons of sugar daily (9 teaspoons for men).

4. DRINK AN 8-OUNCE GLASS OF WATER WITH EVERY MEAL AND SNACK.
"It's a no-brainer way to get most of the water you need," Schwartz says.

Coffee is optional. If you drink it, stick to the recommended 2 to 3 cups per day (don't exceed 400 milligrams of caffeine).

Alcohol isn't recommended during the plan because it's caloric and can cloud judgment. Try to limit yourself to two drinks per week. One drink equals one light beer (12 ounces), wine (5 ounces), or 1 shot of spirits (vodka, gin, rum, Scotch, bourbon).

Got it? Here's a sample of how the guidelines would break out across a day.

Sample 1-Day Menu Plan

BREAKFAST

Each option contains 1 to 2 servings veggies; 1 serving whole grains; 1 serving protein (including 1 serving healthy fat); 1 serving fruit (optional).

Egg over Sweet Potato Hash Browns (page 341)

Bacon and eggs: 2 eggs any style (prepared with 1 teaspoon oil or grass-fed butter), 1 slice turkey bacon, ½ cup cooked spinach (in eggs, if desired), 1 slice whole grain toast

Cereal and fruit: 1 serving whole grain cereal (see the Food Shopping Guide for brands), ½ cup plant milk, ½ cup sliced fruit, 1 ounce nuts or seeds (sprinkled on cereal)

Smoothie: 1 serving, any variety, from the Clean & Green Recipes (pages 337–338) with 1 slice whole grain toast

Almond-Butter Oatmeal: Stir 1 tablespoon almond butter into ½ cup cooked oatmeal; add ½ cup sliced banana, sprinkle with cinnamon.

LUNCH

Each option contains 1 to 2 servings veggies; 1 serving whole grains; 1 serving protein (incorporating 1 serving healthy fat).

Nutty Chicken Salad: Top 1 cup raw baby spinach with chicken salad (prepared with 3 ounces grilled chicken breast, ¼ cup 2% plain Greek yogurt, ½ teaspoon curry powder, and 2 tablespoons chopped celery). Sprinkle with walnuts. Serve with 1 slice whole grain bread.

The Lunch Express: 1 veggie burger on a whole grain roll, topped with spicy brown mustard, onion, lettuce, and tomato. Serve with a salad or roasted or sautéed veggies.

Mediterranean Salad: Toss ½ cup cooked kidney beans with 2 tablespoons each finely chopped onion, tomato, and bell pepper. Add ground cumin and garlic powder to taste. Dress with a lemon juice and olive oil dressing. Serve over ½ cup whole wheat couscous.

Soup and Salad: 1 serving Curried Lentil and Spinach Soup (page 350) with 1 serving whole grain bread or crackers. Add a salad topped with nuts.

DINNER

Each option contains 1 to 2 servings veggies; 1 serving whole grains; 1 serving protein (including 1 serving healthy fat)

Fish Night: Broil 3 to 4 ounces salmon sprinkled with crab-boil seasoning to taste. Serve with a salad and ½ small sweet potato topped with 1 teaspoon grass-fed butter or ghee and dusted with ground cinnamon.

Tofu Night: Stir-fry ½ cup tofu and ½ cup broccoli in 1 teaspoon oil. Stir in ⅓ cup salsa. Serve over ½ cup brown rice.

Chili Night: 1 serving Kidney Bean and Turkey Chili (page 375) over ½ cup brown rice. Serve with 1 cup salad or ½ cup of your favorite cooked veggie—roasted, steamed, or stir-fried.

Meat Loaf Night: 1 serving Turkey Meat Loaf (page 374). Serve with ½ small baked potato topped with 1 teaspoon grass-fed butter or ghee and ½ cup steamed green beans tossed with 1 teaspoon minced roasted garlic, and a dash of sea salt.

SNACKS (2 per day)

Each of these contains 1 to 2 ounces of protein (ideally rich in healthy fat), with 1 serving of whole grain or other whole food, such as a fruit or a vegetable.

- 1 small apple or ½ banana with 1 tablespoon nut butter
- 1 small peach with 1 ounce almonds
- 1 to 2 tablespoons chopped dried fruit with 1 ounce goat cheese
- 1 serving whole grain crackers with 2 tablespoons hummus
- 1 serving whole grain crackers with 1.5 to 2 ounces lean deli turkey
- 1 brown rice cake with 1 tablespoon nut butter

DESSERT (after dinner only, after the Jumpstart)

Remember: Do not consume more than 6 teaspoons of sugar a day.

WEEKS 1 TO 3: CHOOSE ONE OF THESE DAILY, IF DESIRED.

- ½ cup fresh fruit salad
- 4 ounces 2% plain Greek yogurt with ½ tablespoon chopped nuts
- 1 cup air-popped popcorn tossed with 1 teaspoon grass-fed butter or melted coconut oil

WEEKS 4 AND AFTER: ADD THESE TO AFTER-DINNER SELECTION ABOVE.

- 1 serving of any dessert from the "Treats and Sweets" section of the Clean & Green Recipes chapter, or one of the desserts from the Food Shopping Guide (page 403)
- A couple spoonfuls of frozen yogurt or ice cream

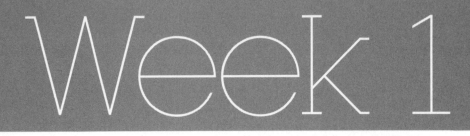

Week 1

"Starting with a daily intention has become a must for me. It sets the tone for the day."

—PANELIST SANDY FRANKLIN

STAY-YOUNG STEPS	GOALS	TO-DO LIST
EAT	Lose the bloat.	Follow the 4-day Jumpstart. Progress to the rest of Week 1's Clean & Green menu plan.
MOVE	Wake up your body.	Ease into morning with the Sunrise Stretch. Optional: Walk or run to stay active and prep for Week 2 cardio.
ENGAGE	Commit to healthy new morning and bedtime habits.	Learn to set an intention. Tweak your sleep schedule and rituals.
GLOW	Reset your skin.	Begin Dr. Jeannette Graf's skin-care routine.

Be Prepared!

- A day or two before you start the program, review the recipes in the Jumpstart menu and make a shopping list. Shop for the food you need and schedule a Batch Day to prep your meals for the week.

- Set your alarm 10 minutes early for your Sunrise Stretch.

- Make sure to buy the six or seven products listed on pages 191–192 for Dr. Graf's skin-care routine. (See our Product Guide on page 407 for brand recommendations.)

- If you can, clear your evening calendar. You will attempt to reboot your sleep schedule this week and will see best results if you can limit your late nights.

EAT

The First 4 Days: The Jumpstart

This 96-hour initiation—a more intense, focused version of the Clean & Green eating plan—helps you shed bloat and water weight so you sail confidently into the program. You'll swap foods, beverages, and spices known to cause belly bloat and fluid retention for a fresh, healthy, whole-foods menu.

Test panelist Sandy Franklin lost 10 pounds during the 4-day Jumpstart. "I had high energy and was always full," she says. Panelist Jen Casper experienced a similar surge of energy: "I felt awesome—and the Jumpstart was much easier than I thought." What else can you expect from the belly-flattening Jumpstart menu?

- **It's light on unhealthy fat.** The Jumpstart includes a high dose of the healthy fats found in olive oil, olives, nuts and seeds, and avocado, and it is light on unhealthy fats (saturated fat, found in animal foods, and trans fat found in processed foods). Also off the menu: fried or fatty foods, which move through your system slowly and can leave you feeling sluggish and bloated.

- **It's low in salt.** When you eat a lot of sodium, your body temporarily retains fluid (water weight) and your face can get puffy. On the Jumpstart, you'll avoid sodium-laden processed foods and boost flavor with salt-free seasoning blends, fresh or dried herbs and spices, and lemon or lime juice (great on fish and chicken, by the way).

- **It's high in healthy veggies.** To flatten your belly during these 4 days, you'll eat mostly cooked veggies for the simple reason that they're easier to digest. Steam them over an inch of water in a pan for 3 to 7 minutes—a shorter period for leafy greens, longer for broccoli, cauliflower, or green beans. You can nuke your veggies, too; just add several tablespoons of water to a microwaveable glass bowl, cover, and microwave on high power for 3 to 5 minutes, or until just tender.

  Some nutrient-dense veggies—beans, Brussels sprouts, cauliflower, cabbage, onions, and peppers—are also off the menu for the next few days, since they're notorious gas producers. They'll show up again after the Jumpstart.

- **It cuts back on fruit.** While fruit is super nutritious, some kinds—such as apples, pears, and honeydew melon—can cause bloat. On the Jumpstart, you can have fruit only once a day, so be selective.

Major Bloaters You'll Nix on the Jumpstart

Several common foods and beverages are so puff-promoting that we eliminated them from the Jumpstart entirely. These include:

- **Alcohol, coffee, tea, and acidic fruit juices.** All of these can potentially irritate your gastrointestinal tract, causing it to swell. Feel free to enjoy coffee or tea (Andie Bernard Schwartz, RD, recommends organic green tea) later this week. If you really need coffee or tea in the morning, stick to one cup. You can add 1 tablespoon of milk (plant-based or dairy) but no sweeteners.

- **Artificial sweeteners.** While the FDA has recognized artificial sugars (aspartame and sucralose) and sugar alcohols (xylitol, sorbitol, and maltitol) as safe, they seriously bloat you up. Sorbitol and xylitol absorb very slowly in the small intestine and can cause gas, cramping, and even diarrhea. Sucralose (Splenda) has been linked to sugar cravings. While you're at it, consider removing them from your diet permanently.

- **Bubbly drinks.** Those tiny gas bubbles like to make themselves heard after you swallow them. But what you don't belch out tends to drift to your middle, where the gas can cause uncomfortable swelling. Plus, many carbonated drinks typically contain either artificial sweeteners or added sugars. Swap fizzy beverages for pure water or our delicious flavored options (see page 170).

- **Gum.** When you chew gum, you swallow air, which becomes trapped in your gastrointestinal tract and causes pressure and belly expansion.

- **Hot herbs and spices.** Spicy foods—along with herbs and spices like black pepper, nutmeg, cloves, chili powder, mustard, and horseradish—can stimulate the release of stomach acid, causing swelling. Stick to the flavor boosters on the "It's low in salt" entry on page 179. You'll avoid onions, too, which contain a carbohydrate called fructan that some people find causes gas and bloating.

What follows are foods and dishes designed to work with our Jumpstart guidelines. Hate mushrooms? Think chia's for Chia Pets? Feel free to swap in an ingredient or meal from another day. But we also urge you to keep an open mind. Our panelists were surprised by the number of foods they came to love that had previously topped their gag lists.

Your Jumpstart Menu Plan

DAY 1 JUMPSTART

Breakfast

Berry Green Smoothie: **In a blender, combine 1 cup plant-based milk, 1 cup spinach, ½ cup strawberries, and 1 tablespoon flaxseed, hemp seeds, or chia seeds. Blend until smooth.**

1 slice whole grain toast with 1 teaspoon grass-fed butter

Mid-AM Snack

1 cup gently cooked or steamed baby carrots with 2 tablespoons hummus

Lunch

Quinoa with Mushrooms and Toasted Almonds: **Prepare ½ cup quinoa according to package directions and place in a bowl. Sauté 1 cup sliced mushrooms and 2 teaspoons fresh grated ginger in 1 teaspoon coconut oil until mushrooms are soft. Top quinoa with mushrooms and sprinkle with 2 tablespoons sliced or chopped almonds.**

Mid-PM Snack

¼ cup nuts of your choice

Dinner

1 serving Salmon with Swiss Chard (page 383) (omit ground black pepper for Jumpstart)

½–1 serving Fast and Fresh Salad (page 361) (omit ground black pepper for Jumpstart)

Dessert/PM Snack

½ cup plain Greek yogurt

DAY 2 JUMPSTART

Breakfast

Green Juice Blend: In a blender, combine 1 cup flat-leaf parsley, 2 stalks celery, ½ avocado, ½ cup chopped cucumber, ½ kiwifruit, and 8 to 10 ounces water. Blend until smooth.

1 slice whole grain toast with grass-fed butter

Optional: If you're still hungry, eat 1 egg, prepared any style, cooked in 1 teaspoon healthy fat.

Mid-AM Snack

Egg Salad: Mix 1 hard-cooked egg, chopped, with 2 teaspoons olive-oil mayo.

½ cup red bell pepper strips

Lunch

1 serving Turkey-Mushroom Burgers (page 358) (omit onions and ground black pepper for Jumpstart)

½ cup carrots, sautéed in 1 teaspoon olive oil

Mid-PM Snack

1 whole wheat pita cut into 4 wedges with 1 to 2 tablespoons hummus

---

A Tip for Smoother Smoothies

WHEN YOU MAKE THE BERRY GREEN SMOOTHIE, if using chia seeds, I'd advise soaking them in the plant-based milk for about 3 minutes before blending so they melt away (otherwise you may wind up with seeds in the smoothie). Also, brown chia seeds will result in a gray smoothie—not appetizing! Golden chia seeds blend in better.

—PANELIST JENNIE DEAN

If Bloat and Water Retention Don't Go Away . . .

BOTH OF THESE ARE SUPER-COMMON CONDITIONS. But if bloat and water retention are persistent or painful, they can signal more serious health problems. See a doctor if you have any of these symptoms.

- Chronic constipation, diarrhea, nausea, or vomiting
- Persistent abdominal or rectal pain or heartburn
- Unintentional weight loss
- Unexplained fever
- Blood in your urine
- Skin that looks stretched or shiny or that retains a dimple after you press it

Seek immediate medical attention if you experience shortness of breath or chest pain or find it hard to draw a breath.

Dinner

Tempeh Stir-Fry: Prepare ½ cup soba noodles according to package directions. Cut 3 ounces tempeh into strips and sauté with 1 tablespoon coconut oil. After 5 minutes, add 1 cup vegetables of your choice (excluding those from the bloat list). Cover 2 to 3 minutes, or until soft. Toss with the noodles and 1 tablespoon reduced-sodium soy sauce, 2 teaspoons rice vinegar, ¼ teaspoon minced garlic, and 1 to 2 teaspoons grated fresh ginger.

Dessert/PM Snack

1 cup air-popped popcorn tossed with ½ teaspoon jerk seasoning and 1 teaspoon melted coconut oil, or one of the snacks on page 177

DAY 3 JUMPSTART

Breakfast

1 serving Banana-Chia Smoothie (page 337)

1 slice whole grain toast with 1 teaspoon grass-fed butter

Mid-AM Snack

2 slices tomato with ¼ avocado, sliced, drizzled with 1 teaspoon olive oil

Lunch

Tuna Salad Wrap: Mix ½ cup water-packed albacore or chunk lighttuna with 2 tablespoons 2% plain Greek yogurt, ¼ teaspoon paprika or salt-free seasoning, and 1 tablespoon diced carrots, celery, or both. Wrap in romaine lettuce (or arrange the tuna on the lettuce).

Mid-PM Snack

2 ounces smoked salmon wrapped around cucumber spears

Dinner

1 serving Oven-Fried Rosemary Chicken Breasts (page 378)

½–1 serving Fast and Fresh Salad (page 361) (omit ground black pepper for Jumpstart)

Dessert/PM Snack

1 ounce walnuts or almonds

DAY 4 JUMPSTART

Breakfast

1 serving Super Green Smoothie (page 338)

1 slice whole grain toast with 1 teaspoon grass-fed butter

Optional: If you're still hungry, eat 1 egg, prepared any style.

Mid-AM Snack

1 cup gently steamed veggies of your choice with 2 tablespoons hummus

Lunch

1 serving Couscous–Bean Salad (page 363) served over 2 cups baby mixed greens

Mid-PM Snack

1 brown rice cake with 1 tablespoon nut butter of your choice

Dinner

1 serving Pecan-Crusted Roasted Salmon (page 385)

½–1 serving Fast and Fresh Salad (page 361) (omit ground black pepper for Jumpstart)

Dessert/PM Snack

1 serving whole grain crackers with 2 tablespoons hummus

DAY 5: YOU'RE READY TO EAT CLEAN & GREEN

To reiterate: You won't need to count calories or grams of *anything* on this plan (that's because we've done the work for you). For a refresher on the foods you'll be eating more of—and those that are off the plate for 8 weeks—see page 158.

Breakfast

Coffee (black or with 1 tablespoon plant-based or organic regular milk) or green tea

1 slice whole grain toast with 1 teaspoon grass-fed butter

From Batching to Brown-Bagging

PREPARING A COUPLE OF MEALS AHEAD on Batch Day will make your morning routine saner. To feel even more on top of things, pack a lunch for work. Women who eat out at lunch, even just once a week, weigh on average about 5 pounds more than those who don't. You'll be extra motivated if you've packed your lunch in a cute reusable container or wrap that doesn't contain any plastic chemicals that can leach into your food. Here are some suggestions.

BEE'S WRAP. This cloth and beeswax version of plastic wrap can be washed and reused. (pack of three, $18; beeswrap.com)

LIFEFACTORY GLASS FOOD STORAGE. A colorful silicone coating protects the glass. ($15; lifefactory.com)

FREEZABLE SANDWICH BAG. Pop this in the freezer and gel liners keep it cool. ($12; packit.com)

LUNCHBOTS TRIO. This stainless-steel carrier has two dividers. ($22; lunchbots.com)

Apple-Cinnamon Oatmeal: Top ¾ cup cooked oatmeal with ½ cup chopped apple, ¼ teaspoon cinnamon, 1 tablespoon chopped walnuts, and 1 to 2 teaspoons ground flaxseed.

Mid-AM Snack

1 cup steamed edamame with ¼ teaspoon coarse sea salt

Lunch

1 serving Turkey and Red Cabbage Slaw Sandwich (page 355)

½ sweet potato coated with cooking spray and baked at 350°F for 20 to 30 minutes, or until cooked through and tender. Season with salt and pepper to taste.

Mid-PM Snack

¼ cup Chickpea Dip with Baby Carrots (page 344) or prepared hummus from Day 1 with 1 cup baby carrots

Dinner

1 serving Broccoli, Mushroom, and Tofu Stir-Fry with Walnuts (page 392)

Dessert/PM Snack

1 serving Blueberry-Ricotta Sundae (page 397)

DAY 6

Breakfast

Coffee (black or with 1 tablespoon plant-based or organic regular milk) or green tea

1 orange

1 serving Egg over Sweet Potato Hash Browns (page 341)

Mid-AM Snack

1 serving Curried Lentil and Spinach Soup (page 350)

Lunch

Spinach Salad: Mix 1 to 2 cups baby spinach with ½ cup cherry tomatoes; ½ cup diced cucumber; ¼ avocado, sliced or chopped; 1 tablespoon sunflower seeds; and ½ cup chickpeas. Use dressing from the Fast and Fresh Salad recipe (page 361). Serve with 1 slice whole grain bread.

Mid-PM Snack

1 cup 2% plain Greek yogurt

Swap Your Coffee-Shop Sugar Bomb for This

WHILE COFFEE COMES BACK ON THE scene on Day 5, you may miss your usual frothy coffee-shop concoction. Try this low-calorie, zero-sugar coffee drink (it only tastes decadent). We used mocha-flavored coffee, but vanilla or hazelnut coffee—or regular brew—tastes just as good. For an icy treat, freeze leftover coffee into cubes and add a few for a flavor boost.

SKINNY ORANGE MOCHACCINO

Makes one ¾-cup serving

½ cup strong mocha-flavored coffee (cold or hot)

¾ cup unsweetened plant-based milk, such as coconut milk or almond milk

½ teaspoon orange extract

Unsweetened cocoa powder

In a pitcher, stir together the coffee, milk, and orange extract. Serve hot or iced. Dust with the cocoa powder before serving.

Dinner

1 serving Shrimp with Orzo and Edamame (page 389)

½–1 serving Fast and Fresh Salad (page 361)

Dessert/PM Snack

1 serving Warm Glazed Oranges with Walnuts (page 398) (omit added sugar until Day 28)

DAY 7

Breakfast

Coffee (black or with 1 tablespoon plant-based or organic regular milk) or green tea

1 serving French Toast with Fruit (page 338)

Mid-AM Snack

1 serving Spiced Sweet Potato Chips (page 342)

Lunch

Whole Wheat Couscous with Carrots, Peas, and Beans: **Bring 1¼ cups vegetable stock to a boil. Add 1 cup whole wheat couscous and remove from the heat. Stir the couscous until it absorbs all the stock. Add 1 cup pinto beans; 1 carrot, diced; 1 stalk celery, diced; ½ red bell pepper, diced; 3 tablespoons chopped parsley; 2 tablespoons chopped fresh mint; ¼ cup peas; ¼ teaspoon ground cinnamon; ¼ cup toasted chopped walnuts; and 3 tablespoons red or white wine vinegar. Mix well and chill for at least 2 hours before serving.**

½–1 serving Fast and Fresh Salad (page 361); add ¼ avocado, sliced or chopped

Mid-PM Snack

1 cup Creole Cauliflower Soup (page 351)

Dinner

1 serving Sweet-and-Sour Red Cabbage with Sausage (page 379)

Dessert/PM Snack

1 serving Baked Pears with Creamy Lemon Sauce (page 396)

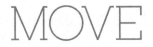

MOVE

Because we want you to focus on the major changes to your eating habits—and they're major, we know—you're starting off the exercise portion of the plan nice and easy this week with a simple Sunrise Stretch (page 288). This 10-minute stretching routine builds movement into your day from the time your feet hit the floor. It also loosens sleep-kinked muscles, helps reduce morning stiffness, and delivers an energy boost that doesn't come from caffeine. You'll be surprised by how quickly it becomes something you look forward to.

If your mornings are chaotic and you can't spare 10 minutes, do the Sunrise Stretch at any time of day, picking a window when you'd most benefit from an activity break. The same moves that wake up your body in the morning also loosen muscles cramped from hours at a desk or help you wind down at the end of the day.

Although we don't begin the cardio program until next week, if you're already walking, jogging, biking, or hitting the gym regularly, keep it up while you integrate the stretch into your mornings.

To review how the exercise plan for the upcoming weeks will progress, turn to the Younger in 8 Weeks Workout, which begins on page 287.

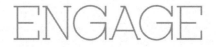

ENGAGE

This week, you'll begin to cultivate two new habits: starting each day with a minute devoted exclusively to you and turning in at a decent hour so you awaken feeling refreshed. Both will lay the emotional groundwork for the next few weeks and infuse your days with energy and purpose.

In the Morning: Set an Intention

This one small step is a huge part of your journey: Setting a daily intention has been shown to help you tap into how you're really feeling and where you most want to go. Both Western psychology and Eastern spiritual traditions emphasize the importance of reflecting on our deepest intentions as catalysts for change. Here's how to do it.

Begin with a "thank-you." Whether or not you're a person of faith, gratitude sets a positive tone for the day. Your thanks might be as simple as, "I'm grateful to have a new day with my friends and family so I can love them and allow them to love me."

Select a focus. Once you've given thanks, pick one area of your life you want to improve or a goal you want to achieve. Then create an intention around it and write it down. (Sometimes the first idea that bubbles up is the one you need most. Go with it.) Here are a few examples.

- Today, my intention is to notice how I feel, physically and emotionally, without judgment.

- Today, my intention is to become aware of any negative thoughts about my age or appearance and to counter them with positive thoughts about myself.

- Today, my intention is to handle frustration and setbacks with patience and calm.

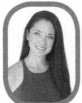

Dr. Vonda Wright says...
SET YOURSELF UP FOR EXERCISE SUCCESS

Week 1—yeah! Beginnings are so exciting. Each year, I take my patients through the Couch to 5K START classes. I look forward to each new group, because in these twice-weekly circuit-training classes, I get to move my patients from their couches or desk chairs to a 5K walk/run in 12 weeks.

At the first class, the "Starters" (as I call them) are shy, filled with nervous energy and more than a little self-doubt: *Can I really do this?* As the music fills the gym, we learn the total-body circuit moves that will eventually give them their lives back. We sweat and sweat. Then we sweat some more. Even on Day 1, know this: If you're sweating, you're succeeding.

I know you can experience the same joy, strength, and reinvigoration that I have seen in so many of my patients. You just need to start. Here's the advice I give my patients as they return to exercise or, in some cases, begin to move for the first time in their lives.

1. If you're overwhelmed by the thought of a multiweek commitment to exercise, start with a smaller goal: finishing just the first workout. Stop for a brief rest if you need to, but promise yourself that you'll jump back in and finish. Then celebrate your accomplishment by telling a friend or putting a sticky note on the refrigerator that says "Yeah me!" I'm not kidding. Getting through that first workout proves that you can do it.

2. If this is your first experience with regular exercise (or if you've been sedentary for a while), you are likely to be out of breath as you move. You may also feel sore for a couple of days. Reframe how you think about this breathlessness or soreness. These sensations aren't negatives. They're positive signs that you're changing your life for the better—so celebrate them!

• Today, my intention is to stick to my food plan and not eat out of boredom or stress.

At Night: Start Turning In Earlier

You won't get very far on your antiaging journey if all you want is a nap. So in Week 1, commit to the recommended 7 to 8 hours of sleep each night to score the energy, calm, and clarity you'll need. Review and use the sleep strategies in the ENGAGE chapter on page 85. Also, take the actions below to troubleshoot your current sleep habits and establish healthier ones, if necessary.

Start a sleep log. Starting on Day 1 and for the next 2 weeks, track the quantity and quality of your previous night's sleep (some activity trackers can do it for you). If you're keeping a journal, you might start each day's entry with your "sleep report." Note what time you turned in, how long it took you to fall asleep, how many times you woke up during the night, and how you felt in the morning (groggy, grouchy, rested, refreshed). Also note what you ate and drank close to bedtime and—beginning in Week 2—how much exercise you did that day. (If you don't currently exercise, you may notice a positive change in your sleep once you start.) Comparing your daily habits with your nightly sleep patterns—and to the sleep strategies in the ENGAGE chapter—can highlight where you need to make changes.

Design (and implement) your chill-out ritual. If you don't already follow a nightly routine to prepare your body for sleep, create one this week. What activities would lull you to sleep—a hot bath, followed by a cup of decaf herbal tea and a good book? Relaxing music, followed by deep breathing or meditation? The activity is up to you, as long as it primes you to sleep. Put your laptop, smartphone, or tablet in another room before you go to bed. The light alone from these devices can impede your body's production of sleep hormones.

GLOW

By now, you should have the six or seven basic skin-care products recommended by Dr. Graf. If you haven't, order them, stat! Here's a quick review of what you need and the order in which to apply them.

A.M. ROUTINE

Cleansing oil or micellar water cleanser

Antioxidant serum

Moisturizer

Broad-spectrum sunscreen

P.M. ROUTINE

> Retinoid cream
>
> Night cream (optional)
>
> Eye cream

We know that's a lot to ring up at once, but these super-effective products will last you for weeks and are key to your full age-defying makeover. Incorporating them each day will reduce lines, erase some discoloration, shrink pore size, and promote your skin's cellular repair so you wake up looking a tiny bit younger than when you went to bed. You'll start seeing changes in the mirror before this date next month—so circle it!

It may feel self-indulgent to spend 10 whole minutes on your skin each day. It may also be confusing if your routine until now has consisted of a splash of water and a face cream. Our panelists had some helpful suggestions for

Renew Right Now

INSTANT GLOW

PLAY UP YOUR SHOULDERS. They're the one body part that is slow to age, so accentuate your shoulders with boatneck tops or wide, scooped necklines. If you have larger breasts, V-necks reveal a hint of collarbone and décolletage, which will help you look less top-heavy. Using a makeup sponge, you can even add a bit of tinted moisturizer or foundation that's two shades darker than your complexion to even out your skin tone, says beauty and style expert Eva Scrivo. (Do this carefully after you've put on your clothes to avoid getting makeup on them. Also be cautious when removing your clothes later.)

SLIMMER IN A MINUTE

FAKE IT WITH SHAPEWEAR. The next-best thing to having the waistline of your twenties is a lingerie drawer that contains shapewear. To flatten and smooth your belly, wear a fitted cami long enough to cover your hips or a high-waisted brief that extends to your bra band (okay, it sounds uncool, but it looks amazing). To slim your thighs, sneak knee-length bike shorts or boyshorts by Wolford under longer skirts, dresses, and trousers. Make sure to look at your back when fully dressed for any bulges around your bra line that can be smoothed with a tight tee worn underneath a blouse or sweater, advises Scrivo.

adapting. Sharon Scheirer was worried she'd forget to use all the products, so she placed them on the bathroom counter where she'd see them, rather than tucking them out of sight. Or try Kate Pelham-Hambly's hack for remembering the order of the routine: "I kept the instructions right on the sink for the first day or two until I got the hang of it."

Pretty soon you may come to view Dr. Graf's skin-care routine as two brief but meaningful moments to give yourself some TLC. You may have an exploding inbox or a to-do list as long as your arm, but for those precious minutes, you're taking care of *you*. And consider the payoff: "My skin is the best it has ever been," says panelist Sandy Fromknecht. "I'll follow this routine for life."

SUCCESS!

Jennie Dean, 44

MY STORY Jennie Dean is only 44, but when she started the Younger in 8 Weeks Plan, she was already worrying about getting old. And her self-assessment validated her concern; Jennie was "aging fast"!

She didn't have the energy to play with her kids. Her joints were hurting. She was preoccupied with thoughts of diabetes and heart disease. And the age spot that appeared for her last birthday wasn't helping.

But now she's worrying less. In fact, Jennie nearly doubled her score on the self-assessment after just 8 weeks. "The first thing people noticed was my skin," she said. "I've been told by no less than 11 people that my skin is 'glowing.'" After just 2 weeks, the pimples that she'd been prone to for 30+ years were gone. The age spot under her eye had vanished by Week 4. And the wrinkles around her eyes and lips had smoothed out by the end of the program. "My skin is so clear that I go completely without face makeup, just a little eye makeup and lip gloss now," she said.

Jennie started to feel inwardly lighter, too, as she embraced the ENGAGE part of the program. Over the past couple of years, Jennie had been withdrawing and neglecting her friendships because she was dealing with chronic pain and depression. It was time to change that.

She started by asking a neighbor to walk. "She'd invited me in the past, but I'd turned her down enough times that she stopped asking." Jennie has since developed a new friendship that's helped her beyond just exercise: "She's been watching my kids for me lately. That was a support I had lost in the neighborhood."

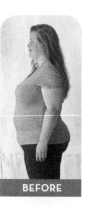

BEFORE

As Jennie's mood improved and the pounds came off, she began dressing up and smiling more. Suddenly, "Everything about me was more positive, and people were attracted to me again. Moms from my kids' school started coming up to me and chatting," she recalled.

This new support finally gave her the confidence to reach out to a close friend. They'd grown apart when her friend started to lead a healthier, more active lifestyle and Jennie had children.

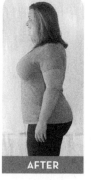

AFTER

When her friend, who lives across the country, returned Jennie's call, they had a tearful 2-hour conversation and are looking forward to a reunion soon. "That was a friendship I missed horribly," Jennie said. "I'm so thankful we reconnected."

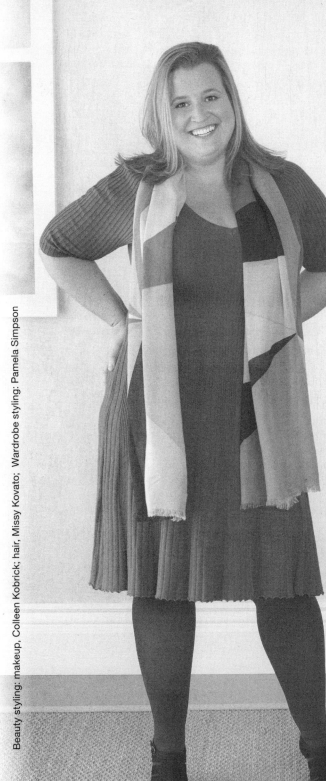

LOOK AT ME

- Lowered high blood glucose level **10 points**

- Reduced high blood pressure **30 points to almost healthy**

- Copes better with stress

- Lost **2.25 inches off thighs**

- Weight lost: **16.6 pounds**

- Inches lost: **7**

Tip BATCH COOK ONCE A WEEK. Cook full recipes that can be reheated easily, but also precook components: Poach a few chicken breasts; boil a dozen eggs; cook up some barley; roast extra veggies.

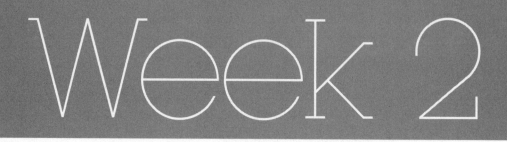

Week 2

"After my first cardio workout, I felt exhilarated.
I found myself thinking, 'I know I can go faster!'"
— PANELIST CINDY CARTER

STAY-YOUNG STEPS	GOALS	TO-DO LIST
EAT	**Continue to eat Clean & Green.**	Follow the Week 2 menu plan.
MOVE	**Ease into exercise and start to get your heart rate up.**	Keep doing the Sunrise Stretch. Begin your workout session with the Dynamic Warmup. Do 10 to 20 minutes of cardio at a steady pace 2 or 3 days this week.
ENGAGE	**Learn to calm and clear your mind.**	Continue to set your daily intention in the morning and work on sleep hygiene at night. Try 10 minutes of mindfulness meditation.
GLOW	**Continue your skin-care routine.** **Focus on hair repair, if you need it.**	Address any skin sensitivity. Follow the steps to lusher, healthier hair. *Splurge!* Treat yourself to a spa facial.

Be Prepared!

- Read through this week's menu plan, review the Food Shopping Guide on page 403, shop for what you need, and schedule your Batch Day.

- Decide on the best days and times for your cardio workouts, and save them to your calendar. (The "best time" is the time you'll do it.)

- Make space in your day for a 10-minute meditation break—in the morning, during your lunch hour, before bed.

- For a splurge, book a facial appointment for the end of the week.

- Buy a clarifying shampoo and a deep-conditioning treatment (or just have some apple cider vinegar and coconut oil on hand).

EAT

Week 2 Clean & Green Menu Plan

DAY 8

Breakfast

Coffee (black or with 1 tablespoon plant-based or organic regular milk) or green tea

1 serving Banana-Chia Smoothie (page 337)

1 slice whole grain toast with 1 teaspoon grass-fed butter

Mid-AM Snack

1 stalk of celery with 1 to 2 tablespoons nut butter of your choice

Lunch

1 serving Zesty Pork Tenderloin Wrap (page 359)

1 serving Roasted Broccoli and Cauliflower (page 372)

Mid-PM Snack

½ cup low-fat cottage cheese

Dinner

1 serving Salmon with Swiss Chard (page 383)

1 small baked potato topped with a mixture of ¼ cup 2% plain Greek yogurt, 1 tablespoon chopped red onion, and 1 teaspoon each of finely chopped fresh dill and minced garlic

Dessert/PM Snack

½ cup sliced strawberries with a dollop of whipped cream

DAY 9

Breakfast

Coffee (black or with 1 tablespoon plant-based or organic regular milk) or green tea

1 serving Muesli with Walnuts (page 336) and ½ cup 2% plain Greek yogurt

1 slice whole grain toast with 1 teaspoon grass-fed butter

Mid-AM Snack

10 baby carrots with ½ cup low-fat cottage cheese mixed with ¼ teaspoon lemon-pepper seasoning

Lunch

1 serving Chicken and Rice Salad with Walnuts (page 368)

Mid-PM Snack

Baked Sugar Snap Peas: Spread 2 cups trimmed sugar snap peas on a cookie sheet lined with parchment paper. Drizzle with 1 teaspoon olive oil and sprinkle with 1 tablespoon shredded Parmesan cheese, ¼ teaspoon garlic powder, ⅛ teaspoon coarse salt, and ⅛ teaspoon red-pepper flakes. Bake at 350°F for 15 to 20 minutes. Makes 2 servings (1 cup each). Save the remaining cup for a Day 11 snack.

Dinner

Rice and Beans Salad: Combine ½ cup cooked brown rice, ½ cup steamed or gently boiled green beans, ¼ cup cooked/canned pinto beans, and 1½ teaspoons almond slices. Sprinkle with 1 tablespoon shredded Cheddar cheese. Top with 1 tablespoon no-sugar-added salsa or pico de gallo and a sprinkle of chopped green chile pepper.

Dessert/PM Snack

1 serving Strawberry Sorbet (page 398)

DAY 10

Breakfast

Coffee (black or with 1 tablespoon organic milk/half-and-half) or organic green tea

1 serving Hummus, Tomato, and Spinach Breakfast Sandwich (page 336)

Mid-AM Snack

Healthy Egg Salad: Gently stir together 2 hard-cooked eggs, finely chopped; ½ cup low-fat plain yogurt; ⅓ cup finely chopped celery; 1 tablespoon mustard; and ¼ teaspoon ground nutmeg. Serve on romaine lettuce with 1 red, yellow, or orange bell pepper, sliced. Makes 1 serving.

Lunch

1 serving Asparagus and Barley Salad and Dill Dressing (page 362)

Mid-PM Snack

½ serving *Homemade Trail Mix:* **Toss together 1 tablespoon raw pecans, 1 tablespoon raw cashews, 1 teaspoon dried cherries or raisins, and ¼ teaspoon coarse sea salt. Makes 1 serving. Save the remainder for a Day 12 snack.**

Dinner

1 serving Tofu-Stuffed Peppers (page 393)

½–1 serving Fast and Fresh Salad (page 361)

Dessert/PM Snack

1 serving Blueberry-Ricotta Sundae (page 397)

DAY 11

Breakfast

Coffee (black or with 1 tablespoon plant-based or organic regular milk) or green tea

Breakfast Scramble with Tofu: **Sauté** ½ cup chopped spinach in 1 teaspoon coconut oil for 2 minutes, or until wilted. Remove from the skillet and set aside. Add 1 teaspoon coconut oil to the skillet. Sauté ¼ potato, grated, in 1 teaspoon coconut oil for 5 minutes, or until crispy and tender. Stir in ¼ teaspoon onion powder; ¼ teaspoon ground turmeric; 1 ounce extra-firm tofu, cubed; and the reserved spinach. Add 1 egg, beaten, and stir for 3 minutes, or until the egg is set.

1 slice whole grain toast

Mid-AM Snack

1 serving Baked Sugar Snap Peas (page 198)

Lunch

1 serving Greek Vegetable Open-Faced Sandwiches (page 354)

½–1 serving Fast and Fresh Salad (page 361)

Mid-PM Snack

1 serving no-sugar-added salsa with healthy crackers (see Food Shopping Guide for recommendations)

Dinner

1 serving Lemon Snapper with Curry-Garlic Cauliflower (page 388)

½ cup cooked brown rice

Dessert/PM Snack

½ peach and 1 tablespoon pecans

DAY 12

Breakfast

Coffee (black or with 1 tablespoon plant-based or organic regular milk) or green tea

1 slice whole grain toast with 1 teaspoon grass-fed butter

¾ cup steel-cut oatmeal with ½ cup berries, 1 tablespoon walnuts, and ½ teaspoon ground flaxseed

Mid-AM Snack

Chickpea Dip with Baby Carrots (page 344)

Lunch

1 serving Vegetarian Sloppy Joes in Romaine Wraps (page 360)

1 cup collard greens sautéed with 1 tablespoon coconut oil and sprinkled with ¼ teaspoon ground cumin and ¼ teaspoon ground red pepper

Mid-PM Snack

½ serving Homemade Trail Mix (page 199) *or* 2 tablespoons hummus with 4 whole grain crackers (see Food Shopping Guide, page 403, for recommendations)

Dinner

1 serving Grilled Trout with Scallion and Dill Sauce (page 386)

1 small baked sweet potato topped with ¼ teaspoon ground cinnamon

1 corn on the cob with 1 teaspoon grass-fed butter

Dessert/PM Snack

1 cup air-popped popcorn tossed with 1 teaspoon grass-fed butter or melted coconut oil

DAY 13

Breakfast

Coffee (black or with 1 tablespoon plant-based or organic regular milk) or green tea

1 serving Southwestern Omelet (page 340)

1 slice whole grain toast with 1 teaspoon grass-fed butter

Mid-AM Snack

1 serving Very Berry Smoothie (page 337)

Lunch

1 serving Beans in Tomato-Basil Sauce (page 394) over ½ cup cooked brown or wild rice

Mid-PM Snack

½ cup cooked edamame sprinkled with coarse sea salt and ground black pepper

Dinner

1 serving Turkey Meat Loaf (page 374)

1 small baked sweet potato drizzled with 1 teaspoon coconut oil and sprinkled with ¼ teaspoon each salt and ground black pepper

1 cup cooked green beans

Dessert/PM Snack

1 serving Cinnamon-Chocolate Ice Pops (page 399)

DAY 14

Breakfast

Coffee (black or with 1 tablespoon plant-based or organic regular milk) or green tea

1 serving (2 pancakes) Blueberry Oat Pancakes (page 199)

Mid-AM Snack

1 small apple with 1 tablespoon nut butter of your choice

Lunch

1 serving Asparagus and Barley Salad (page 362)

Mid-PM Snack

1 brown rice cake with ¼ cup low-fat cottage cheese

Dinner

1 serving Roasted Salmon, Carrots, and Leeks with Penne (page 384)

Sautéed Baby Spinach with Garlic: Sauté 2 cloves garlic, minced, in 1 teaspoon extra virgin olive oil for 2 minutes, or until golden. Add 2 teaspoons extra virgin olive oil and 1 package (5 ounches) prewashed spinach, ¼ teaspoon salt, and pepper to taste. Cook, tossing, until the spinach is wilted. Makes 1 serving.

Dessert/PM Snack

1 serving Double Chocolate Pudding (page 402)

MOVE

Warm Things Up

Last week, you began your days with the energy-revving Sunrise Stretch. This week is about getting into the habit of warming up before your workout to prepare your body for activity.

When you head out for your cardio session, stop at a grassy spot (or near the treadmill at the gym) to do the Dynamic Warmup. These four moves, which will take just 5 to 10 minutes, will prep cold muscles and increase your range of motion and flexibility during your workout. See page 291 for step-by-step images and how-to instructions—and for an at-a-glance chart of your weekly exercise schedule.

Start Your Cardio

This week, you'll also start to do some cardio, but you're going to ease into it. (If you already do regular cardio workouts, just continue with your current routine.) The goal this week is to get up off the couch or away from your desk 2 or 3 days and simply move. You can walk, bike, dance, or use cardio equipment—any activity you'd like. Just do it for 10 to 20 minutes at a moderate intensity, or a 4 or 5 out of 10 on a Rate of Perceived Exertion (RPE) scale (see page 71), meaning you should still be able to carry on a conversation as you exercise. Perform the Dynamic Warmup first, and then finish by slowing your pace for 3 to 5 minutes to cool down.

Keep Moving to Combat Cravings

During the day, don't forget to stand up often if you're parked in front of a computer or TV; you could also get up and walk down the hall to talk to a colleague or family member rather than e-mailing or texting. Frequent movement is not only great for overall health and circulation but also short-circuits cravings. In one study, when active people viewed photos of junk food, the regions of the brain associated with appetite were quieter when compared to those of less active people. That may be because exercise increases sensitivity to leptin, the hormone that regulates appetite.

So if a sugar craving pops up this week, don't cave in! Instead, get up from your desk or the couch and head outside for a brisk spin around the block (or walk inside if you can't get out). "Exercise has become the most effective therapy for me—better than sweets or snacks," says panelist Lisa Boland.

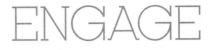

ENGAGE

There's been a lot of change in your life—new foods, more cooking, a new skin-care routine, maybe even a return to exercise. With so much in flux, it's a great time to ground yourself and start a meditation practice. This daily oasis of calm will help quiet your mind and body so you can seek your *duende* and reflect on your vision of how you want your future to unfold.

Calm Your Body, Clear Your Mind

Look back at page 101 in the ENGAGE chapter to review the basic 10-minute mindfulness meditation. Find a quiet, comfortable space with no distractions. There's no need to sit cross-legged with your palms to the sky; sitting on a comfy chair or couch with your hands in your lap will do fine.

Every day this week—and, we hope, during the coming 7 weeks, if not beyond—find 10 minutes to devote to this practice. Not only will you empty your mind and prime your body's relaxation response, but you'll also claim just a little bit more space for yourself. Are you balking at the words *every day*? Try it and see how good it feels. An ideal time to meditate is right after you set your morning intention, when your mind is already focused. Or if that won't fly, find a window during your day that works better (after lunch, say, or just before bedtime).

If you want to go beyond this basic mindfulness exercise, the trio of meditations below, tailored to specific types of stress, can trigger the relaxation response in just 10 minutes.

If you're feeling overwhelmed . . . Stand and feel your feet on the ground, with an even distribution of weight between them. With your eyes open, begin walking at a normal pace. Slow down and notice the sensation of your legs moving up and down. Your mind will wander, but that's okay. When it does, bring it back to those sensations. This will help ground your energy, take your mind off your distractions, and help you feel balanced again.

If you're feeling scattered and unable to focus . . . Sit in a comfortable place, breathe naturally, and settle your attention on your breath. With each inhale and exhale, mentally repeat the words "in" and "out." If your mind wanders, don't worry. Just let go, without judgment of whatever is taking you away from the breath, and bring your attention back to it.

If you're feeling adrift, unsure of what comes next . . . Sit in a comfortable position. Settle your breath, close your eyes, and, as you breathe, mentally repeat the words "I am." Whenever your attention drifts away from the words to other thoughts (which is natural), gently restate "I am." After 5 (or several) minutes, stop repeating and start asking yourself, "What do I want?" Don't feel like you have to answer it—just ask. Repeat the question two to four times, and see what bubbles to the surface. When you take the time to settle down and listen to what your body, mind, and soul are telling you, answers begin to take shape.

GLOW

This week, you should have a handle on the skin-care routine. Your complexion is probably feeling a bit softer and more supple, though you'll score a more visible payoff by Week 3 or 4, as the retinoid cream sloughs away dead skin cells. Meanwhile, the antioxidant serum is quietly battling the aging effects of free-radical damage, while your daily sunscreen is shielding your skin from damaging UV light. And all this in only 10 minutes a day. Feeling some topical sensitivity? The following section is for you.

Pay Attention to Sensitive Skin

If you tend to experience redness, itching, stinging, or burning in response to certain products, you probably have sensitive skin, says Dr. Graf. Ditto if you have a skin condition like acne or rosacea (a medical condition that should be diagnosed by a dermatologist) or sensitivity when you come into contact with certain materials or chemicals. Skin can also become sensitive if you've been overdrying it with harsh cleansers, using too many antiaging products, or exfoliating too zealously.

The products that Dr. Graf selected are all gentle formulations and should be fine for most sensitive skins. But if you're still having issues, visit your dermatologist to see if you might have an allergy. And in general, keep these sensitive-skin guidelines in mind.

- Choose products specifically created and labeled for sensitive skin. Products that say "anti-redness" should be well tolerated, too. (Dr. Graf recommends the Avène line of products for sensitive skin.)

- If your sensitive skin sometimes becomes dry or oily or breaks out, choose a cleanser formulated for sensitive skin that also addresses your other need (acne, oiliness, dryness, and so forth). Look for words such as "nonirritating," "soothing," and "anti-irritating" on the packaging.

- Look for fragrance-free products. "The number-one ingredient that sensitive skin reacts to is fragrance," says Dr. Graf. Don't be misled by "unscented" products (as opposed to fragrance-free). "Unscented products contain masking fragrances because some of the ingredients they contain, like yeast or soy, smell terrible."

Make a Plan for Lusher, Healthier Hair

Although you may be eager to go ahead and get your hair cut and colored (nothing shaves off years like a totally great cut), this week you're going to give your current crop a little love. (Not to worry, your big salon makeover awaits in Week 8!) We tend to shower and shampoo daily without giving our hair's happiness any thought. Review the complete healthy hair advice from Eva Scrivo in the GLOW chapter on page 126 to save yourself from your next bad hair day.

Splurge!

Treat Yourself to a Spa Facial

You're busy getting your new skin-care regimen off the ground, but nothing will jumpstart the skin-renewal process like a spa facial. This youth booster is also a restorative treatment—and good for your overall well-being. A professional facial should always be done by a licensed esthetician (or facialist) with special training in skin care. While every spa has its own techniques, here are the steps that newbies can expect from the experience.

Renew Right Now

INSTANT GLOW

PAMPER NEGLECTED PARTS. It's often your neck, chest, and hands—areas generally neglected when it comes to skin care—that give away your age. With so much focus on facial rejuvenation, women frequently look like 40 above the jawline and 60 below it. For the long run, whatever you slather on your face, put it on your neck, chest, and hands, too, including a retinol night cream, moisturizer, and sunscreen with an SPF of at least 15.

SLIMMER IN A MINUTE

WEAR FITTED STYLES, NOT BOXY. Stick to clothes that are fitted and create shape, such as pencil skirts, A-line shift dresses, and wrap dresses. Designs cut on the bias are slimming to your shape, as well as high-waisted or empire-cut dresses, which make your legs look longer, Scrivo says. Stay away from clothes that are too baggy, like loose sweatshirts. Similarly, avoid clothing that's too tight, which can showcase arm flab, back fat, or muffin tops. Opt for T-shirts one size larger (no more) or A-shape tops and tunics. And remember: Leggings are not pants!

- You'll be "interviewed" about your diet, how much water you drink, the medications and supplements you take, the skin products you use, and your personal concerns about your skin. Give honest answers for more targeted treatments.

- Typically, your hair will be wrapped to get it out of the way while your face is cleansed with pads, wipes, or sponges.

- Your skin will be examined under bright light to assess your skin type and its condition. The facialist will then recommend certain treatments, which you can accept or decline.

- If you have blackheads or whiteheads, your skin may be steamed to soften them for extraction. (If you have sensitive skin, your facialist may skip this step.)

- Your skin may also be exfoliated to slough off dead cells on the surface. Mechanical exfoliants rub off skin cells, while chemical exfoliants, including peels, remove them with enzymes or acids. The solutions that spas use are stronger than what you can find in an over-the-counter product, says Scrivo, and steam makes them even stronger. So if you use topical (applied to the skin) prescription medications on your face, skip them for a week before you get your facial, she says. And don't get a peel at all if you take an oral medication for acne.

- At this point, blackheads or whiteheads may be extracted by hand. It's important to know that improperly done extractions can cause broken capillaries and discoloration. However, this technique may be the only way to get rid of blackheads, Scrivo says. If you choose to have this service, make sure you're at a reputable salon and that your facialist has expertise in this technique.

- A mask targeted to your skin type and condition may be applied. As you relax, you may even be treated to a face, neck, or shoulder massage.

A facial usually starts around $80 at a day spa, but expect a higher price tag at hotel spas, resorts, or major metropolitan areas. Scrivo recommends a professional facial once a month, or at the very least, four times a year, at the end of each season. At summer's end, a facial can remove the buildup of sunblock that can obstruct the pores and cause breakouts. And after a cold, windy winter, a facial can help to replace lost moisture or calm redness or inflammation. Besides, it's more time that you should feel good—not guilty—about setting aside just for you. "Having a skilled professional take care of your skin is not a mere luxury," Scrivo says.

LOOK AT ME   Annie Pearson, 41

- Cut total cholesterol **21 points, lowering it to a healthy level**
- Lost **2 inches from her waistline and hips**
- Better able to focus on the positive
- Smoother skin and fewer lines
- Weight lost: **9 pounds**
- Inches lost: **4.5**

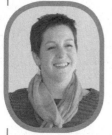

MY STORY: The first few days after starting the Younger in 8 Weeks program—giving up sugar and alcohol—were hard. While Annie's husband munched on potato chips and drank beer, she enjoyed the Fruit Medley with Mint. When he finally asked her where she was getting the willpower, she replied, "I am just so ready for change."

Setting a daily intention also helped. "Taking a couple of minutes each day to think about my own personal goals helps to keep me focused and reminds me why I'm doing this," she said. Sunday intention: I will learn and work the plan as best as I can and not get overwhelmed with all the changes. Monday intention: I will not eat the candy at work! Tuesday intention: I will focus on the things I can control and not obsess over what I can't control.

Each day got easier. "It was no longer about willpower. It was about appreciating the ways I was feeling better and wanting to improve on that," she said. Eating whole foods, fruits, and veggies throughout the day kept Annie satisfied. Cutting out sugar curbed her cravings and the highs and lows she used to experience throughout the day. She also noticed that the belly bloat and tummy troubles she had come to accept as normal were gone.

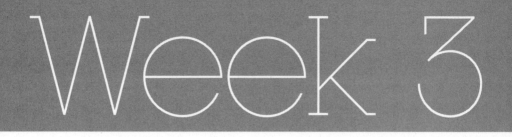

Week 3

"One thing I've noticed is how much less mindless eating I'm doing. I used to just grab things here and there and stuff them in my mouth: crackers, pretzels, kids' leftovers, little tastes while cooking. Now I'm eating my scheduled meals and snacks, and I'm very aware of all the opportunities for snacking that I'm resisting."

— PANELIST KATE PELHAM-HAMBLY

STAY-YOUNG STEPS	GOALS	TO-DO LIST
EAT	Start crafting your own Clean & Green meals. Bonus: Have dinner out!	Use the Meal Builder and incorporate whatever healthy foods you love. Choose a restaurant where you can stay on-plan.
MOVE	Up your cardio game.	Add another day or two of cardio (for a total of 3 to 5) while introducing interval training. Start doing the flexibility stretches to cool down after interval training. *Optional:* Try foam rolling, especially if you have chronic pain points or get achy after working out.
ENGAGE	Connect with others.	Continue with your daily intention and meditation practices. Pick at least one person or group to meet up or mingle with.
GLOW	Continue your skin-care routine. Give yourself a makeover.	Reread "Change Your Makeup" on page 136 of the GLOW chapter to adapt Eva Scrivo's beauty advice to your coloring and skin type. *Optional*: Test-drive an evening look.

Be Prepared!

• This week you're the master chef as you "graduate" to the Meal Builder. Select your meals for the coming week, shop for the food you need, and schedule a Batch Day.

- Make a dinner reservation (or other meal). You've earned it!

- Invest in a foam roller or borrow one from a friend (see page 300 for how to choose one).

- Make sure you have read the GLOW chapter and have purchased the 10 basic beauty products.

- If you chose to test your blood sugar and cholesterol in Week 1, schedule a retest for the end of next week. You'll need those numbers soon.

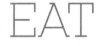

Using the Meal Builder on page 173, you'll design lots of delicious meals that automatically meet our plan's parameters. For ingredients, inspiration, and portion sizes, also review the How to Eat Clean & Green chapter (page 157) and the Food Shopping Guide (page 403).

Dine Out, Lose Weight: Six Strategies to Stay On-Plan

At this point, your soul is probably crying out for a meal prepared and served by anyone but you. On this program, you can eat at your favorite places and attend events or holiday dinners without stressing or starving. Because you won't eat less—you'll eat *smart*. For your restaurant outing this week, use the following strategies.

Know before you go. Most restaurants feature their menus—and often even the calorie counts of sides and entrées—online. If you know which restaurant you'll be dining at, log on and review the menu. Decide what you'll order—say, the broiled fish with stir-fried greens, or the taco salad with grilled chicken, greens, and picante sauce (hold the deep-fried bowl), and stick to your decision once you get to the restaurant.

Order first. That way, you won't be tempted—or derailed—when someone else at the table orders a decadent appetizer or entrée. If you can't order first, choose your healthy meal, close your menu, and hold it in your mind so you can tell your server.

Have it your way. These days, it's totally fine to make special requests when you dine out, even at a chain. So when you place your order, don't be afraid to ask your server to hold the butter, salt, sauce, or gravy; leave the cheese and bacon bits off your salad; put the dressing on the side; or add another order of veggies instead of fries. When asked politely, most restaurants fulfill special requests if they can—and usually, they can.

Eat Clean (Almost) Anywhere

YOUR FAVORITE FARM-TO-TABLE RESTAURANT WOULD BE the perfect place to treat yourself to a healthy, plant-based meal this week. But you can easily stay on plan at any number of chain restaurants, which may be a lot more affordable or suitable if the whole family is tagging along. We cruised these restaurants' Web sites for healthy menus and crunched the numbers, just like you can.

RUBY TUESDAY

Petit Sirloin, grilled zucchini, and baked potato (no toppings) with salt and pepper

PER SERVING: 553 calories, 39 g protein, 57 g carbohydrates, 8 g fiber, N/A g total sugar, N/A g added sugar, 19 g fat, N/A g saturated fat, 863 mg sodium

RED LOBSTER

Broiled Flounder Dinner with fresh broccoli and garden salad with Blueberry Balsamic Vinaigrette

PER SERVING: 620 calories, 78 g protein, 40 g carbohydrates, 9 g fiber, 18 g total sugar, 15 g fat, 1 g saturated fat, 1,110 mg sodium

BOSTON MARKET

Rotisserie Chicken (quarter white, skinless) with fresh steamed vegetables and garlic dill new potatoes

PER SERVING: 390 calories, 48 g protein, 30 g carbohydrates, 5 g fiber, 4 g total sugar, 17 g fat, 4.5 g saturated fat, 790 mg sodium

Be veggie-conscious. Veggies are excellent—so long as they're not drenched in low-quality, inflammation-stoking vegetable oils. Request for them to be sautéed in olive oil (again, don't worry about sounding like a nudge); most restaurants have it.

Wine is fine. Just stick to one glass, and request that it be served with your entrée. If you delay alcohol until dinner comes, you're more likely to keep your mitts out of the bread basket or off the mozzarella sticks. If you'd rather have beer or a cocktail, stick to one and sip it with your entrée.

Follow the two-bite rule of dessert. If you can, satisfy your sweet tooth with fresh berries. If you're angling for the cheesecake, split it with a companion and stick to two bites, which should hit the sweet spot.

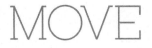

As you prepare to step up the pace, take a moment to congratulate yourself for carving out time to exercise—that's something to be proud of. Then mentally review your daily routine. Can your current workout schedule accommodate an extra session?

If not, tweak it, choosing a time of day you know you can stick with. Whether that's morning, noontime, or early evening, the right fit helps ensure that exercise becomes a regular part of your life. You'll never have to "find time" to exercise because your workouts will be built into your schedule. Now get ready for this week's workout.

Add Cardio Intervals

This week, you'll increase your cardio sessions to 20 to 30 minutes, 3 to 5 days a week. Plus, you'll add heart-pumping intervals—short bursts of higher-intensity aerobic exercise alternated with short recovery periods of lower-intensity activity. As you've read, intervals provide a greater aerobic benefit than going low and slow. Not only will you burn more calories while you exercise, but you'll also boost your metabolism for up to 24 hours after completing a session.

But this isn't just about running faster: You can do intervals with any type of cardio exercise, such as walking, using the elliptical, biking, or swimming.

These interval workouts are separated into Level 1 (beginner) through Level 3 (advanced) options; choose an intensity that feels right to you.

Unless you already do cardio regularly, you should start with Level 1. After 2 weeks (if you feel up to it), move to Level 2. If you're ready to move to the advanced option anytime after Week 4, go for it. You can find all three levels of the cardio interval workouts in the Younger in 8 Weeks Workout chapter, starting on page 297.

Follow with Flexibility Stretches

It's also important to stretch out your muscles *after* you use them. The flexibility stretches, which you'll do after your cardio workout is over, are designed to help your muscles and tendons retain their elasticity and to increase range of motion. The five moves in this short-and-sweet routine on page 298 will cool down your whole body. Don't skip them! Besides, they feel pretty amazing.

Try Foam Rolling

Foam rolling involves rolling tight, tender areas of your body across a log of dense foam. Similar to a deep-tissue massage, this combination of stretching and massage breaks up fibrous tissue and boosts circulation so you're less sore. You can roll targeted areas that are prone to pain (say, calves or IT band) before exercising to reduce muscle fatigue and soreness dramatically enough that workouts feel easier. Or do it after workouts, as part of your cooldown, to reduce postexercise discomfort. You can also just roll out your whole body a couple times a week to keep aches and pains at bay. See page 300 for our seven-move foam-roller routine.

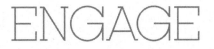
ENGAGE

You've taken great care of yourself for a couple of weeks now—and hopefully, that attention has brought a mounting sense of optimism and well-being. This week, it's time to share that little flicker of light with the world or someone close to you.

Connect with Others

If you haven't yet tried a strategy that engages you with other people or a community or cause you care deeply about, pick a simple one from the suggestions in the ENGAGE chapter on page 84 and execute it this week. Research shows that connecting with others boosts everything from mood to immunity (introverts can keep it one-on-one, if that's your happy place).

Or come up with your own plan. Arrange a Saturday or Sunday night dinner where friends and family prepare a healthy meal together. Call your college roommate. Strike up a conversation with that confident and fun-seeming woman at the dog park. Attend a city or town council meeting to see what's going on beyond your backyard. Join a book group or documentary film club. Or go to the park, tuck your turned-off cell phone in your purse, and greet the parade of humanity passing by your bench.

After the experience, find a quiet moment to reflect on the feelings that it brought up in you. (Use your journal, or just note these feelings to yourself.)

- Were you mentally or physically energized? Did you leave feeling inspired or with a big new idea?

- Were you living more "in the moment"? (While schedules keep us sane and on track, it's good to occasionally lose track of time and enjoy the now.)

- Did the experience prompt feelings of gratitude? (When you appreciate the blessings in your life, you're more likely to give what you have—time, attention, a listening ear—to others. That generosity of spirit can spark meaningful connections.)

GLOW

You're doing great—sticking to the eating plan, making every cardio workout, riding a wave of self-confidence and well-being. And if you've followed Dr. Jeannette Graf's skin-care plan faithfully (especially if you went for that Week 2 facial), you also may be noticing a brighter, more luminous complexion. To accentuate that emerging glow, dip into Eva Scrivo's makeup tips this week.

Makeover Your Makeup

If you tend to go au naturel or wear minimal makeup, you should approach this week with an open mind and a spirit of playful experimentation—a little bit of lipstick or mascara can go a long way. Or if you've been working certain colors or habits since the last millennium, it's time to take a clean-slate approach (and see page 217 for Scrivo's advice on the correct way to remove makeup).

You probably have some of the 10 basic beauty products that Scrivo recommends for daily wear in your makeup bag. These include (in the order of application):

1. Primer
2. Foundation
3. Concealer
4. Powder
5. Eyebrow pencil or powder
6. Eye shadow
7. Eyeliner
8. Mascara
9. Lip color
10. Blush

If you don't own them all, review the color and formulation guidelines beginning on page 138 of the GLOW chapter and then hit the drugstore or department store makeup counter (maybe with a friend in tow). Whether your change will be subtle or sweeping, refreshing your makeup is another step toward the glowier, more youthful self that's beginning to emerge.

Follow Scrivo's steps for application (also in the GLOW chapter, beginning on page 138) at the time you normally put on your makeup. And make sure that you start with clean, moist skin and that you're working in bright, balanced lighting (wall sconces or natural light as opposed to overhead lighting) on both sides of your face.

Day vs. Evening Makeup

The tips in the GLOW chapter focus on daytime makeup. But since this week you'll be splurging on a dinner out, it's the perfect chance to test-drive an evening look, which tends to be darker and bolder. You can even build off your daytime base; just mist with a bit of toner, add new concealer, and dab foundation on spots that might need it. Here are the major differences between your day and night looks.

Day Look: Less Coverage, Subtle Color

For daytime color options keyed to hair and skin tone, see "Change Your Makeup" on page 136.

- **Foundation, concealer, and powder** should be minimal. You want a bit of your skin tone and texture—even a bit of dewiness—to shine through.

- **Blush** should be softer and well blended.

- **Lip color** should be natural—sheer formulations in lighter tones.

- **Eyeliner** should be subtle and blended. Save heavier application for the evening.

- **Brows** should be more natural; use just a touch of pencil or powder, if needed.

- **Mascara** should be applied with a lighter touch; use an eyelash comb to get rid of any clumps.

Night Look: More Coverage, Bolder Color

- **Foundation, concealer, and powder** should provide more coverage. For evening, the goal is a flawless finish.

- **Blush** should be bolder. Deeper colors offer more drama.

- **Lip color** should be bolder, too. Opt for satin or matte formulations and richer colors, such as plums and deep reds for brunettes, darker rose and blue-based reds for blondes, and metallic copper and orange-based reds for redheads.

- **Eyeliner** needs to be heavier, so it's visible in low or diffused lighting. For a more glamorous look, line eyes in black or black/brown.

- **Brows** need a sharper line so they're more defined and "done."

Renew Right Now

- **Mascara** should be darker—black or brown/black. Apply two or three coats to build up fullness.

Remove Your Makeup to Wake Up to More Radiant Skin

We all have slept in our makeup at one time or another. But spending the occasional night in your favorite foundation or mascara is harmless enough provided it isn't happening on the regular—right? Wrong.

Skin, like the rest of the body, functions on circadian rhythms. At night, the skin's most important function is to renew itself. "Wearing makeup and foundation at night prevents the renewal process, causing damage to the skin," says Dr. Graf.

Foundation breaks down during the day, and its by-products can cause collagen damage—and ultimately wrinkles, clogged pores, and acne. Meanwhile, mascara particles can clog and irritate eyelash follicles, says Dr. Graf. The resulting irritation can cause blepharitis (inflammation of the eyelids) and lead to conjunctivitis. Snoozing in your mascara can also cause eyelashes to become brittle and break.

Whether you wear a full face of makeup or just mascara, liner, and blush, Scrivo recommends removing your makeup before you cleanse. "If you're breaking out or your skin looks dull, removing your makeup can help reduce breakouts and brighten your complexion," she says. Here's how to do it.

1. **Remove eye makeup first.** Use a cosmetic wipe made for this purpose or mineral oil applied to a cotton pad dampened with warm water and then squeezed out. (Don't use toilet paper or tissue, says Scrivo. They're made with wood fibers, which are rough on delicate skin around the eyes.) Settle the wipe or pad on your lashes to soften and dissolve mascara and other eye makeup. Wipe gently—no pulling or tugging.

2. **Apply a makeup remover to your entire face, eyes included.** Massage gently to emulsify the makeup, and then remove with cotton pads. Don't skip this step; all cosmetics contain oil that needs to be emulsified first, as oil and water don't mix.

Having properly removed your makeup, you are now ready to cleanse—and to get your beauty rest (literally) so you can put your best face forward each day.

Week 4

"What I'm proudest of so far? Exercising consistently and being able to stop and think before grabbing junk food to soothe myself. Several times, I chose to walk rather than eat as a way to cool off when I was angry."

— PANELIST SHERRY JUBOOR

STAY-YOUNG STEPS	GOALS	TO-DO LIST
EAT	Keep playing around with Clean & Green menu ideas.	Mix in foods outside your comfort zone. *Optional:* Reintroduce treat-size amounts of added sugar.
MOVE	Add muscle to your exercise routine.	Review the moves you'll use in the strength-training routine so they'll be familiar when you begin. *Optional:* Update your playlist to boost motivation.
ENGAGE	Reflect on and celebrate your inner changes.	Practice your daily intention and meditation sessions. Try a challenging ENGAGE activity. At the end of the week, complete the Personal Check-In.
GLOW	Continue your skin-care routine. Use beauty tricks to put your best face forward.	Consider features that need polishing or highlighting. Streamline your beauty space; toss old (and bacteria-packed) cosmetics and skin-care products. *Splurge!* Celebrate your midpoint with a massage.

Be Prepared!

- Choose your favorite meals from the menu plans for Weeks 1 and 2, and use the Meal Builder to design a week of meals. Make a list, shop for the food you need, and schedule a Batch Day.

- Buy a set of resistance bands for the strength routine. Sets of bands (with or without handles) are widely available at sporting-goods stores and online for less than $20.

- One night this week, set aside time to take the Midpoint Self-Assessment (page 230) and "How Old Are You Today?" quiz (page 20). Then settle in a quiet place with a cup of tea and do the Personal Check-In (page 230) to identify the biggest challenges and changes of the past 4 weeks and take stock of whether your vision for your life is coming into focus, in ways small or large.

- Book a massage for the end of the week. You deserve it!

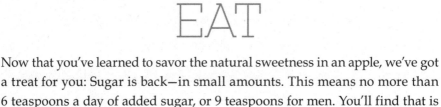

EAT

Now that you've learned to savor the natural sweetness in an apple, we've got a treat for you: Sugar is back—in small amounts. This means no more than 6 teaspoons a day of added sugar, or 9 teaspoons for men. You'll find that is more than enough.

Still struggling to commit the Meal Builder to memory? For details, portion sizes, and meal ideas, see the How to Eat Clean & Green chapter (page 157), the Food Shopping Guide (page 403), and the recipe section (page 333).

Try Something New

In the spirit of experimentation, keep pushing yourself to expand your palate. This week, add a couple of new, healthy foods to your menu. Here are four to consider.

- **Asparagus.** This tasty splurge contains inulin, a type of soluble fiber that works as a prebiotic to promote digestion and good gut bacteria.

- **Edamame.** A Japanese staple, these immature soybeans, harvested while still green and in their pods, are an excellent source of veggie protein. Buy them fresh or frozen.

- **Wheat berries.** This is a delightful name for kernels of whole wheat, and you can enjoy them in veggie-based salads or as a hot-and-hearty breakfast.

- **Steel-cut oats.** More nutritious than highly processed rolled oats, the steel-cut variety digests more slowly, so you feel fuller, longer. Cook them overnight, so you can spoon them up first thing in the morning.

Frozen Meals You Can Feel Good About

IF YOU DON'T HAVE TIME to batch cook one week, go to Plan B: frozen meals that are honestly good for you. These four impressed us for their taste, nutrition, and lack of additives—all are low in added sugars and contain fewer than 450 calories.

EVOL SHREDDED CHICKEN AND CARAMELIZED ONION STREET TACOS. This is microwaveable Mexican done right. Spicy antibiotic-free chicken, roasted tomatoes and corn, and caramelized onions are all combined in a naturally gluten-free corn tortilla (evolfoods.com).

PER SERVING: 230 calories, 17 g protein, 26 g carbohydrates, 2 g fiber, 3 g sugar, 5 g fat, 2.5 g saturated fat, 320 mg sodium

LUVO ORGANIC APPLE COCONUT CURRY BURRITO. This sweet and savory burrito will keep you full for hours thanks to hearty, fiber- and protein-packed lentils. Bonus: It's organic and totally vegan-friendly (luvoinc.com).

PER SERVING: 290 calories, 11 g protein, 47 g carbohydrates, 8 g fiber, 6 g sugar, 7 g fat, 2.5 g saturated fat, 380 mg sodium

AMY'S SINGLE-SERVE LIGHT IN SODIUM SPINACH PIZZA. Pizza minus the guilt—whole wheat crust topped with organic tomato sauce, spinach, feta, and mozzarella that packs a protein punch while ditching pizza's high-sodium reputation (amys.com).

PER SERVING: 440 calories, 19 g protein, 54 g carbohydrates, 3 g fiber, 5 g sugar, 18 g fat, 6 g saturated fat, 390 mg sodium

Bring a Little Sugar Back (If You Want)

As you go back to eating sugar, make sure you keep it measured (literally), rather than losing control. You've gone 3 weeks without the sweet stuff. You're a boss at this!

How you let sugar back into your life is up to you—splurge all at once or ration out a few tiny tastes a day, so long as you don't exceed 24 grams of added sugar or 6 teaspoons. The guidelines below will help you enjoy sugar's return without suffering its worst drawbacks.

Review your sugar math. A teaspoon of sugar is 4 grams and contains 6 calories. So if a ½-cup serving of your favorite premium ice cream contains 24 grams of sugar, you'll know two things: that ½ cup contains

6 teaspoons of sugar and you're at your added-sugar limit for the day.

Read the fine print. Sugar will often show up in foods that don't even taste sweet, like bread, salad dressings, and jarred pasta sauces. When you shop, read a product's nutrition facts label as well as its list of ingredients to suss out the added sugars it contains.

Careful, though. These days, sugar goes by many aliases. To be a good sleuth, get familiar with the list below so you can separate healthy, lower- or no-sugar products from their sneaky, sugar-laden counterparts.

You're Busted, Sugar

MORE OFTEN THAN NOT, IT'S SMART to steer clear of foods that come in bags, boxes, and wrappers. These tend to contain added sugars—not to mention unhealthy fats and loads of salt. If you do decide to buy packaged foods, think twice if one of the words or phrases below appears in a product's first three ingredients. They're all sneaky names for sugar.

Agave nectar	Corn syrup solids	Lactose
Barley malt	Crystalline fructose	Maltose
Beet sugar		Mal syrup
Brown rice syrup	Date sugar	Molasses
Brown sugar	Dextrose	Muscovado sugar
Buttered sugar	Evaporated cane juice	Raw sugar
Cane crystals	Fructose	Rice bran syrup
Cane juice	Fruit juice con-centrates	Rice syrup
Cane sugar		Sorghum
Caramel	Glucose	Sorghum syrup
Carob syrup	High-fructose corn syrup	Sucrose
Castor sugar		Sugar
Coconut sugar	Honey	Syrup
Corn syrup	Invert sugar	Turbinado sugar

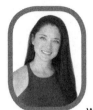

Dr. Vonda Wright says . . .

I KICKED SUGAR FOR GOOD

This week, you have the option to reintroduce small amounts of added sugar to your diet. At this point, I want to share with you the most profound health change I've ever made: I gave up added sugar. Completely. While this may or may not be your choice, I wanted to tell you how this choice has affected me personally.

Not so long ago, I was a sugar and chocoholic. While I always ate healthy meals and snacks, you'd find me with 73 percent dark chocolate in my hand every day at 3 p.m., and at social functions, I ate dessert first (hey, you never know). While I made lots of healthy food choices, this one choice—to sweeten *everything*—predominated.

On December 1, 2013, I stopped adding sugar to my coffee and cereal. I also gave up dessert and began to read food labels to ferret out added sugars.

Two things happened almost immediately. First, I lost the 11 pounds left over from carrying my daughter 8 years ago. Second, my joints felt better. When I got up from the floor after playing with her, I no longer felt achy and old. In fact, I felt like a new woman.

Recently, I let sugar creep back into my diet—wine at dinner, dessert here and there. I cut it out again and *bam*—7 more pounds gone and energy to burn. My joints improved again, too.

I realize that dropping sugar entirely is a struggle for most people. But for me, the choice is no longer a hard one. I'm amazed by the difference in how I feel, and the truth is, I don't even miss it anymore.

Plan your treats. If you know you'll want ice cream every night after dinner, you can have it. Just work it into your food plan. Stick to whole foods for the day and steer clear of the candy dish at work. The pleasure you get from your treat—and the anticipation you'll feel as you look forward to it—will make it easier to avoid other sources of added sugar during the day.

Ditch sugar bombs for just-as-tasty treats. There's no need to blow your whole sugar budget on certain foods when there are lower-sugar alternatives that are just as sweet. To get you started, just search for 22 Smart Sugar Swaps on prevention.com.

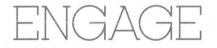

MOVE

Start Your Strength Routine

Ready for more sculpted upper arms, tighter abs, or a more defined waist? This week's a game-changer. You'll be adding a strength routine (page 305) to your cardio workouts. This streamlined sequence, which requires resistance bands (Weeks 4 to 6) and eventually dumbbells (Weeks 7 and 8), takes just 10 to 15 minutes 2 or 3 days a week. The time commitment is small, but the benefits are huge: You'll build muscle—which will shape your body and showcase your weight loss—and improve your overall fitness and health.

You'll ease into the routine, as you did with cardio. This week, you'll begin with simple upper- and lower-body moves using your resistance bands or just your body weight. In later weeks, you'll progress to more challenging variations of the basic moves. This way, you continue to challenge your body but avoid frustration and potential injury.

If you're new to strength training, follow the routines as they appear each week (flip to page 305 for photos and how-tos). This will allow you to progressively master the moves before adding new ones, making the routine manageable and minimizing soreness. You can always repeat a week if you'd like more time to become comfortable with the exercises.

If you currently strength train or have done so in the past year, feel free to introduce each week's exercises more quickly, even doing the full routine (exercises from Weeks 4 to 7) during Week 4. When you need a new challenge, you can switch to the Advanced Workout (page 320), starting as early as Week 6.

ENGAGE

Four weeks into the program, clean-eating and skin-care routines are firmly integrated into your days. Shake things up a bit with a new ENGAGE strategy.

Push Past Your Comfort Zone

This week, try a strategy that you normally wouldn't pick or that you think isn't "you." For example, if you've been focusing on social activities, consider writing in your journal faithfully this week. If most of your connection has been internal, donate a few hours at the local food bank or animal shelter. You don't have to stick with it; just be open to the experience. The idea is to stretch your inner self, just as you stretch your muscles before and after workouts.

This would also be a perfect moment to take a step back and consider whether you're getting any closer to your *duende*. (Remember, that's the term from Spanish folklore that refers to the fire in your soul, or your personal inspiration.) So ask yourself: Are you doing activities that are reinspiring you? Tapping into a vision of your life that you've postponed for too long? If you're dissatisfied at work, is it time to consider what your Second Act could be? Use this week to tackle some of the hard questions on your quest to find your *duende*. Make a list of goals and think about how you can knock them off, one by one. Then, at the end of the week, be sure to take the Personal Check-In at the end of the Midpoint Self-Assessment.

GLOW

At this point in the program, you should definitely be seeing the results of Dr. Jeannette Graf's skin-care regimen in the mirror: Your skin should appear clearer, brighter, and fresher, with visibly smaller pores and fainter fine lines.

Now it's time to level up and focus on individual features that could use extra defining and polishing.

Open Your Eyes

Reduce puffiness. As we age, our eyes tend to recede due to both skin laxity and under-eye puffiness. If the skin around your eyes tends to marshmallow in the morning or after you've eaten certain foods, try the following:

- Review the Week 1 bloat-busting Jumpstart menu to be sure you're avoiding or reducing the bad boys of face puffery, like salt, caffeine, and acidic fruit juices.

- If you've been holding out on switching to an eye cream, start using one. Regular moisturizer, which typically contains water, can puff up the eye area, says Dr. Graf. There are also eye creams that target this problem, containing ingredients like *Asparagopsis armata* marine extract and *Spilanthes acmella* flower extract, which lighten dark circles, tighten skin, and depuff. Products containing caffeine are also effective.

- If the swelling persists and you need to quickly flatten the eye area, try this low-tech trick: tea. The black variety is packed with compounds called tannins, which help deflate and tighten under-eye pouches. Boil a pot of water, add two tea bags, and steep them for 3 minutes to activate their tannins. Let them cool, given them a quick squeeze, and lie down with the damp bags over your eyes for 10 minutes.

Brighten your whites. Try Eva Scrivo's technique for making your eyes appear larger and the whites brighter: Line your inner lash line with a peach or pale blue eye pencil. This is a great addition to a smoky eye to prevent your makeup from looking too dark and appearing to "close in" your eyes.

A trick for hooded lids. Try this: "A few individual eyelashes (three or four) applied to the center of the upper lid helps to open eyes that have narrowed from sagging lids," advises Scrivo.

Smooth Out Upper Lip Lines

Decades of unconsciously pursing your lips (or worse, smoking) can lead to those characteristic vertical wrinkles—called whistle lines—on the skin above your lips. If this is a problem for you, look for lip treatments with peptides, collagen, or retinol to strengthen and tighten the area.

Scrivo suggests the following to prevent lipstick bleed: (1) Apply a cosmetic lip primer; (2) use lip liner; (3) apply loose powder around the outside perimeter of your lips, which will act as a barrier and help prevent bleeding.

Highlight Your Cheekbones

Because it catches the light, a shimmer product can brighten your skin and act as an instant face-lift, says Scrivo. Apply shimmer right after your blush (see page 146 for blush application how-tos). And make sure to match your highlighter formulation to the finish you've chosen—dewy or matte. Always use shimmer sparingly (a little bit goes a long way).

Dewy finish: Touch one drop of liquid shimmer or an oil-based serum to the top of each cheekbone and blend with your fingertips.

Matte finish: Select a highlighter or shimmer powder—a champagne hue for fair skin or a rose gold or bronze for darker skin. Touch a small, clean brush, free of any other makeup, to the powder. Tap off the excess, and then touch the brush high on the cheekbone, about 1 inch under the eye.

Polish and Perfect Your Brows

Eyebrows are so important: They frame and define the eyes and balance out the face. Still, it's easy to forget them in a beauty routine. Take an appraising look at their shape and color.

"If you look at an old photo of yourself, you may be surprised by how your brows have lost definition or color," Scrivo says. This week, follow her recommendations to bring your brows to polished perfection.

Schedule a professional grooming. At least once. If your brows need to be shaped or colored, these tasks are best left to a salon brow artist, says Scrivo. "It's not just about what the artist plucks. It's what she leaves behind."

But don't just stroll into any salon. As with any skill, becoming proficient with eyebrow shaping takes years of experience. Ask a woman whose brows you like who *she* sees, Scrivo suggests. (Chances are, those brows are the work of a professional.) At the appointment, your brow artist can help you decide the shape and color that flatter your facial structure, hair, color, and skin tone.

Do DIY grooming sessions. Once the brow artist's work is done, you may be able to maintain them yourself. (But always have them professionally dyed, Scrivo says.) Her guidelines:

- Tweeze stray eyebrow hairs as they grow in, but that's it. Your goal is to nab strays, not change the shape.

- Don't tweeze when you're rushed, moody, or have had one too many glasses of wine. "Make sure you feel mentally stable and that you have enough time," says Scrivo.

- If you use a magnifying mirror, step away often to look at your brows in a regular mirror. "A magnifying mirror makes eyebrows look a lot furrier than they actually are," she says.

Plump up your brows. If your brows are skimpier than they used to be, add back youthful definition with makeup (see page 141 for the how-tos). Or consider a brow growth serum. Scrivo recommends the prescription drug

Latisse. While it's only FDA-approved for the growth of hair on eyelashes, it works on brows, too.

Out with the Old

NOW THAT YOU'RE USING THE RIGHT products, you don't need those old bottles, jars, and tubes that may still be taking up space in your medicine cabinet or on your bathroom counter. Toss them!

There's good reason to. First, if they're over a year old, their active ingredients have reached the end of their shelf life; the longer they sit, the less potent they become. Worse, they may contain bacteria from repeated finger-dipping that you don't want on your face or near your eyes. Dispose of them (extra points for recycling the glass and plastic). Now you have more room for the products you know *are* working.

Splurge!

Book a Professional Massage

You made it to the midpoint! Nothing says "I earned this" like a massage from a trained professional—whether it's at a local gym or a salon or a resort. And it's legitimately good for your health, reducing stress hormones and boosting the immune system. Are you a newbie? (If so, you'll quickly become a convert.) Here's what you can expect.

Before you begin, you may be asked about your current and past health, lifestyle, stress levels, and medications and any areas of pain (a bad back, an achy knee, and so forth). Your answers help the massage therapist customize the session to your needs.

What type of massage do you want? The Swedish variety, in which you're gently kneaded with oil, is the most common. Aromatherapy massage uses fragrant plant oils (called essential oils) that can energize, relax, or balance you; in a hot-stone massage, heated, smooth stones are placed on certain parts of the body to warm and loosen tight muscles. If you've been diagnosed with fibromyalgia, consider a shiatsu massage, which incorporates traditional

Chinese medicine's acupressure principles. It can improve the pain and sleep issues associated with this condition, a *Journal of Manipulative and Physiological Therapeutics* study found.

Undress to your level of comfort (your therapist will leave the room), and lie down on the padded table (with a face cradle) beneath the sheet.

Do you want music? If you'd rather melt into a puddle of bliss in silence, ask your therapist to turn it off. And don't feel obligated to make chitchat, either, although your therapist may occasionally "check in" to see if you're comfortable.

Choose your oils or lotions (a therapist usually gives you scent options) to reduce drag on the skin. If you're allergic, tell her beforehand.

A massage typically lasts 30 to 90 minutes. (Remember to breathe normally.) After your massage, you'll be left to bask in the afterglow for a few minutes before you arise and dress in privacy. As real life begins again, smile to yourself: You now know what it's like to feel spoiled. Plan to do it again sometime.

Halfway to Your Younger Self: How's It Going?

It's time to assess your progress. For your convenience, we've copied the before-and-after worksheet from the beginning of the book, on the next page.

If you chose to record your weight, measurements, and resting heart rate only, fill in today's numbers. If you decided to get the optional blood pressure reading and cholesterol and blood-sugar tests, fill in those numbers, too. If you've followed the food and workout plans faithfully, prepare for a fist-pump! By the start of Week 4, our test panelists had lost up to 21 pounds.

No matter what the measuring tape and scale reveal, however, bear in mind that your goal is to "lose" years, not just weight. So retake the "How Old Are You Today?" quiz (which begins on page 20) and compare this score with your original score. Then find some quiet time—preferably with your journal in hand—to review the Personal Check-In prompts. In the past 4 weeks, you've adopted a whole lot of habits scientifically shown to promote health, happiness, and longevity. Your results may show that your turnaround is more dramatic than you'd thought!

Week 4: Midpoint Self-Assessment

MEASURE THIS	MY RESULT	WEEK 1
Weight		
Waist measurement		
Hip measurement		
Waist–hip ratio		
Resting heart rate		
Body-fat percentage (optional)		

Week 4: Your Numbers (Optional)

WHAT TO MEASURE	MY RESULTS	WEEK 1
Total cholesterol		
Triglycerides		
HDL cholesterol		
LDL cholesterol		
Fasting blood glucose		
Blood pressure		

"How Old Are You?" Quiz Results: Week 4

My score 4 weeks ago: _____

Were you aging smart, aging well, or aging fast?_____

My score today: _____

What category did your score place you in today?_____

Personal Check-In

All of our panelists mentioned that as much as they loved the changes in their body measurements and on the scale, they experienced internal changes that were just as gratifying. For Kathy McCarthy, that inner transformation comes down to three words: *I'm worth it.* "I am worth the time it takes to shop, plan, and prepare healthy meals and snacks; to exercise each day; and to care for my skin and hair," she says. "I am absolutely worth it, and everyone around me benefits, too." How about you?

Reflect on the past 4 weeks, and then answer the questions below to see where you've made changes that don't show on the outside but that make you feel years younger on the inside.

1. What is the single biggest positive change you've experienced during your 4 weeks on this program? How does that change make you feel more like your younger self?

_____

_____

_____

_____

2. What is the single biggest challenge you've experienced on the program up to this point? Is it physical or emotional in nature? Brainstorm a few ways you might solve this challenge.

_____

_____

_____

_____

3. Imagine yourself 4 weeks from now, at the end of the program. Describe who you see, inside and out. Does your younger self have a long-term goal for the future? It can involve your body, your health, your job, a dream you've wanted to make real all your life. Name that goal, and then describe the steps you'll take in the next 4 weeks—and beyond—to achieve it.

_____

_____

_____

_____

Now that you've assessed your gains and identified your goals, you're ready for the second half of the program. We'll keep building on your progress to EAT, MOVE, ENGAGE, and GLOW, but we'll also troubleshoot some of the most commonplace complaints of aging. Turn the page to see what's in store!

SUCCESS!

Kathy McCarthy, 57

MY STORY "I was mortified," said Kathy, recalling the day she took her self-assessment and found she was "aging fast." "It was a wake-up call."

Kathy had lost 15 pounds a year earlier on Weight Watchers, but the Younger in 8 Weeks Plan showed her how to adjust her diet and workouts for even greater benefits. While she ate fruits, vegetables, and lean meats, her diet still included fat-free, sugar-free, processed, and nonorganic foods. "I'd check food labels for calories or fat once in a while, but I never looked closely at the ingredients list," she admitted. "Now, I'm appalled at some of the things I used to eat."

Cutting out white flour was Kathy's most difficult food change. "I love pasta, and pretzels have always been my go-to snack," she said. She started experimenting with alternatives, such as soba noodles, whole wheat pasta, and edamame and other bean pastas. "One night, I mixed edamame spaghetti with a little olive oil, fresh basil, and roasted tomatoes from the garden—delish! It felt like I was indulging in something I should not have been eating." And now she snacks on crunchy foods like nuts or carrots and hummus so she doesn't miss the pretzels.

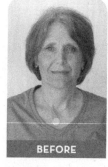

BEFORE

Her exercise plan wasn't up to par either. "I thought my leisurely neighborhood walks or sporadic treadmill visits to the gym qualified as 'getting enough exercise,'" she said.

The fact that she needed to put more effort into exercising became apparent when she started the Younger in 8 Weeks Workout: "Even the early-morning stretches were difficult for me, in particular, the Cobra! My body shook each time I did it." As she became stronger, soon she was holding Cobra and planks for up to 60 seconds. She was also noticing definition in her arms. Feeling confident, she wore a tank top, instead of her usual short-sleeve shirt, out one night. "Two friends separately came up to me to tell me how good I looked," she said.

Kathy saw progress in her cardio workouts, too. "I never exerted myself, and I avoided sweat at all costs," she said. Now she's doubled the length of her cardio workouts to 30 minutes and pushes herself with intervals. "I learned that sweating isn't so bad, and I feel great afterward. If I don't work out one day, I feel off, like something is missing. That's a far cry from the old me!" As a result, the new Kathy is in the "aging smart" category.

LOOK AT ME

- Lowered total cholesterol **27 points**

- Shrank waist and hips by **3¼ inches each**

- Less foot and knee pain

- No more break-outs or bloating

- Weight lost: **7.2 pounds**

- Inches lost: **8.5**

KEEP SNACKS ON HAND. I keep a stash of 100-calorie nut packs, roasted chickpeas, and crackers in my car glove compartment at all times. The worst thing is to be stuck someplace, hungry with no healthy food choices.

Beauty styling: Eva Scrivo; Wardrobe styling: Erin Turon

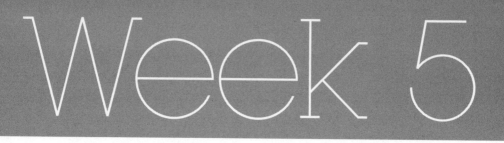
Week 5

"I no longer feel guilty for taking the time to take care of me."
— PANELIST LISA BOLAND

On to the Second Half!

Did you do your midpoint happy dance? By now, you've mastered a plant-based diet. You're feeling stronger and more energetic from your workouts. You've started to find inner peace and outward connections, and your skin-care routine has actually become, well, pretty routine. In other words, *you got this.*

In the second half of the program, you'll continue your baseline plans to EAT, MOVE, ENGAGE, and GLOW. You'll also have a chance to identify and troubleshoot age-related issues that affect your well-being, from hot flashes to hearing loss. Pick the strategies that apply to you now; you'll have the others if you need them in the future.

STAY-YOUNG STEPS	GOALS	TO-DO LIST
EAT	Continue to follow the Clean & Green guidelines.	Keep plugging new foods into your Meal Builder and mastering your weekly Batch Day.
MOVE	Commit to your workout schedule.	Add two new moves to Week 4's strength routine (see page 310 of the Younger in 8 Weeks Workout). Move up a level of intensity in your cardio intervals, if you feel ready.
ENGAGE	Keep finding ways to connect with others and more deeply engage with yourself.	Set your daily intention and make time for meditation. Select and try another new ENGAGE guideline.
GLOW	Continue your skin-care routine.	Reverse hair loss if it's an issue for you.

Keep Up Your Sleep

ARE YOU CONTINUING TO GET THE recommended 7 to 8 hours of sleep per night? Staying on plan is easier when you're well rested. You'll make smart food choices, have the energy to exercise, and sail through stresses and irritations that might derail you if you're sleep-deprived. The most important sleep-hygiene measure: Get up and turn in at the same times, 7 days a week. For a refresher on good sleep practices, flip back to Week 1.

Week 5 Troubleshooting Plan

- Relieve Pain without Meds
- Boost Energy Naturally
- Improve Your Balance
- Reverse Hair Loss

Relieve Pain without Meds

A "no pain, no gain" attitude might have worked for you at 25, but today it can totally backfire. Exercising with a back spasm or tweaked knee will worsen the agony—maybe even causing permanent harm. You'll also get diminishing returns from your workout.

"Now is the time to listen to your body," Dr. Vonda Wright says. "But that doesn't mean sitting still and 'resting' for weeks." If you have a nagging pain that resurfaces when you exercise, see your doctor to be sure it's nothing serious. Then keep moving in any way you can without aggravating the area. "I always tell my patients that even if they have a bum shoulder, they still have a strong core and two good legs to keep moving while the shoulder mends," she says.

If certain parts of your exercise program are causing you pain, try to modify the routine or fix the poor mechanics that are throwing your body off. Check your form in the mirror against the exercise photos in the Younger in

8 Weeks Workout. For instance, if your knee hurts while you're lunging, your knees are probably extending beyond your toes.

And every time you feel a twinge, don't automatically reach for ibuprofen to manage the pain. Chronic use can irritate the stomach. Dr. Wright encourages her patients to fight pain-causing inflammation by turning to the kind of diet you're eating on the Clean & Green plan, cutting out inflaming sugar and processed foods, and consuming more turmeric and green tea. Reach for the NSAIDs only if necessary.

You can also try these natural ways to heal aches, pains, and annoyances.

PAIN POINT: MY LOWER BACK HURTS

Try cold, and then hot. Break out a bag of frozen peas or an ice pack for the first 48 hours after the pain sets in, and use it for 20 minutes a session, a few times a day. After 2 days, switch to a heating pad for 20-minute intervals. Cold shuts down capillaries and reduces bloodflow to the area to ease swelling and thwarts nerves' ability to conduct pain signals. Heat loosens tight muscles and increases circulation, which brings extra oxygen to the area.

Assume the position. Lie on the floor on your back with your feet on a chair or lie on the floor with pillows under your knees, your hips and knees bent. This takes the pressure and weight off your back. But don't stay down for hours on end; your muscles can weaken, which can slow recovery. Even if it hurts, walk around for a few minutes every hour.

Get on up. Stretch, walk, and stand up at your desk periodically to help stabilize your spine and prevent muscle imbalances. Yoga may help ease back pain, too, research suggests.

Downsize your purse. If you can do biceps curls with your handbag, your back may be paying the price. When you tote a heavy bag, you elevate the shoulder carrying the bag, which throws off your spine. Do this every day, and eventually your back muscles will rebel. When fully loaded, your bag should weigh no more than 10 percent of your body weight, according to the American Chiropractic Association. Also, alternate your carrying shoulder from day to day.

Just breathe. The simple "circle breathing" remedy on page 95 can minimize pain right now and—with regular practice—may lower sensitivity to it in the long run.

PAIN POINT: MY KNEE'S THROBBING

Ice it. Whether you suffer an arthritis flash or injure your knee, that bag of frozen peas (or ice) molded around the joint for 20 minutes each hour can reduce inflammation.

Stay active. Regular activity builds muscles that support the knee joint. But don't run or do full leg extensions with a resistance machine. Instead, walk, ride your bike, or do "closed kinetic chain" exercises, in which your foot stays put (like on an elliptical trainer).

Try tai chi. This slow-and-gentle Chinese martial arts practice improves knee osteoarthritis as effectively as physical therapy. In one study that tracked 204 people, half of the participants went to physical therapy for 6 weeks and then continued it at home for another 6 weeks. The rest of the participants went to a tai chi class twice a week. At the end of the 3-month study, the tai chi group's pain relief matched and even exceeded that of the physical therapy group.

Or deep-water walking. This is Dr. Wright's favorite exercise for people with serious knee pain. Get in chest-high water and walk across the shallow end of the pool as fast as you can; without turning around, walk back again, for a total of about 20 minutes. Then shuttle sideways across the shallow end for another 20 minutes.

If You Pop Acetaminophen for Arthritis Pain, Read This

IF THE PAIN OF OSTEOARTHRITIS (the most common form of arthritis) regularly sends you to your medicine cabinet, you should know that acetaminophen doesn't relieve osteoarthritis pain all that well, found a study published in *British Medical Journal*.

When researchers analyzed results from 13 clinical trials on the effectiveness of acetaminophen, they found that it improved patients' hip and knee osteoarthritis pain by an average of just 4 points on a scale of 0 to 100 and was entirely ineffective for lower-back pain.

What *does* work to reverse pain? Regular strength and flexibility exercises: One study found exercise resulted in an average drop of 2.3 points on a 0 to 10 pain scale, nearly five times the impact of acetaminophen in the study.

PAIN POINT: MY ARTHRITIS IS FLARING UP

Make a spicy compress. Ginger doesn't have to be eaten to heal. People with osteoarthritis who placed warm ginger compresses on their midback for 30 minutes a day saw their pain and fatigue reduced by half after a week, a study published in the *Journal of Advanced Nursing* found. Topical ginger seems to warm and relax the musculoskeletal system, which helps mobility. The fix probably works for pulled muscles and achy joints, too. To make the compress used in the study, mix 2 teaspoons ground ginger with 1 cup hot water. Soak a cloth in the mixture and squeeze it firmly to remove excess water. Then apply it to your achy spot.

Boost Energy Naturally

By now, you've hopefully made a serious dent in your personal energy crisis: A healthy diet, regular exercise, and stress management are the go-to trio to beat fatigue. But if you're looking for an instant energy rush, here's a roundup of science-backed strategies to try.

Step outside. Do you conk out like clockwork in the afternoon? To revitalize, take a short, brisk walk. "Boosting your heart rate will rush more blood to your brain and wake you up," Dr. Wright says. Even better if you can walk on the sunny side of the street; light, even afternoon sun, can revivify you.

Change your posture. Lift your head and stand tall, and your mood and energy level may perk up, as well. When you move from poor to good posture, you increase levels of energizing hormones and feel-good serotonin while decreasing the stress hormone cortisol.

If you can, take a catnap. Short midday naps (less than 20 minutes) have been shown to revitalize your brain for the second half of your day, Dr. Wright says.

Brew a cup of tea. A recent report found that pairing caffeine and the amino acid L-theanine, both present in black tea, decreased mental fatigue and improved alertness, reaction time, and memory.

Pop a piece of gum. It may be an icky habit, but save it for when you're fried. In a British study, people who chewed gum for 15 minutes felt more alert than those who didn't. Chewing gum increases heart rate, which increases bloodflow to the brain, the study found. It also stimulates the autonomic nervous system, which can increase alertness.

Massage your ears. This one sounds a little out-there, but try rubbing the edges of your ears between two fingers from the very top all the way to

Suddenly Exhausted? Check Your Heart

IF YOU HAVE EXPERIENCED A SUDDEN drop of energy or have chest pain, anxiety, or trouble concentrating, see a doctor, pronto. She may recommend a stress test or an echocardiogram to screen for heart disease, the leading cause of death in American women—which strikes one in every four.

In a study in the journal *Heart & Lung*, half of all women who had heart attacks said they had trouble sleeping and felt unusually fatigued in the weeks beforehand. Feeling fatigued and breathless when you exert yourself should also raise a red flag. Blocked arteries or a weak heart muscle reduce bloodflow, which prevents your muscles and tissues from getting the oxygen they need to function properly.

the bottom of your lobe a few times. In traditional Chinese medicine, the upper part of the body is associated with more active energies. Massaging the ears increases these energies, which creates a sense of wakefulness.

Improve Your Balance

As we age, our sense of balance can get glitchy. Balance problems can have many causes, including low blood pressure, allergies, infections, or disturbances of the inner ear. Once your equilibrium is off, tripping or falling can cause serious injury that can be hard to recover from.

Many of the exercises in our workout plan build stability, but to stay rocksteady on your feet, do our three-move antiaging balance exercises (see page 316) multiple times a day. The moves take seconds, and you can do them anywhere—standing in line at the bank or while you're brushing your teeth.

Reverse Hair Loss

"There's a lot of emotion around hair loss. Our sense of femininity and beauty is so connected to our hair," says beauty advisor Eva Scrivo. Fortunately, there's a lot you can do to help stem further loss or promote regrowth—once you know what's going on.

It's normal to lose up to 100 hairs to the shower drain or your brush each day. With age, however, the overall density of hair changes and each strand becomes finer. By 50, half of all women will notice some hair loss. The prime culprit: menopause, when levels of hair-friendly estrogen typically decline, increasing the relative levels of androgens (male hormones) normally present in the body. The resulting hair loss, called female pattern baldness, typically affects hair on the top or the crown (back) of the scalp. Unlike men, who often see their hairlines recede, women may notice their part widening close to the forehead.

Another type of hair loss is *telogen effluvium,* often triggered by stress to the body—high fevers, major surgery or illness, crash diets, and medications like birth control pills, beta-blockers, or certain antidepressants—or severe psychological stress, like the death of a loved one or divorce. With this kind of hair loss, some "shock" pushes hair roots prematurely into the resting state, causing hair loss, sometimes by the handful, about 2 months later. Usually this type of hair loss is temporary, and it slows down in 6 to 8 months.

To help identify the type of hair loss you're dealing with, your doctor may look for bulbs on the roots of a fallen hair. (The bulbs mean the hair has gone through a complete cycle of growth, suggesting that either physical or emotional stress accelerated the cycle.) In some cases (say, surgery), hang on—the loss will slow. If medication is the problem, your doctor may be able to lower your dosage or switch you to another drug. If it's stress-related, do your best to relax (easier said than done, we know). And check out the styling options on pages 135–136; there's lots you can do to camouflage the loss, from color to extensions.

If your hair loss is hereditary (look at your mom or dad, or their parents), a

Renew Right Now

INSTANT GLOW

RESTORE FLUSHED CHEEKS. With age, blood circulation to the skin decreases, so you lose that healthy flush you once had. That means you can get a little bolder with your blush. Warm, bright tones like peaches and pinks flatter aging skin better than dusty, muted colors, advises Scrivo. If you suffer from rosacea, opt for a bronzer in place of blush.

SLIMMER IN A MINUTE

GO MONOCHROME. Rather than wear nude panty hose with dark shoes, wear clothes, hose, and shoes in the same color family, from top to bottom, suggests Scrivo. This monochrome palette tricks the eye, making you appear taller and slimmer.

dermatologist can help you consider your options. One is minoxidil, the active ingredient in Rogaine and the only FDA-approved proven ingredient. While it doesn't work for everyone—about 50 percent of women who use it see improvement—minoxidil can enhance the size of the follicle so it produces a bigger strand of hair. Scrivo likes Densifique Minoxidil by Kerastase ($35, kerastase.com), which triggers visible regrowth after about 4 months. (For the first 2 to 8 weeks of use, hair loss may temporarily increase, but don't panic—this stops when your hair starts to regrow.)

Or try the following hair "cocktail" that, in one study, reduced hair loss in 90 percent of the women who took it.

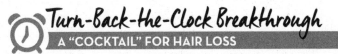

Turn-Back-the-Clock Breakthrough
A "COCKTAIL" FOR HAIR LOSS

In a study published in the *Journal of Cosmetic Dermatology*, a group of 80 healthy women with mild female pattern hair loss took fish oil, black currant seed oil, vitamin E, vitamin C, and lycopene supplements every day for 6 months. The result: Hair density increased for 62 percent of the women, hair became measurably thicker in diameter, and 90 percent of the women reported a decrease in overall hair loss. The researchers believe the fatty acids and antioxidants found in the supplements support the health of blood vessels and cell membranes and promote cell growth and anti-inflammatory activities in and around hair follicles.

Interested? Check with your doctor first. (Black currant seed oil can lower blood pressure further in people who already have low numbers and can slow blood clotting.) Here's what the women in the study took.

FISH OIL: 460 milligrams

BLACK CURRANT SEED OIL: 460 milligrams

VITAMIN E: 5 milligrams

VITAMIN C: 30 milligrams

LYCOPENE: 1 milligram

Several of our panelists tried the cocktail, with positive results. Panelist Jen Casper started the regimen on Day 1. Within days, "my hair felt thicker and healthier and seemed less dry and frizzy," she says. Sandy Franklin, too, reported that her hair feels thicker since taking the supplements. Don't worry if you can only find the supplements in larger doses (especially lycopene and vitamin E)—a little extra won't hurt. Also keep in mind that, like any hair loss treatment, you'll likely need to keep up with the supplement cocktail to maintain the results.

Too complicated? If you'd like to take just one supplement, Scrivo suggests Skin, Nails & Hair by MegaFood. ■

SUCCESS!

Loretta Fredericks, 66

MY STORY Loretta Fredericks had been at peace with many aspects of aging. "Psychologically and emotionally I feel better now than when I was younger," she said. But physically, her weight had been creeping up, and she was noticing the effects. "I used to love riding my bike along the Potomac," she said before starting the program. "But the last time I did it, I felt too pudgy and I stopped riding." When she saw a videotape of herself sitting down, she was shocked. "I looked like a little old lady plopping down into the chair."

Then her doctor diagnosed her with high cholesterol and prediabetes. "I didn't want to go on medication, so I knew I had to lose the weight," she said.

She tried a "metabolism-boosting" diet that required starting her days with a cold-water bath, two cups of coffee, and an intense workout—then waiting another 2 hours before breakfast. While she lost weight, she gained it all back as soon as she stopped.

On the Younger in 8 Weeks Plan, Loretta lost about a pound a week. "It isn't gimmicky. It focuses on healthy foods and the exercise is moderate; I don't have to be a maniac," she said. "I can keep this up."

Loretta's success comes from making some simple habit changes. For example, she now makes sure that two meals a day are plant based instead of meat focused. She has cut back on eating out and instead uses the Meal Builder to create simple meals from healthy staples.

To fit in exercise, Loretta tweaked her morning ritual. Instead of relaxing with a cup of coffee and reading the paper for an hour, she exercises first. "I still have to push myself to do it, but putting my rower in front of my picture window and listening to my favorite music makes it more enjoyable," she said. The cardio combined with the stretching routines and balance exercises has had a significant impact on Loretta's body.

"I'm more limber and flexible. My legs have more power, and I feel more graceful getting in and out of a chair," she said.

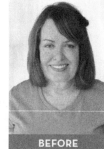

BEFORE

She's also excited that her jeans are zipping up easily and she's fitting back into the size-10 sheath dresses she'd been longing to wear again. And it looks like she'll be able to avoid cholesterol and diabetes medications: Loretta lowered her total cholesterol 24 points and her LDL cholesterol by 25 points. Even better, her blood glucose level dropped enough that she no longer has prediabetes. She even signed up to take ice-skating lessons—an activity that she loved as a kid—and she's eager to get back on her bike in the spring.

Beauty styling: makeup, Colleen Kobrick; hair, Missy Kovato; Wardrobe styling: Pamela Simpson

LOOK AT ME

- More energy

- Lost **3.75 inches from her thighs**

- No more cravings

- Better balance

- Weight lost: **10 pounds**

- Inches lost: **8**

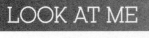 **PICK OUT YOUR EXER-CISE CLOTHES THE NIGHT BEFORE.** I put mine next to my bed so I see them first thing in the morning. This way, I'm reminded of my commitment to start the day with exercise. (Make sure to choose workout clothes that you like, that are flattering and comfortable, and that go with your mood. It makes a difference!)

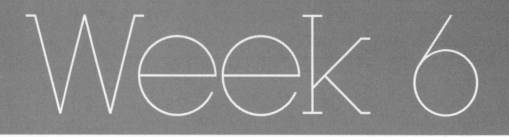

Week 6

"I have never purchased so many awesome veggies and fruits. I am really learning what my supermarket has to offer and have never been so excited to buy groceries and cook."

— PANELIST JEN CASPER

STAY-YOUNG STEPS	GOALS	TO-DO LIST
EAT	Continue to follow the Clean & Green guidelines.	*Optional*: Make over a family favorite using healthier oils, whole grain ingredients, and more veggies.
MOVE	Commit to your workouts.	Ratchet up your strength routine with two new moves (see page 312 of the Younger in 8 Weeks Workout).
ENGAGE	Keep trying new strategies.	Set your daily intention and make time for meditation. Make a new-you move, like registering for a course at a local college or asking someone you'd like to know better to coffee or lunch.
GLOW	Continue your skin-care routine.	*Splurge!* Get products to help you achieve more youthful-looking legs.

Week 6 Troubleshooting Plan

- Boost Your Brainpower

- Lower High Blood Pressure Naturally

- Handle Hot Flashes

- Take Time Off Your Hands

Boost Your Brainpower

With another week of tasty eating and healthy living behind you, you're officially in the home stretch! As your belly continues to shrink and your energy and self-confidence continue to grow, it's time to turn your attention to a body part that's higher up: your brain, the storehouse of memory.

Chances are you've walked into a room and forgotten why, misplaced your keys, blanked on a word. But these occasional brain glitches are almost certainly not some red flag of imminent senility. Much like a computer, your brain places information it judges to be important into "files." When you remember something, you pull up a file—and with age, those files may take longer to retrieve (your brain's version of that spinning wheel on your computer screen).

So rest assured that occasional "senior moments" are perfectly normal, while cognitive decline, experts say, is a slow and subtle process. In one study, adults whose memories were tested at age 55 and again at 81 exhibited only a small difference in the number of items they could remember nearly 30 years later.

The good news is that you're already practicing the basics of a healthier brain and sharper memory—sleep, exercise, meditation, social interaction. To manage the inevitable glitches, review these sharp-brain basics along with some expert-recommended tricks.

Seek out the new. If you don't challenge your brain with new places and information, your memory suffers. Familiar activities allow your brain to laze into autopilot. But novelty—whether you explore a new route to the mall or take up Sudoku puzzles—can stimulate cognition and memory.

Minimize multitasking. Paying undivided attention to something you really need to remember later will boost your recall. In other words, don't listen to the news as you respond to e-mail or text a friend to make a plan while rushing to finish a work presentation. You'll limit your recall of both. Why? We process new information with a part of the brain called the cerebral cortex. But when we multitask, the brain is forced to switch over to using an area called the striatum, and the information stored there tends to contain fewer important details. Less multitasking, better recall.

Give your brain a break. Cortisol—the hormone your body releases under stress—is toxic to the nervous system, and your brain is the motherboard of that network. To keep stress from battering your memory bank, intersperse periods of brain drain with short breaks of relative inactivity or active relaxation (another reason to stick with that meditation habit).

Double-check your meds. Memory lapses can be a side effect of many prescription and over-the-counter drugs. Antidepressants, antianxiety drugs,

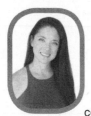

Dr. Vonda Wright says . . .

YOU CAN TRAIN YOUR BRAIN FOR SUCCESS

As a surgeon, researcher, and curious person in general, I consider my brain the best part of me. The ability to concentrate on deep work, create research ideas that change how we think about our health, have rich conversations with other people, and solve problems—whether simple or complex—is a deeply satisfying part of my life. One of my Second Act goals is to become one of those "smart as a whip" old ladies.

Beyond regular exercise—the ultimate brain builder, research shows—and eating the brain-boosting foods included in the Clean & Green plan, I do other things to stay mentally sharp.

1. **I DO CIRCUIT EXERCISES INSTEAD OF MACHINE-BASED EXERCISE.** When you task your brain to focus on complex moves, keep your balance, *and* think about what move comes next, you engage many different parts of it. The more complex the moves, the more they stimulate your brain, studies show.

2. **I PLAY BRAIN GAMES.** I use Lumosity, a phone app that offers tons of brain-training games and exercises. My brain workout of the day makes me feel sharper, and my heart rate even rises as if I'm working out. In our family, we also do crosswords and play chess with our kids, which has become a real challenge!

3. **I SURF THE INTERNET.** Really! In measured doses, it can be good for your brain. When I was a geeky kid, I used to pull an encyclopedia off the shelf, open to a subject, and read. The Internet is the modern way to do this. Some of my recent searches include the top 10 cities for millennials and the research-supported advantages to kids of having a working mother.

antispasmodics, beta-blockers, chemotherapy, Parkinson's medications, sleeping pills, ulcer medications, painkillers, antihistamines, and even statins can all affect your memory. And as you get older, drugs tend to stay in your system for a longer period of time, increasing the likelihood of troublesome interactions. Fortunately, any drug-related impairment will improve as soon as the drug is discontinued. Speak with your doctor if you think your meds are muddling your memory; it may be possible to adjust your dose or switch medications.

Make sure it's nothing worse. Common health conditions associated with aging—such as diabetes, high blood pressure, and high cholesterol—contribute to narrowing of the blood vessels that supply oxygen and nutrients to the brain. And they have a negative impact on memory if they aren't controlled by diet, exercise, and, if necessary, medication. Your doctor can spot this and other reversible causes of memory loss.

Lower High Blood Pressure Naturally

An estimated 20 percent of Americans have high blood pressure and don't know it. While often symptomless, this condition raises the risk of top killers such as heart attack, stroke, and kidney failure.

The *Younger in 8 Weeks* healthy lifestyle changes—a plant-based diet, regular exercise, stress management—have been shown to help reduce high blood pressure or keep it at a healthy level. So job one is to get to a healthy weight. But while you're working on that, add one or more of these science-backed strategies.

Have a red smoothie. Drinking 17 ounces of beet juice can yield a 5-point drop in blood pressure in just 6 hours, a 2012 Australian study found. The crimson root veggie is rich in nitrates, which is thought to relax blood vessels and improve bloodflow.

Indulge in dark chocolate. This tip needed to be first! Dark chocolate varieties contain flavanols that make blood vessels more elastic. In one study, 18 percent of patients who ate it every day saw their pressure decrease. Another study found that dark chocolate helped to keep white blood cells from sticking to artery walls. Dark chocolate, as you know, is totally cool on the Clean & Green plan. Have 1 ounce daily (make sure it contains at least 70 percent cocoa).

Go full-bore vegetarian. A vegetarian diet can lower blood pressure by up to 7 points, about the same drop you'd get from an 11-pound weight loss, one published analysis found. Plant foods are low in sodium—which can raise blood pressure in susceptible people—and high in potassium, long known to lower it.

Check your sodium intake. The average American consumes 3,300 milligrams of sodium a day. Whoa! Dietary guidelines recommend less than 2,300 milligrams a day (equal to about 1 teaspoon of salt), and that's if you're *healthy*. The guidelines recommend reducing sodium intake even lower—to 1,500 milligrams per day—if you're age 51 or over, African American, or have high blood pressure, diabetes, or chronic kidney disease. That's because these groups have been shown to be more susceptible to sodium's blood pressure–raising effects. The great news: Because over 75 percent of dietary sodium comes from packaged and restaurant foods, this plan can help lower your sodium intake automatically.

Leave work at a reasonable hour. People who put in more than 41 hours per week at the office raised their risk of hypertension by 15 percent, according to a study of nearly 25,000 people. While it may be difficult more often than not, clock out at a decent hour so you can get your workout in and cook a healthy meal.

Get a little sun. Low levels of vitamin D are thought to contribute to high blood pressure. In one study, 20 minutes of UV ray exposure helped blood vessels expand, which boosted cardiovascular function and reduced blood pressure independently of vitamin D intake. Of course, don't forget to wear a broad-spectrum sunscreen.

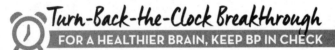

Turn-Back-the-Clock Breakthrough
FOR A HEALTHIER BRAIN, KEEP BP IN CHECK

A healthy blood pressure (BP) benefits your brain as well as your heart. In a study published in the journal *Neurology,* researchers measured the BP of more than 4,000 adults in middle age (around age 50) and again in older age (around age 76). In older age, the participants were given MRIs to assess blood vessel damage in the brain, and memory and thinking ability were tested. Turns out the participants who'd had high BP in midlife actually had *smaller brains*, less gray matter, and lower thinking and memory scores!

Blood vessels are needed to deliver blood and nutrients to the brain, and high BP creates stress that can weaken the vessels over time, the study noted. Unchecked, this condition may eventually send less blood to the brain, leading to tissue damage and loss.

The tactics you're learning in this book—to eat healthfully, exercise, and de-stress—can make a big difference here. In fact, to lower BP, lifestyle changes are as important, if not more important, than medication. ■

Handle Your Hot Flashes

If you occasionally sweat like you're staring into the jaws of hell, then you're familiar with how changing levels of estrogen can create surges of heat lasting between 30 seconds and 10 minutes. Hot flashes affect about 85 percent of women in the years right before and after menopause.

And get this: A recent study revealed that the window for hot flashes is a whopping *7 to 14 years*, rather than the previously believed 3 years. That's some serious sweat time. Fortunately, relief—both natural and, if you need it, pharmaceutical—is at hand.

Relief starts with a healthy diet. In fact, several of our panelists reported that the plan seemed to dial down the heat. "I've definitely noticed a reduction in the number of my hot flashes," Lisa Boland says. "Also—and this is huge—my night sweats have stopped entirely."

But there are other remedies to try. A recent paper published by the North American Menopause Society evaluated the effectiveness of top nonhormonal treatments, including yoga and hypnosis, based on an analysis of rigorously conducted studies. The surprise winner? Cognitive-behavioral therapy (CBT) came out on top, followed by clinical hypnosis. To learn more about CBT and find a specialist, visit the National Association of Cognitive-Behavioral Therapists at nacbt.org. To find information on hypnosis, check out the American Society of Clinical Hypnosis Web site at asch.net.

If you're looking for DIY relief, this trio of strategies (and a last word of advice) can help.

Sip . . . tomato juice? Unexpected but effective, according to a recent study. When 95 women with at least one menopausal symptom—such as hot flashes, anxiety, and irritability—drank just under 1 cup of unsalted tomato juice twice a day, these symptoms were reduced by 16 percent in 4 weeks, halfway through an 8-week study.

Try sage tea. A Swiss study evaluated the effects of a once-daily sage tablet on 71 postmenopausal women and found that the average number of hot flashes dropped by half within 4 weeks and by 64 percent within 8 weeks. Women with severe and very severe hot flashes had even greater benefits: 79 percent and 100 percent, respectively.

Instead of a sage supplement, you can brew the herb into a tasty tea. Use 1 tablespoon of fresh sage leaves or 1 heaping teaspoon of dried sage per cup. Steep for 5 minutes and then strain. Drink a cup two or three times a day. (Because sage may have estrogen-like effects, avoid therapeutic amounts if you've had breast cancer or could be pregnant.)

Whip up a scented cooler. Not to drink, but to spritz. This easy-to-make, herbalist-recommended cooling mist can help soothe night sweats. Mix together 3 ounces of water; 1 ounce of witch hazel extract; and 8 drops each of peppermint, clary sage, and Roman chamomile essential oils in a

4-ounce dark-glass spray bottle. At the first flash, spritz away and breathe deeply. Herbalists say that clary sage and Roman chamomile essential oils help balance mood swings, while peppermint can chill hot flashes.

If hot flashes continue to plague you, see your doctor. There are effective new drugs, including one nonhormonal medication, Brisdelle (paroxetine), which is FDA-approved to treat hot flashes. And transdermal estrogens—in the form of a gel, lotion, spray, or patch—are not metabolized by the liver and therefore have safety advantages over oral estrogen products (since oral estrogen can up your risk of blood clots and other problems).

Take Time Off Your Hands

You've spent more than a month pampering the skin on your face (and hopefully you've been caring for your neck, too!). Don't neglect your hands, though, which can vividly show the effects of sun damage and natural aging—yes, wrinkles and brown spots—as early as your thirties and forties. Here's how to make caring for your hands and nails part of your regular routine. (As always, you can find brand recommendations in the Product Guide, page 408.)

Moisturize. A recent survey found that 70 percent of us wash our hands at least seven times a day. Such hygiene, commendable as it is, can really dry out hands (and soap does extra damage). Carry a moisturizing hand cream and reapply it regularly throughout the day. For major triage, there's a bedtime trick to return rough, scaly mitts to smooth overnight. First, slough off rough skin with a gentle scrub. Then, smooth on a hand cream that contains such moisturizing ingredients as hyaluronic acid, glycerin, lanolin, mineral oil, and petrolatum. (Products that contain silicone or simethicone leave hands soft without feeling greasy.) Finally, don cotton mittens and keep them on for a couple of hours while you watch TV or even overnight.

Erase brown spots. Age spots are the result of too much sun exposure and can show up as early as one's forties among reformed sun worshippers. Get into the habit of smoothing on a dime-size dab of hand cream with SPF 30 before heading out the door each day—especially if you drive, as UV penetrates windows. Reapply after you wash your hands or every 2 hours if you're exposed to even a little sunlight.

Tackle existing spots with an OTC fade cream with 2 percent hydroquinone. Test it out on a small patch of skin first, since hydroquinone can create

Three Ways to Score Healthier, Younger-Looking Nails

LIKE THE REST OF YOUR HANDS, your nails can age prematurely if you don't care for them. These tips can help with the most common age-related nail challenges.

FADE THE STAINS. First, figure out why your nails are turning yellow or brown. If the discoloration persists or is accompanied by pain, it's likely a fungal infection; check with your doctor ASAP to treat it.

If your doc says the problem isn't fungal, the discoloration is likely a harmless side effect of things like psoriasis medication or wearing dark polish. Buff your nails with a lemon wedge, or soak them in—wait for it—denture cleaner for 15 to 20 minutes to remove stains. Also make sure to apply a base coat before you reapply your favorite dark lacquer.

ADD STRENGTH. Water or chemical exposure, seasonal weather changes, and even genetics can lead to brittle nails. Taking a 2.5-milligram dose of the B vitamin biotin improves nail strength and reduces brittleness after 6 to 9 months, a study published in the *Journal of Cosmetic Dermatology* found.

UPDATE YOUR MANI. Nail shapes and shades are in constant flux, and keeping up with nail trends can help hands look more youthful. Right now, shorter nails are the norm; keep nails no longer than ¼ inch beyond your fingertips. Bonus points if you follow up with flattering shades of polish that make your hands look modern and draw attention away from wrinkles or spots. Eva Scrivo recommends pale neutrals, like cream, taupe, or the palest pink, which appear to elongate the fingers.

spotting on some browner skin tones. Darker age spots may need a 3 percent solution, but you'll need a dermatologist's prescription—and guidance—to give this a try. These whiteners target the skin's uppermost layers—not the pigment cells producing the brown spots—so you must continue the treatments indefinitely, even after seeing improvement.

Hide veins. You can invest in high-tech vein removal that runs $2,000 a session. But a more sensible plan is to tone down the color of large, raised, or unsightly blue veins with a covering foundation made to erase imperfections

Renew Right Now

on the legs and body. You'll have to reapply after washing your hands, but it still beats surgery. You can also find hand-treatment creams that plump up and smooth thinner skin with ingredients like hyaluronic acid.

Splurge!

Get Younger-Looking Legs

While your short-shorts days may be behind you, it *would* be nice to bare your legs every now and again—but cellulite or spider veins can force them under wraps. While you may not be prepared to spend thousands on treatments that offer lasting improvements, these less-expensive splurges can give your legs a temporary reprieve.

SMOOTH DIMPLES

More than 85 percent of women have cellulite, even women in their twenties, so it's not just a factor of age. But as skin's connective tissue weakens over time, the dimples and ripples tend to worsen. (But you already knew that, right?)

The fast fix: "Sea salt scrubs that contain minerals and algae are detoxifying, and rubbing them over the dimples will help make your legs appear at least a *little* smoother," says Dr. Jeannette Graf. Or splurge on an over-the-counter cream that contains caffeine, which enhances fat metabolism and reduces puffiness by flushing out excess fluids. You might also try a high-end self-tanner to camouflage cellulite and spider veins, suggests Scrivo. Follow the instructions on the label. For a smooth and even application, there are two musts: Shave your legs before you apply the self-tanner, and do your knees last, using only the product left on your hands. (See the Product Guide on page 410 for cellulite creams and self-tanners.)

The serious-money solution: It's pricey—$300 to $1,200 per session—but endermologie combines high suction and massage to break up the fibrous bands that cause the lumpy appearance and clear out the lymphatic fluid that builds up in cellulite. While the procedure won't completely remove all of the cellulite, you can expect to see anywhere from 20 to 75 percent improvement in appearance.

REDUCE SPIDER VEINS

About half of women over age 50 have these small, dilated blood vessels just beneath the skin's surface that give off a serious road-map vibe. This age-related skin annoyance typically is caused by genetics. But if you're overweight, on your feet a lot, or always crossing your legs, spider veins can get you, too.

The fast fix: The immediate solution is temporary but effective: Use a tinted leg spray or a brush-on waterproof body makeup.

The serious-money solution: The gold standard for spider-vein treatment (and varicose veins, too) is sclerotherapy, an in-office procedure in which each vein is injected with a solution that causes it to collapse. Treated veins typically fade within a few weeks; however, bear in mind that treatment for both legs can take up to four $275 to $400 sessions spaced 6 to 8 weeks apart. If you have severe varicose veins, see a vascular specialist for further treatment options, like laser ablation.

SUCCESS!

Lisa Ham, 51

Lisa never imagined something as simple as taking a stroll could provide such amazing benefits. "I never thought walking was a workout!" she said. "When I was walking for the program, I could feel my muscles working, and I was sore the next day."

Exercise was never a priority, and as Lisa got older, she recognized how out of shape she was. Even though she wasn't overweight, Lisa was often out of breath and constantly tired. Now, she has the energy to wake up an hour earlier to exercise, stretch, and practice yoga.

Completing the exercises on the Younger in 8 Weeks Plan also gave Lisa the confidence to do something she says she would have never done before. She walked with her daughter's high school marching band in a Labor Day parade and finished the entire thing. "I walked 7,000 steps that day, and I'd never done that," Lisa said. "I thought I'd have to sit out, but I finished. I felt so accomplished."

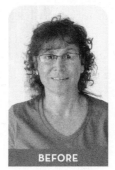

BEFORE

This program not only taught Lisa how to live a healthier lifestyle, but it allowed her to teach her 15-year-old daughter an important lesson. "I showed her it's okay to take care of yourself instead of always putting others first, something we both struggle with," Lisa said.

By sneaking vegetables into meals and eliminating many processed foods from her diet, Lisa was able to switch her previous diet of meat, pasta, and potatoes to a vegetable-based meal plan, one that satisfied her whole family. Her husband ate (and enjoyed!) all of the healthy meals and saw improvements in his own health as a result.

"I try not to eat any canned or bagged foods," Lisa said. She chooses her vegetables based on the season. In the summer, there are always tomatoes in the garden. "There's nothing like fresh tomatoes." And during the winter, Lisa adds parsnips and turnips into her beef stew. She transforms other fattening favorites into powerhouse meals by swapping half of the noodles in lasagna for zucchini and baking sweet potatoes in olive oil instead of eating greasy fries. By cooking this way, her delicious meals are bursting with nutrients.

"Losing weight wasn't the main goal. I needed to do this because I wanted to be fit and healthy and someday see my grandchildren," Lisa said. "Eight weeks is really just the start. You have to maintain it, and over time it's all going to be worth it."

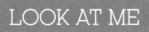

LOOK AT ME

- Lost **3 inches off waist**

- Eliminated processed sugar

- Improved sleep

- Lost **5.75 inches total**

- Lost **4.8 pounds**

Tip SATISFY YOUR CRAVINGS THE HEALTHY WAY. When I'm hungry for pizza, I make a vegetable pizza pie. I puree tomatoes from my garden for pizza sauce and pile spaghetti squash and cauliflower on top of a wrap. Then I sprinkle it with part-skim mozzarella cheese and throw it in the oven. Now I have a nutritious alternative!

Beauty styling: makeup, Colleen Kobrick; hair, Missy Kovato; Wardrobe styling: Pamela Simpson

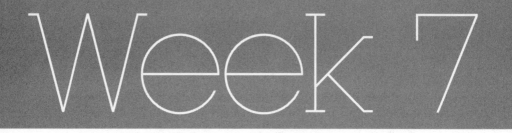

Week 7

"I'm not as stiff as I was, and if I do wake up stiff, the Sunrise Stretch helps me work out the kinks."

— PANELIST CINDY CARTER

STAY-YOUNG STEP	GOALS	TO-DO LIST
EAT	Continue to follow the Clean & Green guidelines.	*Optional*: For extra telomere lengthening, try dropping red meat and chicken entirely this week.
MOVE	Commit to your workouts.	Add two new moves to your strength routine (see page 314 of the Younger in 8 Weeks Workout). Move up a level of intensity in your cardio intervals, if you feel ready.
ENGAGE	Take a step toward finding your duende.	Set your daily intention and make time for meditation. Ponder your career and take one decisive action: Revamp your résumé; work your LinkedIn connections; register for a course that lets you sample a new passion.
GLOW	Keep up your skin-care routine.	*Troubleshoot*: Address two skin conditions that can hit at midlife: adult acne and rosacea.

Be Prepared!

• Make sure you have a set of dumbbells for this week's strength routine (see page 305 for advice on choosing weights).

• Schedule a hearing or eye test if you're due for either.

Week 7 Troubleshooting Plan

• Sharpen Your Senses

• Settle Your Stomach

• Stop Springing Leaks

• Handle Hormonal Skin Problems

Sharpen Your Senses

It's easy to take sharp vision and hearing for granted—until the day you struggle to read a menu or hold up your end of a conversation. Some dulling of the senses is normal, but more significant declines in hearing or vision can cut us off from the world, leading to potentially painful social isolation. So this week, if you choose, focus on the health and upkeep of these vital senses.

PROTECT YOUR HEARING

Here's the thing about hearing loss: It's so subtle and gradual that you may not realize there's a problem until you notice how hard it is to follow a conversation or how often you ask people to repeat themselves. An estimated 18 percent of Americans ages 45 to 64 and 30 percent ages 65 to 74 have some degree of hearing loss. Now's the time to protect your hearing or seek treatment. These steps can do a lot.

Live clean. The same healthy lifestyle that promotes health protects hearing. On the flip side, uncontrolled high blood pressure, cholesterol, and blood sugar can damage blood vessels in the ears and lead to hearing loss.

Avoid ear blasters. Not since the industrial age, when almost everyone with a job reported for duty at a factory, have we been so exposed to incessant noise. This aural assault can cause the loss of high-frequency hearing registered by the sensory cells closest to the eardrums. We don't regenerate these cells, so once they're gone, that's it.

Plug up. If you're regularly in environments where you have to strain to hold a comfortable conversation—a café or noisy public space—pick up a pair of earplugs. Try the custom kind, which are made to fit your ears (about $40), or just regular over-the-counter earplugs ($3 to $11).

Ease up on OTC painkillers. Women who took ibuprofen (e.g., Advil) 2 or more days a week experienced up to 24 percent more hearing loss than those who used painkillers just once a week, one study found. Acetaminophen's effect on hearing loss was almost as high. It could be that these drugs damage the cochlea, the spiral structure in the inner ear that's essential for hearing. Ibuprofen seems to reduce bloodflow to the area (just as it reduces bloodflow elsewhere in the body to ease inflammation), while acetaminophen might deplete the antioxidants that protect against oxidative damage.

Always use the lowest possible dose of OTC painkillers for the shortest duration. If you regularly take these meds, work with your doctor to get a firm diagnosis of the cause of your pain. Then you can discuss options that may help reduce or eliminate your need for pills.

Request a test. To ensure your hearing is up to snuff—or if you suspect you've had some loss—call your doctor. Most likely, you'll be referred to a specialist. An otolaryngologist (a specialist in ear, nose, and throat disorders) can investigate the cause, while an audiologist can perform a hearing test to assess the type and degree of loss.

If you do need a hearing aid, there are lots of good options. For mild to moderate hearing loss, traditional analog aids amplify sound via a thin tube that sits in or behind the ear. Many newer aids are so small they can be snugged into the ear canal or discreetly behind the ear. More powerful digital aids can separate background noise from speech with startling clarity; these are also smaller and less conspicuous than they used to be.

While most insurance plans don't pick up the entire tab for a hearing aid, some pay a portion of the cost. Do find out—a hearing aid is an investment in your future, and it's lovely to hear a whispered "I love you" loud and clear.

SAVE YOUR SIGHT

An estimated 17 percent of Americans ages 65 and older report diminished vision. Fading eyesight can make driving more dangerous, and it can suck the joy out of the simple pleasures of life—devouring a book or enjoying a movie or gorgeous view. Left untreated, it can also lead to social isolation. Here's what you can do now to stay eagle-eyed.

Get your eyes examined. Even if you think your vision is fine, schedule an eye exam every 1 to 2 years after age 40. An ophthalmologist can look for diseases such as glaucoma, cataracts, diabetes-related changes, or macular degeneration (see the "Five Eye Symptoms to Mention to Your Doctor" box on page 260).

Know your family's eye health history. Many eye diseases or conditions are hereditary, and this information can determine if you're at higher risk.

Continue your Clean & Green eating. Research has found that a diet rich in fruits and vegetables (dark leafy greens, in particular) and fish high in omega-3 fats, such as salmon, sardines, and halibut, promotes eye health. Eating healthy also keeps weight down, which in turn manages conditions like diabetes that can cause vision loss.

Wear your sunnies. Sunglasses may be a style statement, but their most important job is to protect your eyes from the sun's ultraviolet rays. Be sure to get a pair that blocks out 99 to 100 percent of both UVA and UVB radiation.

Settle Your Stomach

A cranky digestive system can really put a damper on the active, energetic life you're seeking. But sadly, heartburn, constipation, gas, or other tummy troubles can become more common with age. You might even have intolerances to certain foods (or components of food) that you never had before.

The Clean & Green plan alone may be making a difference with your digestive issues. Panelist Vesta Ackernecht's abdominal pain, nausea, and bloating from irritable bowel syndrome (IBS) was significantly reduced. "I used to leave my home daily with fear and anxiety; I couldn't go anywhere without medication," she says. "Since I started the diet change, I have no need to take IBS medication. I have none of the previous symptoms, absolutely none."

Living well, minimizing stress, and eating a diet high in fiber can all improve the health of your gastrointestinal system, Dr. Vonda Wright says. "The loads of leafy greens and elimination of processed foods suggested in this book all increase the fiber content through the gut and allow for more rapid passage of food, so it doesn't settle in as noxious sludge."

Even if you're not struggling with an acute digestive issue, a gut tune-up can't hurt. As you know, the eating plan includes regular doses of prebiotics and probiotics to balance your microbiome.

If you still struggle with discomfort or queasiness after eating, these strategies can help.

ZERO IN ON FOOD INTOLERANCES

Food allergies can be life-threatening. An intolerance to dairy, gluten, or other food isn't. Yet it can cause bothersome symptoms like gas and bloating, as well as mystery symptoms like brain fog, breakouts, and joint pain.

There are several types of food intolerances. Abdominal bloating, cramps, diarrhea, gas, or gurgling sounds in your belly after a glass of milk or a meal containing dairy products are symptoms of lactose intolerance. People who have it are unable to digest the sugar in milk, called lactose, because they lack the digestive enzyme lactase. You may also be sensitive to food additives, such as the flavor enhancer MSG (monosodium glutamate) or sulfites in wine.

Five Eye Symptoms to Mention to Your Doctor

WITH AGE, THE RISK FOR A number of vision problems goes way up. Call your doctor if you experience the following symptoms.

FREQUENT CHANGES IN HOW CLEARLY YOU SEE. This may be a sign of diabetes or high blood pressure, which can damage the tiny blood vessels in the retina—the light-sensitive layer at the back of the eye. This damage can cause permanent vision loss.

YOUR "FLOATERS" COME WITH FLASHES. Typically, those images of particles that float in the fluid of the eye are harmless. But call your doctor ASAP if you see more than normal, and if they're accompanied by flashes. This may signal impending retinal detachment (a tear of the retina), which requires immediate treatment.

YOU'RE LOSING YOUR PERIPHERAL (SIDE) VISION. This may be a sign of glaucoma, which occurs when the optic nerve is damaged and no longer transmits all visual images to the brain.

STRAIGHT LINES LOOK WAVY, OR YOU HAVE A BLIND SPOT. Age-related macular degeneration affects the part of the retina responsible for central vision, the macula, and causes a blind spot in the middle of your vision. Fortunately, regular eye exams can catch it early.

YOUR VISION'S GONE BLURRY, COLORS SEEM NOT AS BRIGHT, OR IT'S HARDER TO SEE AT NIGHT. You may have cataracts, a clouding of the eye's naturally clear lens that's common with age. People with dark eyes had a 1.5 to 2.5 times greater risk than lighter-eyed folks, a study published in the *American Journal of Ophthalmology* found. While everyone should protect their eyes from the sun's ultraviolet rays, take special care if you have dark eyes to wear shades and a brimmed hat.

Celiac disease, another possible cause of food intolerance, is triggered by eating gluten, a protein found in wheat and other grains. While celiac disease involves the immune system, and so shares some features of a food allergy, it's surprisingly rare and its symptoms are mostly gastrointestinal. If you suspect your symptoms stem from a food sensitivity, here's what to try.

Adjust your dairy habits. Yogurt or hard cheeses, which contain less lactose, can be easier to tolerate than milk. If you love milk, pair it with food to slow the digestive process and potentially reduce symptoms.

Double-check your plant-based milk. Even plant milks can cause digestive issues if they contain carrageenan, a seaweed-based emulsifier. While it's added to make plant milks thicker and creamier, it may spark intestinal inflammation, research suggests. Stick to the carrageenan-free plant milks in the Food Shopping Guide (page 405).

Know your FODMAPs. Though you wouldn't know it from the gluten-free craze, only 1 percent of the population is sensitive to gluten, according to data from the Centers for Disease Control and Prevention. What's more, if you don't have celiac disease, gluten probably isn't the cause of your digestive woes. It's more likely to be FODMAPs—fermentable, poorly absorbed short-chain carbohydrates, such as breads, beer, pastries, and pasta—a study published in the journal *Gastroenterology* suggests. Talk to your doctor. You may be sensitive to FODMAPs, not gluten. The good news: A low-FODMAP diet is less restrictive than a gluten-free one. (And many of these foods are verboten on the plan, so eating Clean & Green may resolve the issue.)

Don't self-diagnose gluten sensitivity. If you have abdominal pain or discomfort at least 3 days a month that feels better when you pass gas or stool, you may have IBS. Some people with the condition have constipation, some get diarrhea, and still others get both. Once diagnosed, you'll be prescribed diet and lifestyle changes that offer relief.

COOL HEARTBURN

Often, that burning pain under your breastbone has causes unrelated to aging, like chronic stress, extra pounds, and lack of sleep—culprits you're chipping away at on this plan. As you steer clear of flame-fanning fare—such as spicy foods, citrus, tomato-based foods, raw onions, and (alas) chocolate—give these strategies a try.

Think about your drink. Carbonated beverages, alcohol, and coffee contribute to heartburn by relaxing the esophageal sphincter, which allows acid to come up into the throat. But do drink lots of water, especially with meals, to wash stomach acids from the surface of the esophagus back into your stomach. Dr. Wright recommends looking for nonacidic or "alkaline" water, which can be found in many convenience stores.

Don't eat, then sleep. Heartburn tends to hit when you overeat and then lie down. Wait at least a couple of hours to go to sleep after eating, or take an H2 blocker before you go to bed on the nights you eat late.

Lift your head in bed. If heartburn wrecks your sleep, consider placing wooden or concrete blocks under the headboard of your bed. Raising the head of your bed 6 inches, so you're on an incline, makes it harder for stomach acid to reach the esophagus.

Call your doctor if your heartburn doesn't respond to healthy lifestyle changes and you pop over-the-counter heartburn remedies two or more times a week. You may have gastroesophageal reflux disease, which occurs when stomach acid flows backward from the stomach into the esophagus.

EASE CONSTIPATION

On our fiber-packed eating plan, constipation—the infrequent and/or difficult passage of stool—should resolve. But if it hasn't, check your meds. Lots of medications—including pain medications (especially narcotics), antacids that contain aluminum or calcium, antidepressants, and calcium channel blockers for high blood pressure and heart conditions—can turn bowels sluggish. Here's how to perk them up.

Go like clockwork. Hit the bathroom at the same time every day, preferably 15 to 45 minutes after breakfast. Eating stimulates movement in the colon.

Pop some prunes. There's a reason why these sticky snacks, aka dried plums, have long been the go-to for this issue: Prunes and prune juice contain sorbitol, a sugar alcohol that draws water into the small intestine and, in turn, makes it easier to go. People who ate 50 grams of dried plums every day for 3 weeks had more weekly bowel movements than those who simply upped their fiber intake, a study in the journal *Alimentary Pharmacology & Therapeutics* found. Five prunes a day ought to get the job done.

Sip two constipation-busting beverages. If you're not following our "water with every meal" guideline, consider this: In one study, low liquid consumption was a better predictor of constipation than low fiber intake. So drink up! Increasing your water consumption may be a simple way to get things moving. If heartburn isn't an issue, coffee can get things moving, too; caffeine can stimulate muscle activity in your colon. One cup should do the trick.

Try a kinder, gentler laxative. If a high-fiber diet and exercise don't lead to relief, taking a laxative is an option. But start with a milder one, such as Miralax, which draws water into the bowel and washes it out, rather than a stimulant laxative, which triggers bowel contractions.

Call your doctor if lifestyle changes don't help, you see blood in your stool, you're having serious stomach pains, or you're losing weight without trying.

Also make the call if you've had abdominal pain or discomfort at least three times a month for the last 3 months without any explanation. You may have IBS. A specific type, called IBS with constipation (IBS-C), is a common cause of constipation. IBS is treated with diet, probiotics, and medications. Sometimes talk therapy or mindfulness training is part of treatment, too, since IBS may have a psychological component, research suggests.

DEFLATE GAS AND BLOATING

Passing gas in public is bad enough, but it's even worse when gas causes painful cramps or explosions you can't control. These tips can help keep the lid on your digestive system.

Give up gas producers. Flip back to the Jumpstart plan (page 178) and refresh your memory on foods that can lead to gas and bloating. Giving up fizzy drinks and foods like cauliflower, broccoli, beans, and bran—which ferment in your gut—may help deflate you.

Cool it on the fruit. Fruits like apples, grapes, and watermelon (as well as certain vegetables, like asparagus, peas, and zucchini) are high in fructose, a naturally occurring sugar that's often poorly absorbed by the small intestine—resulting in abdominal pain, gas, and diarrhea. If you notice that fructose-rich fruits tend to give you the rumbles, opt for varieties that contain less of the stuff, like blueberries or strawberries.

Call your doctor if you're experiencing watery diarrhea and abdominal cramps or weight loss along with gas and bloating. You may have small intestinal bacterial overgrowth (SIBO), an increase in the number of bacteria (or a change in the type of bacteria) in the small intestine. SIBO is usually related to diseases or disorders that damage the digestive system or affect how it works, such as Crohn's disease or diabetes.

Stop Springing Leaks

About one in four women has experienced that embarrassing *Did I just . . . ?* moment when coughing, laughing, sneezing, or exercising. The main culprit: a weak pelvic floor, often caused by childbirth, extra pounds, and pelvic surgery or radiation treatments.

One proven fix: Kegel exercises, named for the physician who first promoted them more than 50 years ago. But targeting the right muscles can be tricky. The next time you have to pee, stop urinating midstream. Feel that? That's the area you want to target with Kegels. Start with 4 or 5 repetitions two or three times a day. When you start, try to hold the squeeze for 2 seconds and increase your hold time each week. (If you suffer from pelvic pain, Kegels may exacerbate it, so try the next option.)

Yoga may also be an effective (and relaxing) remedy, evidence suggests. In one study, women who participated in a yoga-therapy program for 6 weeks experienced a 66 percent decrease in their incontinence frequency. If leakage is a problem for you, do some of the simple yoga moves from that study—including Malasana, Legs Up the Wall, and Reclined Bound Angle at least three times a week for 30 minutes at a time. See page 318 for photos and the how-to.

Handle Hormonal Skin Problems

After 7 weeks of Dr. Jeannette Graf's skin-care routine, your complexion may feel softer and look glowier than it has in years. But two skin conditions that commonly hit in midlife, adult acne and rosacea, require extra care and sometimes the help of a dermatologist.

TREAT (AND PREVENT) ADULT ACNE

Pimples and crow's-feet, on the same face? Yes, it's possible. Adult-onset acne is most common among women going through menopause. "Perimeno-pausal acne tends to be more superficial than teenage acne, with drier skin as well as flushing and rosacea being common culprits," says Dr. Graf. Other causes include:

Fluctuating hormone levels. Around menopause, a spike in male hormones (androgens) relative to lower estrogen levels can raise oil production, which in turn can cause clogged pores where *P. acnes* bacteria can grow, leading to inflammation and blemishes.

Stress. When we're under chronic stress, our bodies produce more cortisol in addition to the androgens, stimulating the oil glands and hair follicles in the skin and leading to acne.

A family history of acne. Research suggests that some people may have a genetic predisposition for acne and are more likely to get adult acne.

To keep your skin calm, Dr. Graf recommends these strategies.

- Always remove your makeup before bed. We told you about this back in Week 1. If you haven't started doing it, see page 217.

- Don't pick or pop. Your skin will take longer to clear, and you increase the risk of scarring.

- If you typically break out on your forehead (say, under your bangs), carry astringent pads to wipe away sweat or excess oil, suggests Dr. Graf. Consider the styling products you use on your hair, as well.

- Along with following a plant-based diet with plenty of leafy greens, drink lots of water.

- If these tips don't quell breakouts, or if over-the-counter acne products aren't working, consider scheduling an appointment with a dermatologist, says Dr. Graf. "They can suggest prescription or in-office treatments that can be very helpful."

SOOTHE THE STING OF ROSACEA

Does your skin seem ruddier than it used to be? Or do your "breakouts" refuse to clear, no matter which pricey acne products you try? You may have rosacea, a chronic skin condition that causes a wide variety of skin issues—including bumps that resemble acne but aren't.

Rosacea typically begins after age 30 as redness on the cheeks, nose, chin, or forehead that comes and goes. Over time, the redness tends to linger, and visible blood vessels may appear. Left untreated, rosacea then progresses to bumps and pimples. Skin may also be very sensitive, or burn or sting.

Rosacea is most common in fair-skinned and menopausal women—indeed, hot flashes associated with menopause may bring on a flare-up.

If you suspect rosacea, don't ignore your symptoms. The condition can get worse over time, so consult a dermatologist if you suspect it. Dermatologists commonly recommend prescription antibiotics, topical (applied to the skin) medications, and light treatments, depending on the severity of the symptoms.

If you're diagnosed with rosacea, good management can help minimize flare-ups. Here's what to do.

Learn your triggers. Common ones include stress, alcohol (especially red wine), caffeine, extremely hot or cold temperatures, and spicy foods.

Apply sunscreen daily. Sun exposure breaks down the supportive structures, like collagen, around blood vessels, exacerbating redness. Sensitive skin often can't tolerate chemical UV blockers in some sunscreens, like avobenzone, but physical blockers, such as titanium dioxide and zinc oxide,

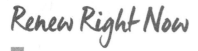
Renew Right Now

INSTANT GLOW

SMOOTH AWAY "CHICKEN SKIN." Regular use of a body scrub, which sloughs dead cells from the skin's surface, can help rub out keratosis pilaris, the rough, bumpy skin on the backs of your upper arms. KP is a buildup of dead cells around individual hair follicles. To keep follicles in the clear, use a lotion with an exfoliator, such as salicylic acid or alpha hydroxy acid, every day.

SLIMMER IN A MINUTE

CAMOUFLAGE WITH CARDIGANS. Slip a long cardigan over your blouse. Wispy, waterfall sweaters that are longer in front are particularly slimming. Make sure the sweater skims your midthigh and covers your butt but won't overwhelm your frame. (If you're tall, you can pull off a longer, more voluminous style.) Wear it open like a jacket to create a chic, lean line when worn with slim pants, a fitted sheath dress, or straight-leg jeans. If a cardigan feels too dowdy for a dress, Eva Scrivo suggests sporting a shrug, which is basically a small sweater with only the arms (dancers use it to keep warm but still be able to move freely).

protect without irritation. Dr. Graf recommends EltaMD sunscreen for patients with rosacea.

Select products for sensitive skin. The chemicals used in most skin-care products and makeup will irritate rosacea. While not chemical-free, products for sensitive skin usually have fewer and less-aggravating chemicals, like fragrances.

Do a test. Before you use any product on your face, try it on your neck first. If you have a reaction, avoid the product and note the ingredients.

To camouflage flare-ups, Scrivo recommends a green-tinted under-foundation concealer (see page 140). The green combines with any red in your face and neutralizes it completely.

Week 8

"I'm not just my husband's wife or my children's mother. I am me. Who do I want to be?"
— PANELIST SHERRY JUBOOR

STAY-YOUNG STEPS	GOALS	TO-DO LIST
EAT	Avoid menu ruts—find new ways to eat Clean & Green.	Push yourself to try a healthy food you've never tasted (daikon radish? kamut?). Dine out to celebrate your last week on the program and the start of your new, healthier life.
MOVE	Keep challenging your body to maximize results.	Push your intervals a little harder—cross the finish line with momentum! Try the Advanced Strength Workout, if you haven't yet graduated to it.
ENGAGE	Renew your spirit—find a get-happy strategy that can last.	Try one more new ENGAGE strategy, or go back to a favorite one. Complete your "after" profile and calculate how much younger you've grown in 2 months.
GLOW	Stay committed to your skin-care routine and get ready for your big reveal.	*Splurge!* Finally! Celebrate the new you with a transformative haircut and a more youthful hue.

Be Prepared!

- Book a salon day for your haircut and color, and gather magazine photos to show to your stylist.

- Make a doctor's appointment to retest your cholesterol and blood sugar, if you're tracking those things (and you didn't get to it last week).

- Snap an "after" photo and print it out (or post it to your Facebook profile).

The Finish Line Is in Sight!

Two months ago, you started this program for a reason. To recapture your old glow. Build up new reserves of energy and strength. Shore up failing health. Shake up a life that ran more on habit or obligation than on joy. Whatever your motivation, you've now reached the end of this path. But at the same time, you're on the brink of a whole new life—healthier, happier, with more perspective on where you've been and what you want next.

After this week, the program's training wheels come off, but it'll be okay. Even if you still have pounds to drop, you're ready to EAT, MOVE, ENGAGE, and GLOW solo. Because now you know that the "secret" of youth is no secret at all. It's all about eating nourishing foods, pushing yourself physically, taking care of yourself and others, and always setting new, fun, achievable goals.

This week, along with transforming your hairstyle (and perhaps color), you'll do your last assessment and learn how far you've come since Week 1. You'll also learn ways to keep the happiness you've reclaimed. Because it truly *is* in your hands. Experts attribute 50 percent of happiness to genetics and another 10 percent to circumstances like where we live, how much we earn, and how healthy we are. That leaves 40 percent of your happiness very much within your control—and that's major!

This week you'll add to the stash of happiness boosters already in your antiaging tool kit, like exercise and meditation. One science-backed fact: Our happiness increases when we do for others. But do go ahead and try our one last recommended splurge to remind yourself of how important it is to take time for yourself.

Get (and Stay) Happy for Good

You're on the runway to your "forever life"—renewed health, radiance, and positivity. So in this last week, give some thought to how you'll keep a welcome "side effect" of the plan: happiness.

When researchers who study positive psychology talk about happiness, they're referring to a sense of deep contentment. To achieve that, you can take three routes, and the most satisfied people pursue all three, according to happiness researchers.

One is the pleasant life, full of pleasure, joy, and good times. The second is the engaged life, in which you lose yourself to some passion or activity. And the third is the meaningful life; it may not have many high moments of bliss, but it is packed with purpose. Here are six ways to travel all three of these routes.

LEARN TO SAVOR LIFE, LIKE CHOCOLATE

You know how you enjoy every mouthful of a particularly delicious meal, from the first toast of wine to the last bite of dessert? Now try doing that with life itself. It's proven to boost happiness.

Here's some evidence: In a New Zealand study a few years back, researchers asked roughly 100 women and men to keep diaries for 30 days. They recorded "pleasant events" and how much they savored or squelched them. At the end of the study, savorers had recorded more pleasure because they stopped to focus on a good experience, tell someone else about it, or even scream or laugh in delight. Wet-blanket types killed the joy by carping that a given experience could have been better, that they didn't deserve it, or that it was almost over. Ultimately, adept savorers got the biggest happiness boost out of pleasurable moments.

The skill set for savoring is one part wild abandon (you hoot, holler, jump up and down) and one part wisdom (you stop to smell the roses while you can). Some of us are better at one part of that, some at the other. To hone your skills, plan a "savoring adventure"—a walk in the woods, a trip into a city, cooking a meal you love. Then do three things.

1. *Before* your experience, spend some time looking forward to how wonderful it will be.
2. During your adventure, focus on the sensations and emotions you're experiencing. Don't judge them; just feel them. If you're with someone, share what you're feeling. If you're alone, write them down when you get home.
3. *After* your savor-worthy experience, mine every detail. Share it with someone. Reminiscing is a key aspect of savoring.

Do you need to book hotels or overheat your Visa for this? Nope. You can adapt this strategy to what you might call mindful savoring. Simply give yourself permission to pause and get lost in the wonder and beauty of the moment.

CELEBRATE THANKSGIVING EVERY SINGLE DAY

Not with a meal—with gratitude. Studies have shown that 90 percent of people say expressing gratitude made them happier, and more than 75 percent said it reduced stress and depression and gave them more energy.

To start, make a conscious effort to thank people more often. When you've got that down, begin to count your blessings—literally—at least once a day for 30 seconds. Need some suggestions? Be thankful for your health, your food, your family, and friends. Once you start, you begin to feel thankful for things most people overlook—a glass of clean water from your tap, fresh berries on your oatmeal, even the big feet that carry you over streets and paths on your daily walk. (Be grateful you *can* walk!)

LET THE DUST SETTLE WHERE IT MAY

Yes, cobwebs on the walls and dust bunnies under the bed can be stressful. But so can housework when it's performed after-hours, a study published in the *Journal of Family Psychology* found. Researchers measured participants' cortisol levels—a marker of stress—as they did a variety of after-work activities (chores, TV, a walk). The more time women spent on folding laundry and cleaning, the less their cortisol levels recovered. So unless housework really lights you up, give your dust bunnies a temporary reprieve and go have some fun.

GO WITH YOUR FLOW

In the state of consciousness researchers call flow, you lose yourself in an activity that fully engages your mind and your creative juices. In this mind-set of intense focus—think athletes describing being "in the zone"—self-consciousness and distractions fade, and you "come to" hours later, refreshed and recentered.

Flow begets *duende*. To find yours, think beyond traditional R&R. Flow states typically involve some level of skill and a challenge that's stimulating but not frustrating. Flow states are highly individual, so let your personality be your guide. You might find flow as you plan and cultivate a garden, take photographs, hike, play chess, write, or knit.

GIVE OUT KINDNESS LIKE DAISIES

People who engage in kind gestures become happier over time. Why? When you're kind to others, you feel more moral, optimistic, and positive. Here are a baker's dozen of ways to do good for someone—and get happier in the process.

- Surprise a coworker with her favorite drink on your next coffee run.

- On the highway, let someone merge into your lane.

- Offer to stay late and help clean up at your friend's party.

- Smile and make eye contact with people in the grocery store.

- Pay the toll for the person in the car behind you.

- Babysit for your neighbor's kids while she takes a nap.

- Make small talk with the cashier at your dry cleaner.

- Let someone go ahead of you in line at the movies.

- Visit family members you haven't seen in a while.

- Volunteer to run an errand for a busy coworker.

- Drive a friend to the airport.

- Give someone a sincere compliment.

- Overtip your server.

MAKE YOUR OWN MEANING—AND LIVE IT EVERY DAY

One key conclusion from the science of happiness: Meaningful social connection is the surest way to improve our own health and well-being, as well as the world around us. In fact, a study conducted at the University of California at Los Angeles found that, compared to women who were less engaged, women who set out to lead a meaningful existence had greater activity among the natural killer cells their immune system produced to fight cancer.

In other words, if your life feels empty or lonely, make an impact in someone else's. Teach illiterate adults to read. Deliver Meals on Wheels to elderly people who can't leave their homes. Write a letter to your local paper about an issue you're passionate about. Or create your own personal mission—for example, to make everyone you meet, every day, feel special in some way. Slowly but surely your purpose will emerge, and your life will never be the same.

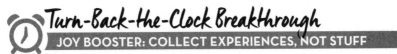

Turn-Back-the-Clock Breakthrough
JOY BOOSTER: COLLECT EXPERIENCES, NOT STUFF

What will make you happier, a new pair of shoes or a day trip? Bet you got this one right: Experiences, rather than objects, are actually more valuable and make us 51 percent happier than tangible material items, a study in the *Journal of Positive Psychology* found. ■

Final Self-Assessment

You've dreamed of this week: your last on the program. How do you look? How do you *feel*? You'll actually measure those qualities as you complete your last assessment. By Week 8, our panelists had trimmed an average of 1.67 inches (and as much as 3.5 inches) from their waists and had lost an average of 10 pounds (and as much as 25). As you can see from their "after" photos throughout the book, they've dropped years from their appearance.

If you chose to record your weight, measurements, and resting heart rate only, fill in today's numbers. If you took the optional blood pressure reading and cholesterol and blood-sugar tests, fill in those numbers, too. Then retake the "How Old Are You Today?" quiz (page 20), compare this score with your original score, and reflect on the questions below. If you're not quite where you want to be, press on. In our book, life isn't a marathon. It's a ride in a hot-air balloon—you never quite know where you'll land, but you sure do enjoy the view. Happy landings!

Week 8: Your "After" Profile

MEASURE THIS	MY RESULTS	WEEK 4	WEEK 1
Weight			
Waist measurement			
Hip measurement			
Waist–hip ratio			
Resting heart rate			
Body-fat percentage (optional)			

Total pounds lost: _____

Total inches lost: _____

Total percentage of body fat lost (optional): _____

Change in resting heart rate from Week 1 to Week 8: _____

Week 8: Your Numbers (Optional)

WHAT TO MEASURE	MY RESULTS	WEEK 4	WEEK 1
Total cholesterol			
Triglycerides			
HDL cholesterol			
LDL cholesterol			
Fasting blood glucose			
Blood pressure			

Change in total cholesterol and triglycerides from Week 1 to Week 8: _____

Changes in HDL/LDL cholesterol from Week 1 to Week 8: _____

Change in fasting blood glucose from Week 1 to Week 8: _____

Change in blood pressure from Week 1 to Week 8: _____

Your Quiz Results: Week 8

Retake the "How Old Are You Today?" quiz, which begins on page 20.

My score today: _____

My score in Week 4: _____

My score in Week 1: _____

What category did your score place you in today? _____

Personal Check-In

This is the time to reflect on the positive highlights of the program for you—and to brainstorm fresh strategies to keep your momentum. As you look back over the entire 8 weeks, answer the questions below (either on the page or in your journal) to see how far you've come since Week 1, and identify the changes that made the most impact.

1. What has been the most significant change you've experienced in these 8 weeks? Perhaps it's in your physical health (improvements in blood sugar, blood cholesterol, fitness level)? Your energy level or appearance? The way you've reconnected with your youthful dreams, goals, plans? List the most

dramatic change (or changes), and then jot down how they've helped you reclaim your younger self.

_____

_____

_____

_____

2. What single biggest challenge remains? Is it physical in nature, or does it stem from old thoughts, feelings, and beliefs about age? List a few ways you might tackle this challenge as you move forward.

_____

_____

_____

_____

3. Think back to the long-term goal you set in Week 4. Have you taken any steps toward achieving it? If not, list that first step here.

_____

_____

_____

_____

4. Have any negative views about age changed as you progressed through the program? Which negative views have you tossed out? Which positive views have you embraced?

_____

_____

_____

_____

5. Which guidelines and tips have you used most consistently? Jot them down. How have they helped you on your journey to age smart?

_____

_____

_____

_____

Splurge!

The Big Reveal—Salon Day

You've booked the appointment, leafed through tons of magazines, and pondered how daring you want to be. Now get ready for what we call "the big reveal": the end-of-program cut, color, and makeup session that totally transforms your appearance.

We planned this splurge at the end of the program for a reason. Whether you've lost weight, improved your skin, or are rocking a new inner confidence, it's *now* that a new look will make maximum impact. Besides, this last splurge is more than a treat. It's an event—a celebration of your hard work and dedication. You earned it.

Before you head out, keep these tips in mind.

- Bring the photos of the styles you've picked out so your stylist can see what you're going for. For guidance, review Eva Scrivo's four antiaging cuts in the GLOW chapter on pages 128–130.

- If you've decided on hair color, flip back to GLOW and review the sections on selecting the perfect color and formulation for you— temporary, demi-permanent (for less than 50 percent gray), and permanent (for more than 50 percent gray).

- Read up on highlights, too. Even if you've decided against all-over color, a few subtle highlights around your face may light up your complexion. Ask your colorist what she thinks.

- While you're at it, consider getting a professional makeup lesson (many salons offer it upon request). You can read more about what you'll get out of that experience on page 143 of GLOW; if ever there was a moment to go for it, it's now. Otherwise, bring your makeup bag to the salon so you can use the techniques you've been practicing over the last 8 weeks to put your best face forward.

- Want even more inspiration? Turn the page for a look at the amazing transformations that Scrivo performed on five of our test panelists.

Five Women, Transformed

There's no better way to kick off your Second Act than with a professional makeover. We whisked five of our panelists to New York City for their big reveal, courtesy of Eva Scrivo Salons. Scrivo, who worked with her team for an entire day, transformed the panelists' "befores" into these stunning "afters." "All of them were in awe of the process, which featured a precision cut, corrective color, and makeup," Scrivo says. We hope their changes inspire you to throw the new you a similarly dramatic "coming-out party."

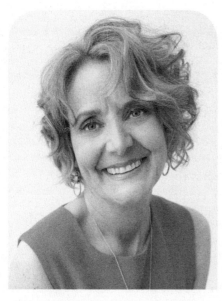

KATHY MCCARTHY
(see page 232 for the "before")

Haircut: McCarthy's beautiful cheekbones, small nose, and well-defined jaw made her a great candidate for short hair. Her new style—cut in a graduated layering pattern—builds height in the crown and removes bulk around the nape of her neck. The shorter style also brings out her hair's natural wave.

Hair color: McCarthy's medium-brown box color was too dark and made her skin look pale and tired. A demi-permanent golden light brown allows some of her natural grays to peek through; highlights catch the light and help illuminate her face. McCarthy's eyebrows got a makeover, too. As brows fade, a woman loses the framing of her eye, which makes her look older. Dyeing McCarthy's brows two shades darker than her natural brow coloring makes her eyes look larger and brighter.

Makeup: While balancing her hair color brightens McCarthy's light-to-medium skin, bronzer, peachy-pink lipstick, and rose blush warm it even more. Taupe shadow and dark-brown liquid eyeliner enhance her blue eyes.

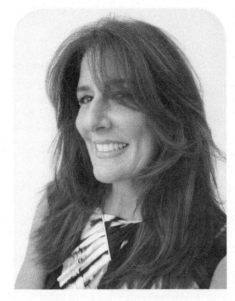

SANDY FRANKLIN

(see page 116 for the "before")

Haircut: Franklin has beautiful hair—thick and slightly coarse—but its length was dragging down her face. Cutting 4 to 6 inches of length returned its bounce, while triangular layers added height at the top of her head, and bangs helped to direct the eye upward. To add even more fullness, her hair was styled using a jumbo round brush.

Hair color: Franklin's natural dark-brown hair was almost black from years of at-home color buildup, and its intense hue made her skin look pale. To warm her skin, her overall color was lightened to chestnut brown, and highlights were added to catch even more light and enhance the shape of the cut. Because Franklin's hair tends to frizz, a salon-smoothing treatment, Goldwell's Kerasilk, was used to smooth the hair's cuticle and add shine.

Makeup: Franklin's sallow skin needed a warmer makeup palette. Bronze eye shadow and a chocolate-brown eye pencil give her eyes definition. Her brows were shaped for more lift and dyed two shades darker.

LISA BOLAND

(see page 148 for the "before")

Haircut: The length of Boland's hair concealed its slight wave and made it flat on top. The solution was to cut 4 inches of length and add square-shaped layers (which give midlength styles an edginess) as well as fullness on the sides and height on top. This style also slims Boland's face, and the bangs balance her tall, strong frame.

Hair color: Boland's too-light color washed out her porcelain skin. Highlights and lowlights create dimension and add fullness, while an overall glaze resulted in a warmer blonde, the perfect tone for her pale skin.

Makeup: Boland's makeup draws attention to her large eyes and full lips. Because longer bangs can hide the eyes, a dark, smoky eye—a combination of midnight-blue and black eye shadow—puts them in the spotlight. However, longer, softer bangs also emphasize a woman's mouth, and a bright, rich, blue-based red lipstick plays up Boland's lips. Darkening her eyebrows completes her transformation.

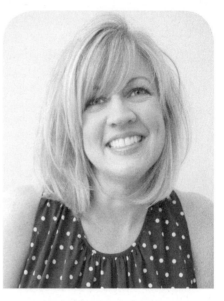

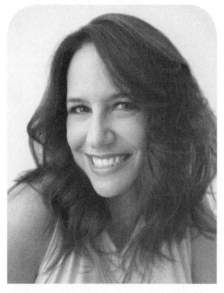

KATE PELHAM-HAMBLY
(see page 62 for the "before")

Haircut: Pelham-Hambly wanted to keep her straight hair on the longer side. This "lob," or long bob (a flattering midlength style), was cut to 2 inches below her collarbone. Soft square layers give her hair a modern shape while keeping an overall one-length feeling. A 1.5-inch barrel curling iron was used to style her hair, adding wave and bounce.

Hair color: Pelham-Hambly's dark-brown/black box color was washing out her skin, which has yellow undertones. A deep, warm auburn with copper highlights adds radiance to her skin and brings pink to her cheeks.

Makeup: The pale pinks and other blue-based colors she favored did not flatter her light olive complexion. A foundation a shade darker than her own and a deeper blush with brown undertones brightens and warms her skin, while a combination of bronzer and shimmer further defines her bone structure. To give her makeup a youthful feel, Pelham-Hambly is wearing a catlike eyeliner in a deep brown/black, some individual lashes, and a shimmery lavender gloss on top of a deep rose (not too blue) lipstick.

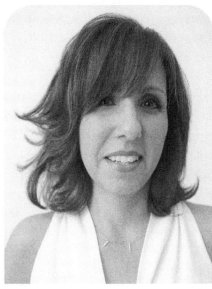

VESTA ACKERNECHT
(see page 328 for the "before")

Haircut: Ackernecht usually wore her naturally wavy hair pinned up because she didn't like the way it looked down. This is usually the case when a woman is searching for height at the crown but fears going shorter. Cutting 3 to 4 inches of length and giving her triangular layers builds more fullness into the sides and crown. The deep side-bang creates softness around her face and strengthens her cheekbones.

Hair color: Scrivo formulated a rich medium chestnut brown base color and cinnamon-toned highlights. She then added a glaze to further blend the highlights and add shine.

Makeup: A palette of warm browns, cinnamon bronzer, and rose-toned blush warms Ackernecht's sallow skin and balances its green/olive undertone, while a deep cherry lip color gives her skin an overall glow. A smoky eye makeup of midnight blue and chocolate brown brings out the depth of her eyes, and a few individual false lashes applied to the center of her eyes make them appear larger.

The End of One Journey, the Start of Another

After a recent spin class, at the beginning of her stretch session, Sandy Franklin tried to touch her nose to her knee—and, for the first time ever, succeeded. Eight weeks before, "they were 2 feet apart!" she says.

We hope your trajectory included similar "I did it!" moments. When you're young, life has lots of them, and it's likely that you're ending the plan feeling a whole lot better than when you began—not just in body, but in spirit.

Eight weeks ago, you hoped for a slimmer body, a flatter belly, improvements in your health and appearance. Then you converted that hope into action. Every healthy food choice made and exercise session kept, every step outside your comfort zone taken, every goal set and met—those successes are all you.

And if your journey turned out like our panelists' did, you got more than you bargained for. A renewed sense of purpose and positivity. A return of that "damn-I-feel-amazing" morning energy that stays with you all day. A sense that your health and happiness matter, and that there really are second acts and second chances.

Perhaps you have come to honor where you've been and are homing in on where you want to go. With every healthy choice made, you learned that age is just a number, and youth a gift you can give to yourself.

At some point in the program, Lisa Boland stopped being so hard on herself when she looked in the mirror. "What I discovered is that when I appreciate where I am now and take pride in each little achievement, I am more inspired to work to get where I want to be, physically and emotionally," she says. "It's so much easier for me to make good choices when I make them out of love for myself."

Our panelists' consistent self-care had far-reaching benefits.

"I remember looking in the mirror and saying, 'Welcome back, Cindy,'" said panelist Cindy Hafner at the end of the program. Ann Raines discovered a seemingly inexhaustible reserve of energy—"I feel fueled to accomplish the near-impossible." Sharon Scheirer, who survived breast cancer years ago but lost the sense that she directed her life, regained that take-charge attitude. "I'm back in the driver's seat and responsible for my well-being, life, and destiny," she says.

Now, so are you. Do tomorrow what you did today, and strive to exceed it. If you stray off-course, the Stay-Young Steps will lead you back. On this path,

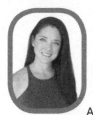

Dr. Vonda Wright says . . .

KEEP THE GREATNESS GOING!

You made it! I'm thrilled for you, and I hope to hear all about your amazing gains and plans for your Second Act adventures. (Connect with me at vondawright.com or via e-mail at Vonda@vondawright.com.)

Now you're at a crossroads: You can keep going, or you can stop. I know which path I'd take. So do you. To keep the physical gains you've made and press forward, I suggest a few options.

1. Intensify Weeks 4 to 8 of the workout routine—add an extra set of exercises, perform them a little longer. Strive for one more interval, one more set, even one more repetition.

2. Take your new exercise confidence public, and join an exercise class or running club.

3. Try the 6-month plan in my second book, *Dr. Vonda Wright's Guide to THRIVE*, or the "20 Minutes to BURN" exercise series in my third book, *Fitness after 40*.

How to keep your inner gains—your newfound self-confidence, joy, and hunger for new experiences? Again, I have a suggestion: Make a "life list."

Remember the exercise I described earlier in which I had started to keep a list of everything I'd done this decade? You could do something similar in order to reflect on the last 8 weeks. Read through your journal, if you've been keeping one during the plan, and reflect on what you loved, what worked, what you'd still like to improve on. Use these to set goals for the next 8 weeks. Then, keep up the list. It's a simple way to continually engage yourself and shape the rest of your life.

I plan my Second Act every day, even as I take my first steps into it. My goal is to move toward it in a mindful and purposeful way and embrace it fully. You can do that, too. The first step is to keep the gains you've made. The second is to strive to surpass them.

there's no going back, only forward. "Until my last breath, I'll be eating healthy, moving, glowing, and engaging in life," Franklin says. "This is my life now." May it be yours, too.

SUCCESS!

Jen Casper, 36

MY STORY No, we didn't forget to list Jen Casper's weight loss. And, yes, she did lose weight. We are respecting Jen's decision to not know what the number on the scale is. When Jen's weight started to fluctuate during the first weeks of the program, she hid her scale under her bed and hasn't taken it out since. "It's the best thing I ever did," she said. "If you get hung up on a number, you're missing the beauty of the journey."

This was a big turning point for Jen. As a spiritual guide and intuitive coach, Jen empowers others to redefine and recreate their lives so they can begin living their dreams. Until she started the Younger in 8 Weeks Plan, she wasn't doing this for herself. "I'm always putting others first," she said. "My needs—whatever they were—were not being met."

When Jen stopped engaging with the number on the scale, she was better able to engage with herself, figure out her needs, and start to meet them. She started blocking off Fridays. One week, she gifted herself a massage. Another Friday, she slept in and stayed in her pj's until noon. "By setting boundaries and doing more for me, I love me more," she said.

That attitude has allowed her to stop being so hard on herself and start appre-

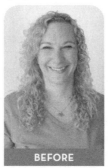

BEFORE

ciating her body. When Jen slipped on the fun exercise clothes she'd bought to inspire her to be more active, she didn't like what she saw. But instead of beating herself up, she shifted her thinking to, "I do look okay, but what if I looked better?" She reminded herself she'd have to work at it. Then she went for a walk with her 10-year-old daughter and fiancé. That was the beginning of her walking habit.

Jen also found that she started to eat intuitively. "I'm more aware of foods that don't do well for my body," she said. Instead of fast food and takeout, she discovered that she likes food better when she prepares it—this coming from the woman who used to be "allergic to the kitchen." Now she's craving foods like steel-cut oatmeal with fruit and nuts, yogurt, apples with almond butter; she even likes salmon now, which had long been on her yuck list. "By being grateful for my body, for feeding it what it needs, it gives me more back," Jen said. "I am getting stronger, braver, and pushing past my ceiling of limitations."

And she's celebrating every little victory along the way. "I wiggled out of my jeans without unzipping them. I'm buying smaller bras. That is more awesome than any number on the scale."

Beauty styling: makeup, Colleen Kobrick; hair, Missy Kovato; Wardrobe styling: Pamela Simpson

LOOK AT ME

- Lowered high blood glucose level **14 points into the healthy range**

- Reduced blood pressure **18 points**

- Shrank two sizes

- Inches lost: **8.75**

Tip

GET OUT OF YOUR WAY.
Your attitude, your mind-set, and your desire to create a new life are what stand between your today and your tomorrow.

PART

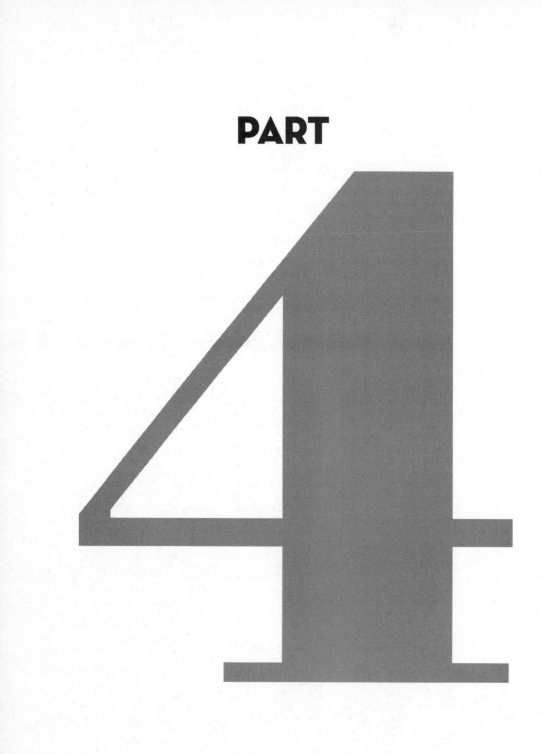

THE YOUNGER IN 8 WEEKS WORKOUT

Getting Started

I t's time to get a MOVE on! Our muscle-building, metabolism-boosting workout—which includes routines for cardio, strength training, flexibility, and balance—will help you slim down and tone up so you look and feel amazing.

Working out regularly will help you stay on plan, too. Many of our panelists said exercise helped curb their cravings, or reduced their stress so they didn't eat to feel better. Invite a friend to join you and reap the benefits of *two* Stay-Young Steps: ENGAGE and MOVE. Don't let the I-can't-do-its stop you. Perfection isn't the goal—consistency is. Sooner than you think, the moves will be second nature and your body will show it.

A reminder: We ramp things up slowly—starting with just a little stretching in the morning to help you ease your body into action. If morning isn't convenient, do these stretches any time of day—in the afternoon for a midday tension release or in the evening to unwind. Do them regularly and you'll start to feel tension and achy joints melt away. If the exercises seem too easy, feel free at any point to add exercises from the following week(s). You can even skip straight to the Advanced Workout in Week 8. The more you put into your workout, the more you'll get out of it.

Before you begin, it's worth skimming Weeks 1 through 8 so you have a clear idea of how the plan progresses and as a reminder of the equipment you'll need. Now, let's start moving!

WORKOUT	HOW-TO	DURATION	FREQUENCY
Sunrise Stretch	See below	5–10 min.	Daily

Sunrise Stretch

Some people can bounce right out of bed as if they were hooked up to an IV coffee drip overnight. If you're not one of them, try this short stretch routine for a decaffeinated morning energy surge—plus, you can do all of these moves in your pj's. Also, make sure to do these exercises barefoot.

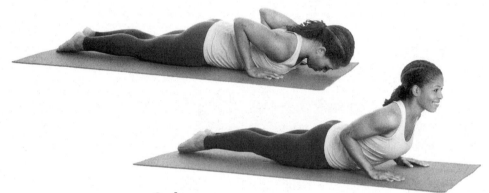

Cobra

Lie facedown with your hands on either side of your rib cage and your forehead resting on the bed (if you have a firm mattress) or floor. With your legs together and toes pointed, press the tops of your feet into the bed or floor and reach back through your toes, lengthening your legs. Evenly press into your hands as you draw your elbows close to your rib cage.

Using your back (not your arms), lift your head and chest off the bed or floor. As you lift, slide your shoulder blades down your back, creating as much space as possible between your ears and shoulders.

Hold as you take three to five long, deep, even breaths. Then gently lower, turning your head to one side. Do this move two or three times. (If you prefer, you can do more repetitions, holding for only one or two breaths.)

Make it easier: **Keep your elbows and forearms on the floor and hold in that position. Your elbows should be beneath your shoulders.**

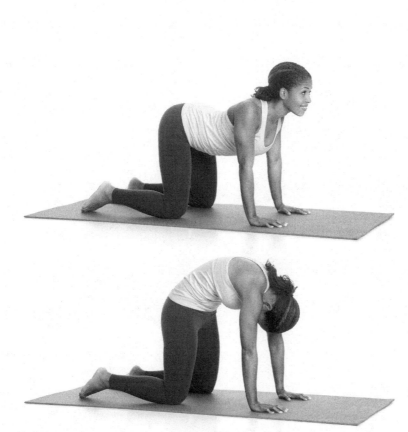

Cow/Cat

Get on all fours on your bed or floor. Place your hands beneath your shoulders and knees under your hips. Keep your spine neutral, your head in line with your spine, and your eyes on the bed or floor, a few feet in front of you.

Inhale as you look up, lifting your tailbone toward the ceiling and dropping your belly toward the floor so your back arches slightly. Keep your shoulder blades down, your chest lifted, and your shoulders open.

Then, exhale as you round your back, pulling your belly button in toward your spine, dropping your chin toward your chest, and tucking your tailbone.

Repeat, alternating between Cow and Cat about 10 to 15 times.

Make it easier: **Make the movement smaller so you are not arching and rounding your back as much. You can also do this move while standing with your hands on your bed or a dresser.**

Sunrise Stretch (cont.)

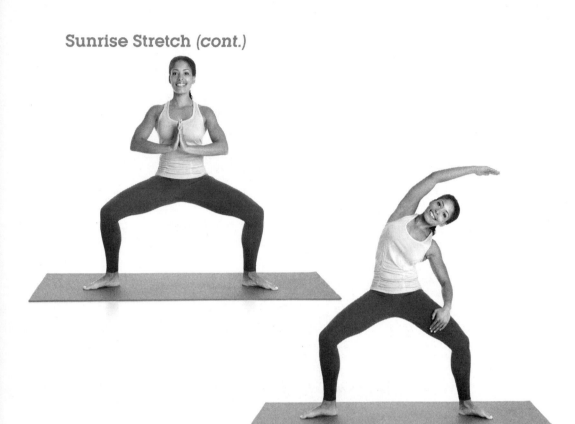

Squat & Reach

Start with your feet wider than shoulder width, toes turned slightly out. Bend your knees and lower into a squat with your palms pressed together like you're in prayer. Hold for three to five deep breaths.

Slowly straighten your legs halfway to a standing position, reaching your right arm overhead as you lean slightly to the left. Keep your hips facing forward, and don't allow them to turn as you reach over-head. Hold for three to five deep breaths.

Lower to a wide-stance squat with palms together. Hold for three to five deep breaths.

Slowly straighten your legs to a standing position, reaching your left arm overhead as you lean slightly to the right. Keep your hips facing forward. Hold for three to five deep breaths

Repeat this entire series at least once more. (If you prefer, you can do more repetitions, holding for only one or two breaths.)

Make it easier: **Bend your knees only about halfway so you are not squatting so low.**

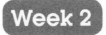

Week 2

WORKOUT	HOW-TO	DURATION	FREQUENCY
Sunrise Stretch	page 288	5–10 min.	Daily
Dynamic Warmup	see below	5–10 min.	2–3 days
Cardio (steady-paced)	page 295	10–20 min.	2–3 days

This week you'll start to get into the habit of warming up to prepare your body for activity. Take a few minutes before starting your walk or treadmill session to do the Dynamic Warmup, which will prep cold muscles and increase your range of motion and flexibility during your workout. These four moves will take just 5 to 10 minutes.

This week, you'll also begin to do some easy cardio. (If you already do regular cardio workouts, just continue with your current routine.) The goal is mainly to get up off the couch or away from your desk 2 or 3 times a week and just move. You can walk, bike, dance, or use cardio equipment—any activity you'd like. Do it for 10 to 20 minutes at a moderate intensity, or a 4 or 5 out of 10 on a Rate of Perceived Exertion (RPE) scale (page 71)—meaning you should still be able to carry on a conversation as you exercise. Finish by slowing your pace for 3 to 5 minutes to cool down.

Dynamic Warmup

These moves will get your muscles ready for action! Perform them in order before each cardio and/or strength workout. If you are doing cardio and strength workouts back-to-back, you only need to do the Dynamic Warmup one time at the start of your session.

To make any of these moves easier, perform them using a small range of motion. For example, don't twist as far or don't swing your leg as high.

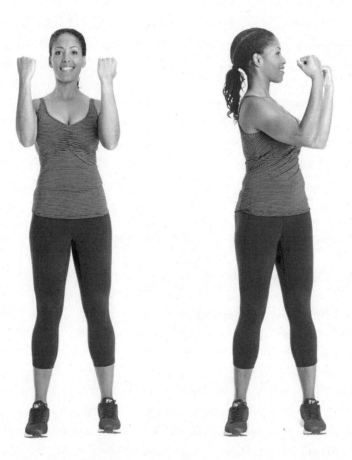

Trunk Rotation

Stand with your feet hip-width apart and your arms bent in front of your chest, like a boxer. Slowly twist your torso to the left and then the right. That's 1 rep. Do 10 reps.

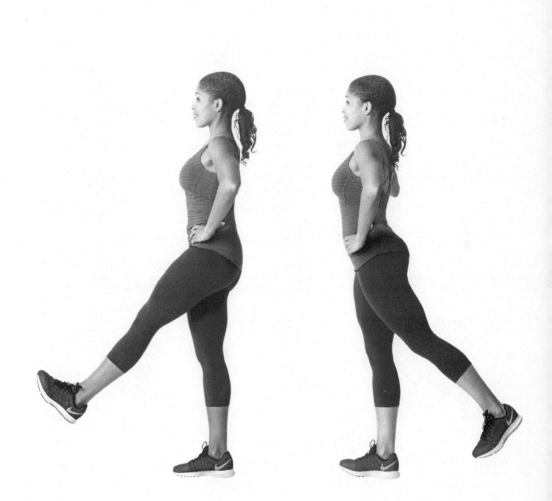

Leg Swing

Stand next to a wall or chair and lightly hold onto it with your right hand for balance. With your left foot flexed, swing your left leg forward and back. That's 1 rep. Keep your toes pointed forward and lift up out of your pelvis so your foot doesn't hit the floor as you swing. Do 10 reps with each leg.

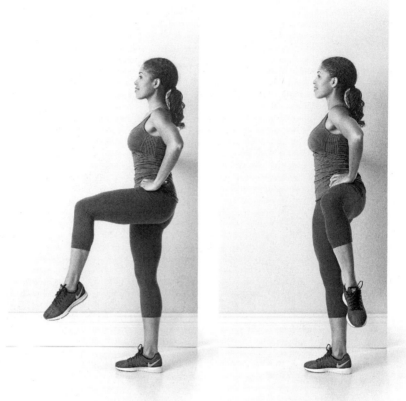

Hip Rotation

Stand with your feet together and lightly hold on to a wall or chair for balance.

Raise your left leg up in front of your body to hip height. Engage your core to steady your balance. Then rotate your leg out to the right and back in a circle. (Imagine you are drawing a circle with your knee.) Do 10 circles and then repeat with your right leg.

Switch legs again and do 10 more circles with each leg in the opposite direction. (Raise your left leg up to the side and rotate forward.) Repeat with your right leg.

The Activator

Standing with your feet hip-width apart, slowly bend from the hips and place your hands on the floor a few inches from your feet.

Walk your hands out to the pushup position. Your body should form a straight line from your heels to your head. Then walk your feet in toward your hands as close as possible. That's 1 rep. Continue by walking your hands out and then walking your feet in toward your hands. Do 8 reps.

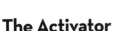 *Make it easier:* **You can bend your knees if needed to get your hands on the floor.**

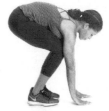

Cardio

Easy does it! Do any cardio you like (walk, run, bike, swim) at a moderate pace for 10 to 12 minutes.

Week 3

WORKOUT	HOW-TO	DURATION	FREQUENCY
Sunrise Stretch	page 288	5–10 min.	Daily
Dynamic Warmup (before cardio)	page 291	5–10 min.	3–5 days
Cardio (intervals and steady-paced)	see below	20–30 min.	3–5 days
Flexibility stretches (after cardio)	page 298	5 min.	3–5 days
Optional: Foam rolling	page 300	5–15 min.	as needed

This week, you're going to build your endurance by upping your total cardio sessions to 3 to 5 days and intensifying your workout with cardio intervals on 2 or 3 of those days (for a total of no more than 5 days).

You'll also start doing the flexibility stretches after every cardio session (and eventually after your strength sessions, starting next week).

Finally, if tight muscles or pain are an issue for you, try the optional foam-roller routine. You can roll one or two pain points before a workout to loosen them up or afterward to prevent soreness. It feels amazing and will help your body recover.

Interval Cardio

Interval workouts alternate between bouts of high-intensity activity to get your heart rate up and lower-intensity activity to recover. You can do intervals with any type of cardio exercise, such as walking, running, using the elliptical, biking, or swimming. These workouts are separated into beginner, intermediate, and advanced options.

Start with the Level 1 option (unless you're regularly exercising and doing a cardio workout already). After 2 weeks (and if you feel ready), move to Level 2. If you feel ready to move to the Level 3 option anytime after Week 4, go ahead. It's best to be conservative when you start a new workout and build your way up slowly. (See the MOVE chapter for methods of evaluating how hard you're working out to ensure that you get the best results possible.)

Level 1: Beginner

TIME	ACTIVITY	RPE*
5 min.	Warmup	2–3
10 min.	Moderate	4–5
9 min.	Intervals (1 min. hard, 2 min. easier) 3 times	6–7 hard 4–5 easy
6 min.	Cooldown	2–3
Total Time: 30 min.		

* RPE refers to Rate of Perceived Exertion, the level of effort you feel on a scale of 1 to 10. See page 71 for how to measure it.

Level 2: Intermediate

TIME	ACTIVITY	RPE*
5 min.	Warmup	2–3
8 min.	Moderate	4–5
12 min.	Intervals (1 min. hard, 2 min. easier) 4 times	6–7 hard 4–5 easy
5 min.	Cooldown	2–3
Total Time: 30 min.		

* RPE refers to Rate of Perceived Exertion, the level of effort you feel on a scale of 1 to 10. See page 71 for how to measure it.

Level 3: Advanced

TIME	ACTIVITY	RPE*
5 min.	Warmup	2–3
8 min.	Moderate	4–5
12 min.	Intervals (90 sec. hard, 90 sec. easier) 4 times	6–7 hard 4–5 easy
5 min.	Cooldown	2–3
Total Time: 30 min.		

* RPE refers to Rate of Perceived Exertion, the level of effort you feel on a scale of 1 to 10. See page 71 for how to measure it.

Flexibility Stretches

The best time to stretch to increase flexibility is after a workout, when your muscles are warm and pliable. Perform these moves after every cardio and strength workout. If you're doing cardio and strength workouts back-to-back, you only need to do the flexibility stretches one time at the end of your session.

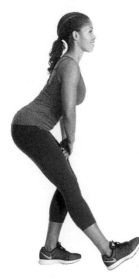

Standing Hamstring Stretch

TARGETS: Back of thighs

Extend your right leg out in front of you with only your heel on the floor and your toes up toward your shin. Bend your left knee slightly, sit back, and lean forward slightly, keeping your chest lifted. Don't lock your right knee. Hold for 30 seconds. Repeat on the other side.

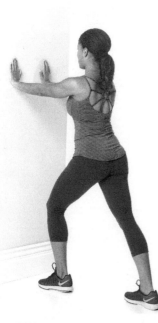

Standing Calf Stretch

TARGETS: Calves

Stand facing a wall and place your hands on the wall at about chest height. Put your right foot about 12 to 18 inches behind you and bend your left knee. Make sure your feet are pointing straight ahead. Lean forward as if you are trying to bring your hips toward the wall while pressing your right heel into the floor. Hold for 30 seconds. Repeat on the other side.

Quad Stretch

TARGETS: Front of thighs and hips

Rest your right hand on a table, chair, or wall for support. Bend your left knee, bringing your left foot toward your buttocks. Hold your foot with your left hand (or use a strap or belt if you can't reach your foot). Aim your bent knee straight down toward the floor and tuck your pelvis. Hold for 30 seconds. Repeat with your right leg.

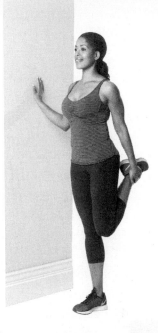

Chest Stretch

TARGETS: Chest and arms

Stand in a doorway with your legs staggered. Stretch your arms out to the sides, elbows bent, and place your forearms and palms on the doorframe. Lean forward to feel a stretch in your chest and arms. Hold for 30 seconds.

Back Stretch

TARGETS: Upper, middle, and lower back muscles

Lie on your back with your legs bent, feet on the floor. Bring your knees toward your chest and grasp them with your hands. Pull them in until you feel a stretch. If you'd like more of a stretch, tuck your chin in and slowly bring your head up to meet your knees. Hold for 30 seconds.

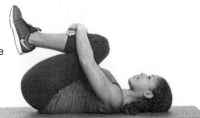

Foam-Roller Routine

Not only will foam rolling help ease your aches and pains, but it will also help you work out better and longer—and it will help keep you injury-free. You can roll out any problem areas before exercise to reduce muscle fatigue or afterward, as part of your cooldown, to limit soreness. Each week, if you wish, aim to do this 15-minute foam-roller routine a minimum of two or three times. If you find an area of increased discomfort during any of these foam-roller exercises, pause for 15 to 20 seconds on the hot spot.

Foam rollers are pretty easy to find these days. Most sporting-goods and big-box stores sell them, and they usually cost $20 to $30. While foam rollers come in many sizes, it's best to get a longer one (about 36 inches) so it gives you enough coverage. The harder the roller, the more intense the pressure on the muscle, so for those just starting out, try a softer roller first. (Note that for the last rolling exercise, you'll need a tennis ball.)

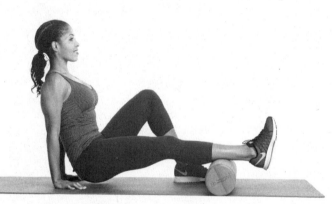

Calf Roll

TARGETS: Calves

Sit on the floor with your left knee bent, your left foot flat on the floor, and your right leg extended so your calf is resting on the foam roller. Lift your butt and shift your weight forward and back to move the roller up and down your calf. Make sure not to go past your ankle or too close to the back of your knee (and never roll over a joint, only muscle). Continue rolling for 30 to 60 seconds. If you find a spot of increased pain or discomfort, pause on that area and rotate your ankle. Switch sides and repeat. (Alternate position: You can also do this move with both legs extended, rolling both calves at the same time if you'd prefer.)

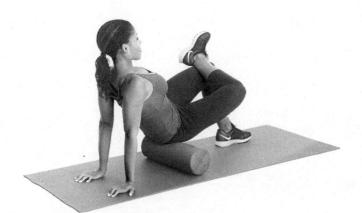

Hip Rotator Roll

TARGETS: Glutes, outer thighs, and hips

Sit on the foam roller with your knees bent, feet flat on the floor. Lean your torso back and place your right hand on the floor, shifting your weight into your right hip and crossing your right ankle over your left thigh. Place your left hand on your left thigh, or keep both hands on the floor if that's more comfortable. Use your supporting foot and hand to roll from the bottom of your glutes to your pelvic bone. Keep rolling back and forth for 30 to 60 seconds. Switch sides and repeat.

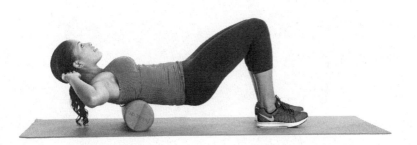

Upper Back Roll

TARGETS: Upper back, rear shoulders, and chest

Lie on the floor with your knees bent, your feet flat on the floor, and the foam roller positioned under your upper back. Place your hands behind your head. Roll from the upper part of your back to your mid-back, being careful not to roll onto your neck or lower back. Continue rolling back and forth for 30 to 60 seconds.

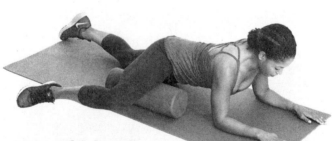

Quad Roll

TARGETS: Quads

Start in a forearm plank position with your quads (tops of thighs) resting on the foam roller. Starting at the top of your quads, move the roller up and down your thighs, making sure to stop about 2 inches before the hip and knee joints. Continue rolling back and forth for 30 to 60 seconds.

Inner Thigh Roll

TARGETS: Inner thighs and hips

Lie facedown with the inside of your right thigh resting on the foam roller. Keeping your core tight, move the roller back and forth along your inner thigh, stopping a few inches before you reach the knee. Continue rolling back and forth for 30 to 60 seconds. Switch sides and repeat. If you find an area of increased discomfort, pause for 15 to 20 seconds on the hot spot, flexing your foot, straightening your knee slightly, and rotating your hip to work that area.

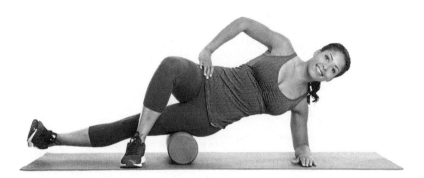

IT Band Roll

TARGETS: IT band and outer quadriceps

Lie on your left side and place your left hip on the foam roller. Put your hands on the floor for support, if needed, or on a hip if you can balance. Cross your right leg over your left, with your right foot flat on the floor. Roll your body toward your left arm until the roller reaches your knee. Then roll back and forth for 30 to 60 seconds. Switch sides and repeat. If this becomes too easy over time, place your supporting leg on top of the other instead of bracing it on the floor.

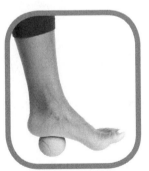

Roll Your Soles

TARGETS: Soles of the feet

While standing next to a wall or chair for stability, place a ball underneath the arch of your foot. Slowly roll your foot from side to side so the ball crosses your arch. Then roll the ball along the length of your foot from heel to toe. Roll for 1 to 2 minutes. Repeat on the other foot.

This exercise requires a tennis or golf ball instead of a foam roller.

Weeks 4 to 7

WORKOUT	HOW-TO	DURATION	FREQUENCY
Sunrise Stretch	page 288	5–10 min.	Daily
Dynamic Warmup (before cardio and/or strength)	page 291	5–10 min.	3–7 days
Cardio (intervals and steady-paced)	page 295	20–30 min.	3–5 days
Strength training	page 305	10–15 min.	2–3 days
Flexibility stretches (after cardio and/or strength)	page 298	5 min.	3–7 days
Optional: Foam rolling	page 300	5–15 min.	3–7 days
Optional: Balance	page 316	5 min.	3–7 days
Optional: Yoga	page 318	5 min.	3–7 days

Now you're going to add the final element of the workout program—strength training. This week, you'll start with four basic moves. Over the next 3 weeks, you'll add two new moves to your routine each week—if you're ready. You can always repeat a week once or twice if you need more time to feel comfortable with the exercises before moving on.

If you already strength train or need a greater challenge, you can add moves to your workouts more quickly. If that still isn't enough, try the Advanced Strength Workout on page 320.

There are also some optional routines that will be introduced over the next few weeks. If you're not as steady on your feet as you'd like to be, you can improve your stability by doing the optional balance routine in Week 5. And in Week 7, there's an optional yoga routine that you may be interested in if you suffer from incontinence—or would simply like some relaxing postures.

Strength Training

Do the Dynamic Warmup before it and flexibility stretches after it. Strength can be done on cardio days.

Here are a few things to keep in mind as you start your strength-training routine.

- The word *rep* is short for repetition. Each time you lift and lower a dumbbell or roll your upper body off the floor and then back down, you've completed 1 repetition. A specific number of repetitions is called a *set*.

- The amount of weight you start with depends on how fit you are. If you can breeze through a set without fatigue, your weights are too light. The last 2 or 3 reps should be difficult to do with perfect form. If you can't keep proper form at any point, you should move to a lighter weight. You may need different weight amounts for different exercises—and as you progress over the weeks, you should increase the weight gradually if those last couple of reps start to feel too easy. Beginners might start with 3- to 5-pound weights; for those who already do weight training, 5 to 8 or 10 pounds might be a better range.

- Perform the moves slowly and with focus. Take 3 seconds to lift or push a weight into place, hold the position for 1 second, and take another 3 seconds to return to your starting position.

- Don't hold your breath. This can cause changes in blood pressure, especially for people with heart disease. Rather, inhale slowly through your nose and exhale slowly through your mouth.

- Exhale as you lift or push, and inhale as you relax.

- Use smooth, steady movements. To prevent injury, don't jerk or thrust weights into position or lock your knees and elbows.

- Take a day of rest between workouts so that your muscles have time to repair themselves.

Week 4: Strength Training

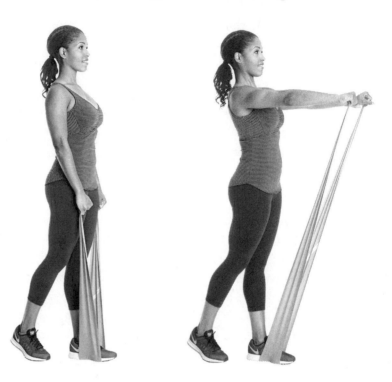

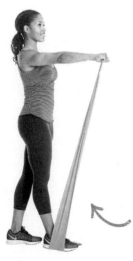

Forward Flexion

Stand tall with your feet staggered. Place the center of the band under your front foot, and hold each end with your hands down by your thighs, palms facing you.

Keeping a slight bend in your elbows, slowly raise your arms up to shoulder height, palms facing the floor.

Pause at the top before slowly lowering back to the starting position.

Do two sets of 10 reps, resting 60 seconds between sets.

No resistance band? You can substitute dumbbells or water bottles.

Make it easier: **Hold only one end of the band and adjust it under your foot so you have more slack. Then do the reps one arm at a time.**

Make it harder: **Slide your hands down the band so it's shorter, providing more resistance. Or use a stronger resistance band or dumbbells (so that the last 2 reps are hard but doable with perfect form).**

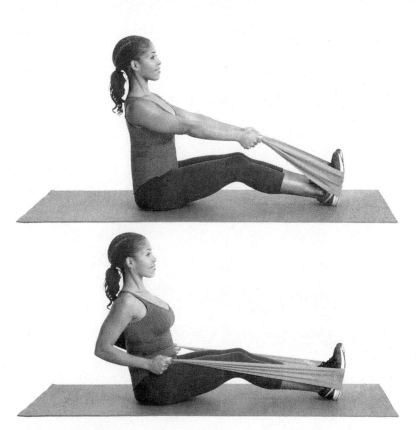

Row with Band

Sit on the floor with your legs extended. Place the center of the band around your feet, and hold each end with your arms extended.

Squeeze your shoulder blades together, bend your elbows back, and pull the band toward your chest.

Pause, and then return to the starting position.

Do two sets of 10 reps, resting for 60 seconds between sets.

No resistance band? Do a standing bent-over row with dumbbells or water bottles. Stand with your feet staggered and lean forward from your hips. Place one hand on a table or chair for support. Hold a dumbbell in the other hand so your arm hangs below your shoulder. Then bend your elbow toward the ceiling and pull the weight toward your torso. Pause, and then slowly lower. Do one set, switch arms, and repeat.

Make it easier: **Slide your hands closer to the end of the band or bend your knees more so you have more slack.**

Make it harder: **Slide your hands down the band toward your feet so it's shorter, providing more resistance. Or use a stronger resistance band. You can also do standing bent-over rows with heavier dumbbells.**

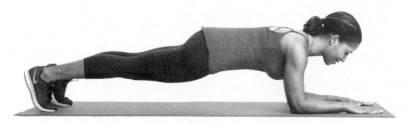

Elbow Plank

Start on all fours.

Place your hands, forearms, and elbows on the floor. Extend one leg at a time back, and balance on the balls of your feet and forearms.

Lower your butt until your back is flat and your body is in a straight line from your ankles to your shoulders. Engage your core by pulling your belly button toward your spine.

Hold this position as long as possible—aiming for 1 minute total. You can come down and take a break as often as needed during that 1 minute. As you become stronger, you will need fewer breaks and will be able to hold it for longer.

Rest for 60 seconds, and repeat once more (only do Elbow Plank twice).

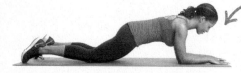

Make it easier: **Bend your knees and place them on the floor so you are balancing on your knees, elbows, forearms, and palms.**

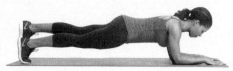

Make it harder: **Lift your left foot a few inches off the floor and balance on your right leg. Aim for 30 seconds with each leg.**

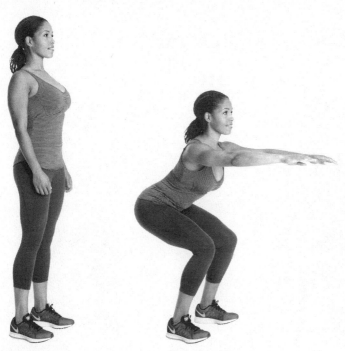

Squat

Stand with your feet shoulder-width apart, arms down at your sides.

Bend at your hips and knees, sticking your butt out and sitting back. Keep your weight in your heels and your chest lifted. Allow your arms to rise up in front of you to help you stay balanced. Make sure that your knees stay behind your toes so that you can see at least the tips of your toes if you look down. Lower until your thighs are as close to parallel to the floor as possible.

Pause, and then stand back up. Do two sets of 10 reps, resting for 60 seconds between sets.

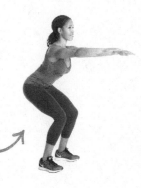

Make it easier: **Lower only halfway.**

Make it harder: **Do squats while holding dumbbells down at your sides.**

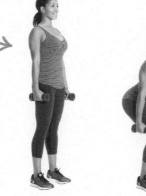

Week 5 Additional Moves

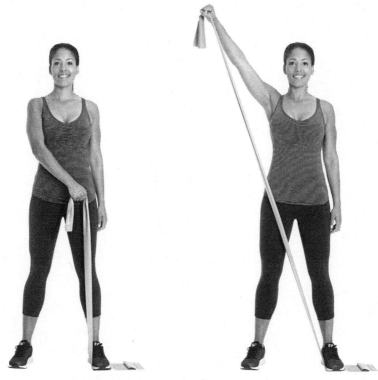

Cross-Arm Abduction

Stand with your feet shoulder-width apart. Place the end of the band under your left foot, and hold the other end in your right hand, positioning your right hand by your left thigh.

Raise your right arm up and out in an arch, crossing your body as if you were drawing a sword.

Pause at the top before returning to the starting position.

Do two sets of 10 reps, resting 60 seconds between sets. Switch sides and repeat.

No resistance band? You can substitute light dumbbells or water bottles.

Make it easier: **Adjust the band under your foot so you have more slack.**

Make it harder: **Slide your hand down the band so it's shorter, providing more resistance. Or use a stronger resistance band or hold light dumbbells along with the band.**

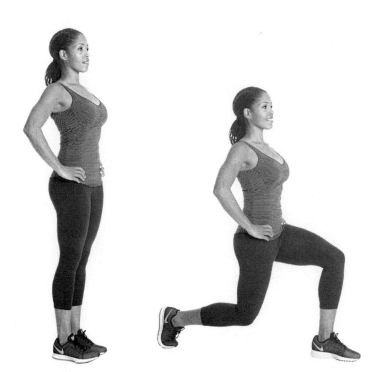

Back Lunge

Stand with your feet together. Step your right foot backward onto your toes.

Slowly lower your body straight down until your left thigh is parallel to the floor. Don't lean forward.

Push into your left heel and off of your right foot to stand back up, bringing your feet together. That's 1 rep.

Do 10 reps with your right side, and then switch to the left, stepping back with your left foot. That's one set total. Rest for 60 seconds, and then complete another set.

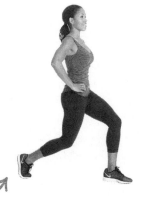

Make it easier: Lower only halfway. If that's still too challenging, start with your feet apart and do stationary lunges, simply lowering and pressing back up without stepping backward and forward.

Make it harder: Do back lunges while holding dumbbells down at your sides.

Week 6 Additional Moves

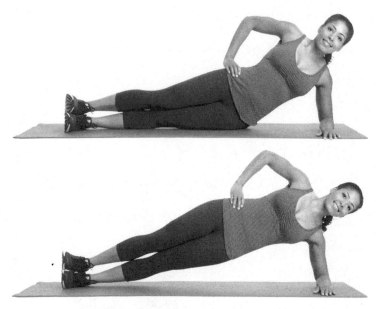

Side Plank

Lie on your side, with your legs extended and stacked. Raise your upper body onto your elbow. Place your weight on your forearm and the side of your lower foot.

Engage your core, squeeze your butt, and raise your hip and leg off the floor. Your body should be in a straight line from your ankles to your shoulders.

Hold this position on one side for as long as possible—aiming for 1 minute total. You can come down and take a break as often as needed during that 1 minute. As you become stronger, you will need fewer breaks and will be able to hold it for longer. Rest for 60 seconds, and then repeat on the opposite side (do once on each side).

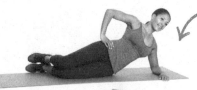

Make it easier: **Bend your legs and do the Side Plank balancing on your bottom knee. If it's more comfortable, you can extend your top leg.**

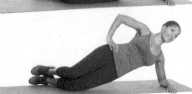

Make it harder: **Lift your top leg off of the bottom one, holding it midair.**

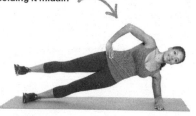

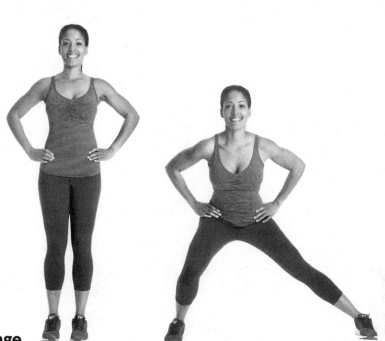

Side Lunge

Stand with your feet slightly apart. Step your right foot out to the side, wider than shoulder width.

Bend your right knee, hinge at your hips, and sit back into a squat. Keep your left leg straight. Slowly lower until your right thigh is about parallel to the floor.

Push into your right heel and stand back up, bringing your feet together. That's 1 rep.

Do 10 reps to the right side, and then switch to the left, stepping out to the side with your left foot. That's one set total. Rest for 60 seconds, and then complete another set.

Make it easier. **Lower only halfway. If that's still too challenging, start with your feet wide apart and do stationary lunges, simply lowering and pressing back up without stepping side to side.**

Make it harder. **Do side lunges while holding dumbbells down at your sides.**

Week 7 Additional Moves

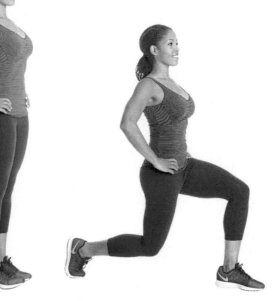

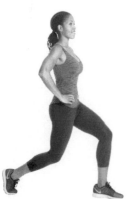

Front Lunge

Stand with your feet together. Step your left foot forward, letting your right heel come off the floor.

Slowly lower your body straight down until your left thigh is parallel to the floor. Don't lean forward.

Push into your left heel to stand back up, bringing your feet together. That's 1 rep.

Do 10 reps on your left side, and then switch to the right, stepping forward with your right foot. That's one set total. Rest for 60 seconds, and then complete another set.

You can now combine all of the lunges into one move. Start by lunging forward with your left foot, and then return to the center. Next, lunge to the left side with your left foot, and then return to the center. Then lunge backward with your left foot and back to the center. Repeat, lunging with your right foot. That's 1 rep.

Make it easier: Lower only halfway. If that's still too challenging, start with your feet apart and do stationary lunges, simply lowering and pressing back up without stepping backward and forward.

Make it harder: Do front lunges while holding dumbbells down at your sides.

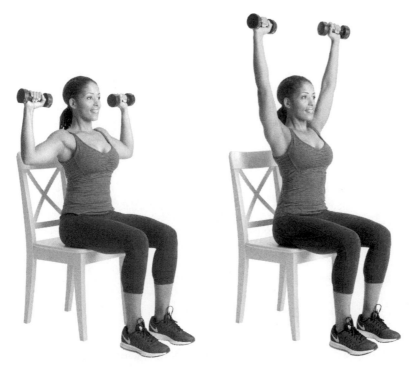

Overhead Press

Sit on the edge of a chair with your feet hip-width apart. Hold dumb-bells by your head with your palms facing forward and your elbows bent about 90 degrees.

Slowly press the dumbbells straight up overhead.

Pause, and then slowly lower the dumbbells back to the starting position.

Do two sets of 10 reps, resting for 60 seconds between sets.

Make it easier: Use lighter weights.

Make it harder: Use heavier weights and do the presses while standing with your feet together.

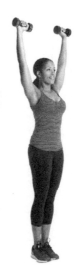

Antiaging Balance Workout

Starting in Week 5 (or whenever you wish), perform these moves multiple times a day as you chat on the phone, do the dishes, or brush your teeth, or do them during your workouts as you rest between sets. If you feel unsteady, do them with a sturdy chair next to you or nearby, so you can grab it if you need to.

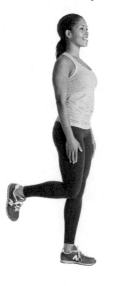

The Stork

TARGETS: Quads, butt, and core

Stand tall with your feet slightly apart and your arms down at your sides. Contract the core muscles in your abdomen, back, and buttocks. Raise one foot behind you and balance on the other foot. Keep your shoulders relaxed. Hold for 30 seconds. Switch legs and hold for another 30 seconds.

When you can hold for 30 seconds on each side, do the move with your eyes closed. For even more of a challenge, stand on a less-stable surface, like a cushion from your couch, or hold light weights or full bottles of water as you swing your arms back and forth.

Tip: **Pick a point on the wall and stare at it to help you balance.**

Heel-to-Toe

TARGETS: Legs

The same sobriety field test cops give drunk drivers also improves balance. Place the heel of one foot just in front of the toes of your other foot. Your heel and toes should touch or almost touch. Choose a spot ahead of you. Focus on it and take a step, placing your heel just in front of the toe of your other foot. Repeat for 20 steps.

Tip: **Keep your chest and shoulders lifted and your gaze upright.**

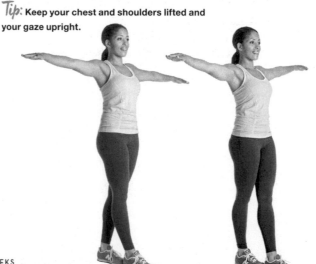

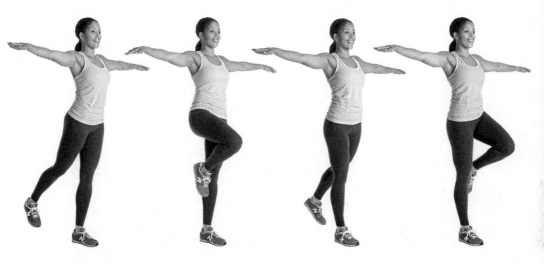

The Stare-Down

TARGETS: Quads, butt, hamstrings, and core

Raise your arms to your sides at shoulder height. Choose a spot ahead of you. Focus on it and walk forward in a straight line. As you walk, lift your back leg behind you. Pause for 1 second and then step forward, bending your knee and raising it up in front of you before landing on the floor. Repeat for 20 steps, alternating legs.

To increase the challenge, look from side to side as you walk. (If you have inner-ear problems, skip this step.)

Tip: **Squeeze your butt as you lift your back leg.**

Four Yoga Moves for Pelvic Strength

If leakage is a problem for you, yoga can help. In particular, one remarkable study showed that women who participated in a yoga-therapy program for 6 weeks experienced a *66 percent decrease* in their incontinence frequency. Starting in Week 7 (or whenever you wish), do the following four moves (the first three are from the study) three times a week.

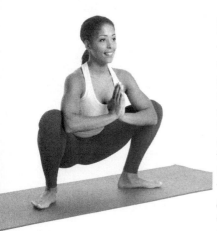

Malasana

This pose lengthens the pelvic floor, which allows it to contract more forcefully.

Stand with your feet shoulder-width apart. Bend your knees and lower into a squat. Separate your thighs slightly wider than your torso and press your elbows against your inner thighs, bringing your palms together in front of your chest. Lengthen your spine, moving your tailbone toward the floor and lifting the crown of your head toward the ceiling. Breathe deeply. Hold for 1 minute.

Make it easier: **Sit on the edge of a chair with your legs wide, toes and knees pointing out to the sides. Place your hands on your knees and gently press out.**

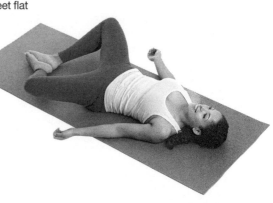

Reclined Bound Angle

Your inner thighs help stabilize your pelvic floor. When they're flexible, you're able to activate your pelvic muscles more deeply.

Lie on the mat with your knees bent and feet flat on the floor. Bring the soles of your feet together and allow your knees to fall out to the sides. Rest your arms by your sides, palms up. Close your eyes and breathe deeply. Hold for 1 minute.

Make it easier: **You can place pillows or folded blankets under your knees to support your legs if needed.**

Legs Up the Wall

The change in gravity puts pressure on your diaphragm, which allows you to breathe more deeply and to fully relax the pelvic muscles without any fear of leakage.

Sit on the floor with one side of your body grazing the wall. Swing your legs up against the wall and slowly lower your back and head to the floor, keeping your legs straight. Allow your hands to fall out to your sides, palms facing up. Close your eyes and breathe deeply, relaxing into the pose. Hold for 1 minute.

Child's Pose

To be strong, your pelvic floor also needs to be flexible. This pose opens up your lower back so your pelvic floor expands and stretches with each inhale.

Kneel with your knees wide apart and your toes touching. Walk your hands forward and lower your torso between your thighs, resting your forehead and nose on the mat. Extend your arms and press your palms into the mat and your hips toward your heels. Close your eyes and breathe deeply. Hold for 1 minute.

Make it easier: You can place a rolled towel between your legs if you're not able to come all the way down to your heels.

Week 8

WORKOUT	HOW-TO	DURATION	FREQUENCY
Sunrise Stretch	page 288	5–10 min.	Daily
Dynamic Warmup (before cardio and/or strength)	page 291	5–10 min.	3–7 days
Cardio (intervals and steady-paced)	page 295	20–30 min.	3–5 days
Advanced Strength Workout (or the basic one if you prefer)	see below	10–15 min.	2–3 days
Flexibility stretches (after cardio and/or strength)	page 298	5 min.	3–7 days
Optional: Foam rolling	page 300	5–15 min.	3–7 days
Optional: Balance	page 316	5 min.	3–7 days
Optional: Yoga	page 318	5 min.	3–7 days

This week, you can keep doing what you've been doing unless you're looking for a new challenge. If you're feeling really strong when you strength train—like you could keep doing reps long after you've completed your sets or need heavier weights or a more resistant band—you can try the Advanced Strength Workout. Don't worry if you're not up to it, though! You can progress to this routine at any time. Remember, even though the official 8-week program is wrapping up, you want to keep on going. And having a new workout to look forward to can help you stay motivated.

Advanced Strength Workout

Here's a combo workout that combines upper- and lower-body exercises for a challenging total-body workout. It can be used during the 8-week plan for those who need more of a challenge. Or it can be something to work toward following the 8 weeks.

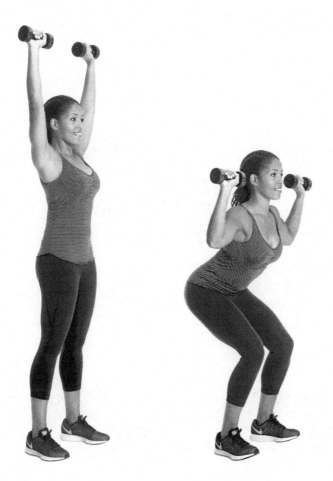

Squat with Overhead Press

Stand with your feet shoulder-width apart and your arms extended overhead, palms facing forward.

Bend at your hips and knees, sticking your butt out and sitting back. Keep your weight in your heels and your chest lifted. Make sure that your knees stay behind your toes. As you lower, bend your elbows and bring the dumbbells down toward your shoulders with your palms facing forward and your elbows pointing down. Lower until your thighs are as close to parallel to the floor as possible.

Pause, and then stand back up, pressing the dumbbells overhead.

Do two sets of 10 reps, resting for 60 seconds between sets.

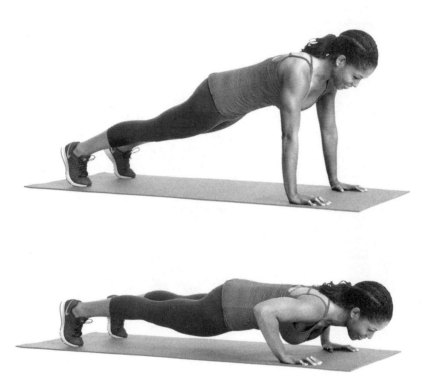

Pushup

Get into a plank position, balancing on your palms and the balls of your feet.

Bending your elbows out to the sides, lower your chest toward the floor. Keep your abs tight and your body in a straight line from your head to your heels.

Pause, and then press back up to the starting position.

Do two sets of 10 reps, resting for 60 seconds between sets.

Make it easier: **If you can't complete all of the reps on your toes, you can put your knees down and finish with kneeling push-ups. Or do kneeling pushups for all of your reps if this move is too challenging.**

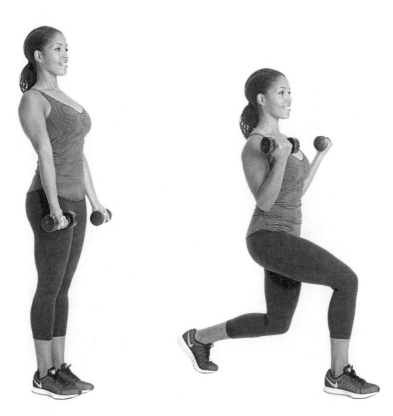

Front Lunge with Biceps Curl

Stand with your feet together, holding dumbbells down at your sides with your palms facing forward.

Step your right foot forward, letting your left heel come off the floor.

Slowly lower your body straight down until your right thigh is parallel to the floor. Don't lean forward. As you lower, bend your elbows and curl the dumbbells up toward your shoulders.

Push into your right heel to stand back up, bringing your feet together and slowly lowering the dumbbells. That's 1 rep.

Do 10 reps on your right side, and then switch to the left, stepping forward with your left foot. That's one set total. Rest for 60 seconds and then complete another set.

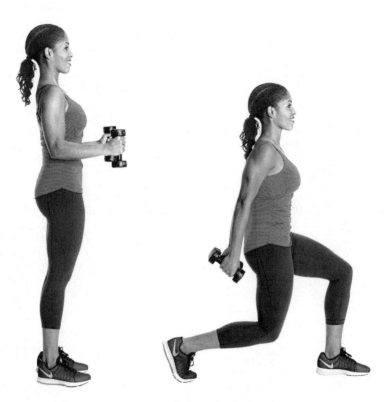

Back Lunge with Triceps Kickback

Stand with your feet slightly apart, holding dumbbells at your sides with your arms bent and palms facing in.

Step your right foot backward onto your toes. Slowly lower your body straight down until your left thigh is parallel to the floor. Don't lean forward. As you lower, straighten your arms, pressing the dumbbells behind you.

Push into your left heel and off your right foot to stand back up, bringing your feet together and bending your arms. That's 1 rep.

Do 10 reps on your right side, and then switch to the left, stepping back with your left foot. That's one set total. Rest for 60 seconds, and then complete another set.

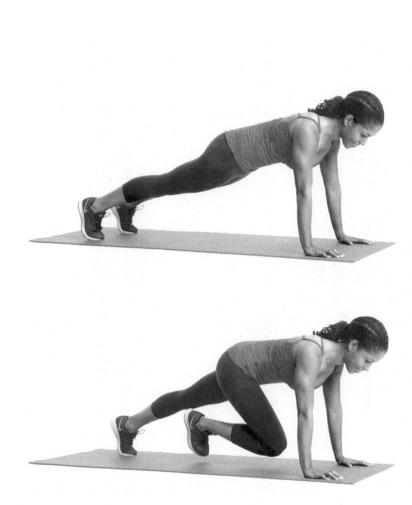

Plank Crunch

Get into a plank position, balancing on your palms and the balls of your feet.

Lower your butt until your back is flat and your body is in a straight line from your ankles to your shoulders. Then bend your right knee and pull it in toward your chest.

Pause, and then return to the starting position. Repeat with your left leg. That's 1 rep.

Do two sets of 10 reps, resting for 60 seconds between sets.

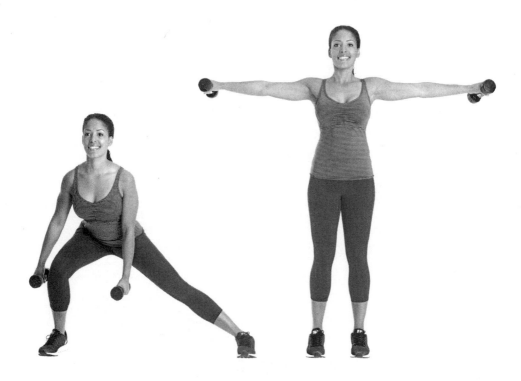

Side Lunge with Lateral Raise

Stand with your feet slightly apart, holding dumbbells down at your sides with your palms facing in.

Step your right foot out to the side, wider than shoulder width.

Bend your right knee, hinge at your hips, and sit back into a squat. Keep your left leg straight. Slowly lower until your right thigh is about parallel to the floor.

Push into your right heel and stand back up, bringing your feet together. As you come up, raise your arms out to your sides, bringing the dumbbells to shoulder height. That's 1 rep.

As you do your next rep, lower the dumbbells as you lower into the lunge.

Do 10 reps on the right side and then switch to the left, stepping out to the side with your left foot. That's one set total. Rest 60 seconds and then complete another set.

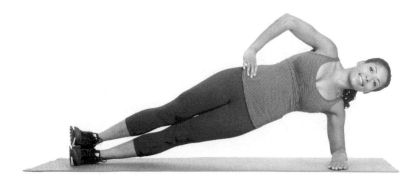

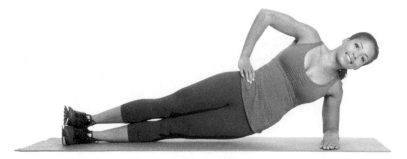

Side Plank Dip

Lie on your side with your legs extended and stacked. Raise your upper body onto your elbow. Place your weight on your forearm and the side of your lower foot.

Engage your core, squeeze your butt, and raise your hip and leg off the floor. Your body should be in a straight line from your ankles to your shoulders.

Slowly lower your bottom hip toward the floor. Then lift back up without touching the floor.

Do two sets of 10 reps on each side, resting for 60 seconds between sets.

SUCCESS!

Vesta Ackernecht, 46

MY STORY For the past 5 years, Vesta Ackernecht's stomach hurt all the time. "No lie, *every day*," she said. The culprit: irritable bowel syndrome, or IBS. The pain, bloating, nausea, and diarrhea would usually strike after eating. Even prescription medication wasn't helping. "IBS had negatively affected my life," Vesta said. "I was anxious and fearful of symptoms every time I ate. I was depressed. I thought that I'd have to live with the horrible symptoms of IBS forever."

But after just 1 week on the Younger in 8 Weeks Plan, Vesta was feeling better. Midway through the program, she reported that 90 percent of her digestive issues had resolved. "I have had to take my meds for IBS only twice. My stomach feels so good that I want to continue to eat right."

Vesta is convinced that cutting out processed foods, sugar, salt, fatty foods, and fried foods did the trick. "It cleansed my system," she said, adding that she used to think she was being careful by staying away from spicy foods. Now she knows the real triggers. "When I eat fatty, fried, or sugary foods, my IBS symptoms return full force."

With results like that, Vesta was very motivated to follow the diet plan to a T. But it was challenging on days she worked. "I do 12-hour shifts at the hospital," she explained. "I rarely sit. I rarely have a half-hour for lunch, and I rarely eat. I end up eating everything in sight at 8 o'clock at night when I get home." Now, she comes to work prepared, often bringing soup and cut-up veggies that she can eat on the run. And she cooks meals in advance, so all she has to do when she gets home is reheat and eat. For quick breakfasts, she assembles smoothie ingredients into baggies ahead of time and then just dumps them into a blender for a quick, nutritious meal.

"I feel the best I've ever felt," she said. So good, in fact, that she joined her 24-year-old daughter to go stand-up paddleboarding—something she would not have done before the program. "I was so proud of myself. I didn't fall off, and I paddled across the lake and back, keeping up with my daughter. When I saw the pictures, I thought I looked pretty darn good for my age." Next up: Vesta wants to try kayaking, whitewater rafting, and zip-lining.

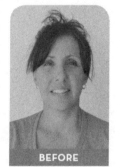

BEFORE

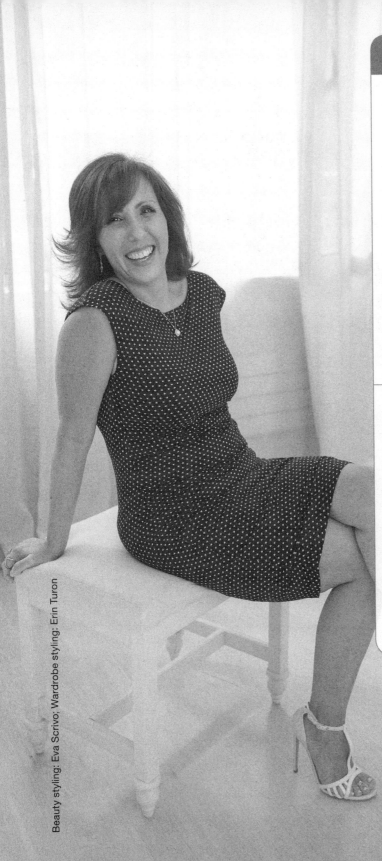

LOOK AT ME

- More muscle definition in her arms
- Increased energy **4 points (80 percent)**
- Dropped two sizes
- More active sex life
- Weight lost: **9.8 pounds**
- Inches lost: **7**

Tip EASE INTO IT. When I started the program, I could do only 15 minutes on the elliptical at Level 2. Now I can go for 30 minutes at Level 7. Each time I'd push myself to a new level, it made me so happy. Celebrate what you can do and don't worry if it isn't perfect.

Beauty styling: Eva Scrivo; Wardrobe styling: Erin Turon

PART

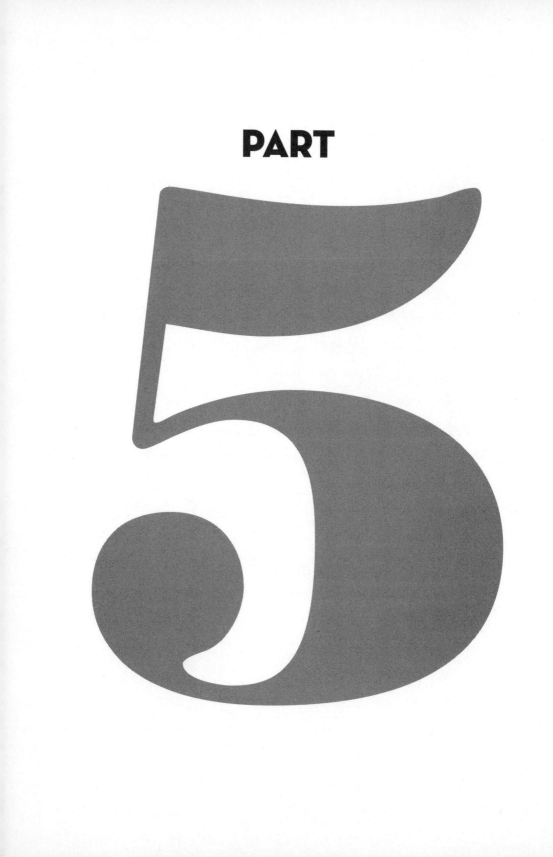

TURN-
BACK-THE-
CLOCK
TOOLS

Clean & Green Recipes

In this section, you'll find 76 recipes for wholesome, healthy, and delicious dishes and desserts. The recipes are organized in the following categories so you can browse each section and mark recipes you'd like to try. *Note:* If you're cooking for one or two or you don't like lots of leftovers, halve the ingredients in the recipes to make fewer servings.

VEGETABLE FRITTATA

Make it ahead!

Makes 4 servings

PREP TIME: 10 MINUTES | TOTAL TIME: 1 HOUR + COOLING

2 teaspoons extra virgin olive oil

1 onion, chopped

1 large red bell pepper, chopped

16 ounces brown mushrooms, sliced

1/4 cup water

2 omega-3-fortified eggs

2 egg whites

1 1/2 cups 2% small curd cottage cheese

2 tablespoons ground flaxseed

3/4 teaspoon mustard powder

1/4 cup shredded low-fat, extra-sharp Cheddar cheese

1/3 cup chopped fresh flat-leaf parsley

Hot-pepper sauce (optional)

1. Preheat the oven to 350°F. Coat a 10" pie plate with cooking spray.

2. In a large nonstick skillet over medium-high heat, warm the oil. Cook the onion, pepper, mushrooms, and water, stirring occasionally, for 7 to 10 minutes, or until the vegetables are soft and all the liquid has evaporated.

3. Meanwhile, in a food processor or blender, combine the eggs, egg whites, cottage cheese, flaxseed, and mustard powder. Puree until very smooth. Transfer to the skillet. Add the Cheddar and parsley. Stir just to combine. Pour into the pie plate.

4. Bake for 35 minutes, or until the frittata is set and lightly browned. Let it sit for 5 minutes before cutting into 4 wedges.

5. Serve with hot-pepper sauce, if desired.

PER SERVING: 221 calories, 20 g protein, 17 g carbohydrates, 3 g fiber, 8 g total sugar, 9 g fat, 2.5 g saturated fat, 424 mg sodium

NOTE: *For instant breakfasts, bake the frittata on a weekend or weeknight. Cool the frittata completely. Cover tightly with plastic wrap and refrigerate for up to 5 days. A single serving can be eaten at room temperature or placed on a microwaveable plate, covered with waxed paper, and microwaved on medium power for 1 to 2 minutes, or until warmed.*

BLUEBERRY OAT PANCAKES

Make it ahead!

Makes 6 servings

PREP TIME: 5 MINUTES | TOTAL TIME: 35 MINUTES

1¼ cups quick-cooking oats

½ cup whole wheat pastry flour

2 tablespoons ground almonds

½ teaspoon baking powder

¼ teaspoon baking soda

Dash of fine sea salt

1 cup buttermilk

1 omega-3-fortified egg

1 egg white

1 tablespoon coconut oil, melted

1 teaspoon freshly grated lemon peel

1½ cups fresh or frozen unsweetened and thawed blueberries

1. In a large bowl, combine the oats, flour, almonds, baking powder, baking soda, and salt.

2. In a medium bowl, combine the buttermilk, egg, egg white, oil, and lemon peel. Pour into the oat mixture, stirring until just moistened. Gently fold in the blueberries with a rubber spatula. Set aside for 10 minutes.

3. Heat a large nonstick skillet or griddle coated with cooking spray over medium heat. Spoon ¼ cupfuls of the reserved batter into the skillet or griddle, making as many pancakes as possible without them touching. (You'll need to do several batches.) Cook for 2½ to 3 minutes, or until the tops begin to bubble slightly. Turn the pancakes and cook for 2½ to 3 minutes, or until golden and cooked through. Transfer to a platter.

4. Repeat with the remaining batter.

PER SERVING (2 PANCAKES): 180 calories, 7 g protein, 26 g carbohydrates, 4 g fiber, 6 g total sugar, 6 g fat, 2.5 g saturated fat, 169 mg sodium

NOTE: *You can make a double or triple batch of pancakes. Cool the pancakes on a rack. Pack between small pieces of waxed paper in a plastic storage container and refrigerate for up to 3 days. To eat, remove the pancakes you need and heat in a toaster oven.*

MUESLI WITH WALNUTS

Make it ahead!

Makes 10 servings

PREP TIME: 5 MINUTES | TOTAL TIME: 25 MINUTES + COOLING

4 cups steel-cut oats or regular oats

½ cup chopped walnuts

1 cup ground flaxseed

1. Preheat the oven to 375°F.

2. Spread the oats on a rimmed baking sheet or shallow roasting pan. Bake, stirring occasionally, for 10 minutes. Stir in the walnuts and bake for 7 to 10 minutes, or until lightly browned. Scrape into a large bowl and let cool completely.

3. Stir in the flaxseed. Refrigerate in a tightly sealed container for up to 1 month.

4. Serve over yogurt topped with fresh berries or sliced banana.

PER SERVING: 226 calories, 9 g protein, 26 g carbohydrates, 7 g fiber, 1 g total sugar, 11 g fat, 1 g saturated fat, 3 mg sodium

NOTE: *Sometimes served after soaking in milk, this dry muesli is a simpler version of granola. If you prefer, you can skip toasting the oats and instead simply toast the walnuts in a dry skillet.*

HUMMUS, TOMATO, AND SPINACH BREAKFAST SANDWICH

Makes 1 serving

PREP TIME: 5 MINUTES | TOTAL TIME: 5 MINUTES

1 whole wheat or multigrain English muffin, split

3 tablespoons hummus

1 thick slice tomato

¼ cup baby spinach

Toast the muffin. Spread the hummus on the bottom half of the muffin. Top with the tomato, spinach, and the muffin top.

PER SERVING: 216 calories, 8 g protein, 36 g carbohydrates, 7 g fiber, 8 g total sugar, 6 g fat, 0 g saturated fat, 491 mg sodium

BANANA-CHIA SMOOTHIE

Makes 2 servings

PREP TIME: 5 MINUTES | TOTAL TIME: 5 MINUTES

2 cups cold unsweetened almond milk or coconut milk

1 large frozen banana, cut into chunks

1 cup baby spinach

2 tablespoons natural nut butter (such as almond, peanut, or cashew)

2 teaspoons chia seeds

1/2 teaspoon ground cinnamon (optional)

6 ice cubes

In a blender, combine the milk, banana, spinach, nut butter, chia seeds, cinnamon (if using), and ice cubes. Blend until smooth and creamy.

PER SERVING: 213 calories, 6 g protein, 22 g carbohydrates, 6 g fiber, 9 g total sugar, 13 g fat, 1 g saturated fat, 219 mg sodium

VERY BERRY SMOOTHIE

Makes 2 servings

PREP TIME: 5 MINUTES | TOTAL TIME: 5 MINUTES

1 cup baby spinach

1/2 cup frozen unsweetened strawberry halves

1/2 cup frozen unsweetened wild blueberries

3/4 cup fat-free plain yogurt

1 teaspoon flaxseed oil or ground flaxseed

2–4 tablespoons water or plant-based milk, as needed

In a blender, combine the spinach, berries, yogurt, and flaxseed. Blend until smooth and creamy. Drizzle in a few tablespoons of the water or milk, if needed, to thin slightly.

PER SERVING: 95 calories, 4 g protein, 17 g carbohydrates, 2 g fiber, 11 g total sugar, 2 g fat, 0 g saturated fat, 52 mg sodium

SUPER GREEN SMOOTHIE

Makes 2 servings

PREP TIME: 5 MINUTES | TOTAL TIME: 5 MINUTES

1 cup 2% plain Greek yogurt

3/4 cup cold coconut water

1 banana, cut into chunks

1/2 cup baby spinach

1/2 cup chopped kale leaves

In a blender, combine the yogurt, coconut water, banana, spinach, and kale. Blend until smooth and creamy.

PER SERVING: 155 calories, 11 g protein, 24 g carbohydrates, 2 g fiber, 16 g total sugar, 3 g fat, 1.5 g saturated fat, 70 mg sodium

FRENCH TOAST WITH FRUIT

Makes 1 serving

PREP TIME: 5 MINUTES | TOTAL TIME: 15 MINUTES

1 omega-3-fortified egg, beaten

1/3 cup unsweetened almond milk

1/2 teaspoon almond extract

1/2 teaspoon ground cinnamon

2 slices whole wheat or whole grain bread

1/4 cup 2% plain Greek yogurt

1/2 cup frozen unsweetened wild blueberries, thawed

1. In a large bowl, whisk together the egg, milk, almond extract, and cinnamon. Dip the bread slices in the mixture, turning to coat them completely.

2. In a large skillet coated with cooking spray over medium heat, cook the bread slices for 6 to 8 minutes, turning once, or until browned.

3. Place the toast on a plate and top each slice with the yogurt and blueberries.

PER SERVING: 340 calories, 18 g protein, 48 g carbohydrates, 11 g fiber, 16 g total sugar, 9 g fat, 2.5 g saturated fat, 372 mg sodium

Make it ahead! **CINNAMON-BERRY FLAXSEED MUFFINS**
Makes 6

PREP TIME: 15 MINUTES | TOTAL TIME: 35 MINUTES

¾ cup almond meal or almond flour

⅓ cup ground flaxseed

1 teaspoon baking powder

1 teaspoon ground cinnamon

2 omega-3-fortified eggs

¼ cup unsweetened applesauce

¼ cup 2% plain Greek yogurt

1 tablespoon olive oil

1 tablespoon vanilla extract

½ cup blueberries or raspberries

1. Preheat the oven to 350°F. Coat a nonstick 6-cup muffin pan with cooking spray or line with paper liners.

2. In a medium bowl, whisk together the almond meal or flour, flaxseed, baking powder, and cinnamon.

3. In a separate medium bowl, whisk together the eggs, applesauce, yogurt, oil, and vanilla. Stir in the berries and the flour mixture. Divide the batter among the muffin cups.

4. Bake for 18 minutes, or until a wooden pick inserted into the center of one of the muffins comes out clean. Transfer to a rack to cool completely before storing in an airtight container for up to 1 week.

PER MUFFIN: 175 calories, 8 g protein, 9 g carbohydrates, 4 g fiber, 3 g total sugar, 13 g fat, 1.5 g saturated fat, 118 mg sodium

SOUTHWESTERN OMELET

Makes 1 serving

3 omega-3-fortified eggs

2 tablespoons unsweetened almond milk or coconut milk

1 teaspoon olive oil

1 small red bell pepper, chopped

1/2 cup shredded kale

1 tablespoon chopped fresh basil

1. In a medium bowl, whisk together the eggs and milk.

2. In a small nonstick skillet over medium-high heat, warm the oil. Cook the pepper and kale, stirring occasionally, for 4 to 5 minutes, or until softened.

3. Add the egg mixture and tilt the skillet to spread the mixture across the bottom. Cook, pushing in the edges with a spatula to let the uncooked egg flow underneath, for 3 minutes, or until just set.

4. Fold the omelet in half and slide it carefully onto a plate. Top with the basil.

PER SERVING: 294 calories, 23 g protein, 11 g carbohydrates, 2 g fiber, 3 g total sugar, 20 g fat, 5 g saturated fat, 293 mg sodium

EGG OVER SWEET POTATO HASH BROWNS

Makes 1 serving

PREP TIME: 10 MINUTES | TOTAL TIME: 20 MINUTES

1/2 teaspoon coconut oil or extra virgin olive oil

2 slices extra-lean turkey bacon, coarsely chopped

1/2 small sweet potato, cut into 1/2" pieces

1/2 green bell pepper, chopped

1/4 small onion, chopped

1 omega-3-fortified egg

1. In a large nonstick skillet over medium-high heat, warm the oil. Cook the bacon, potato, pepper, and onion, stirring occasionally, for 8 to 10 minutes, or until the bacon is crisp and the vegetables are tender. Transfer to a plate.

2. Coat the skillet with cooking spray. Cook the egg for 2 to 3 minutes, or until the white is set and the yolk is still runny.

3. Serve over the hash browns.

PER SERVING: 206 calories, 12 g protein, 14 g carbohydrates, 3 g fiber, 4 g total sugar, 12 g fat, 4.5 g saturated fat, and 371 mg sodium

SPICED SWEET POTATO CHIPS

Makes 2 servings

Make it ahead!

PREP TIME: 5 MINUTES | TOTAL TIME: 20 MINUTES

1 large sweet potato, very thinly sliced

1 tablespoon coconut oil, melted

½ teaspoon ground cumin

¼ teaspoon chili powder

1. Preheat the oven to 375°F. Coat a large baking sheet with cooking spray.

2. Lightly coat the potato slices with the oil. Arrange in a single layer on the baking sheet.

3. Bake for 7 minutes, or until the slices start to brown. Remove the baking sheet and turn the slices. Bake for 7 to 10 minutes, or until browned. Transfer the slices to a large tray.

4. Meanwhile, in a small bowl, combine the cumin and chili powder. Sprinkle over the chips. Toss well and serve.

PER SERVING: 120 calories, 1 g protein, 13 g carbohydrates, 2 g fiber, 3 g total sugar, 7 g fat, 6 g saturated fat, 42 mg sodium

NOTE: *Cool and refrigerate the chips in a tightly sealed container for up to 5 days. Serve at room temperature.*

CARAMELIZED ONION AND LENTIL SPREAD

Make it ahead!

Makes 12 servings

PREP TIME: 10 MINUTES | TOTAL TIME: 1 HOUR + COOLING

- 2 teaspoons extra virgin olive oil
- 3 onions, chopped
- 3 tablespoons + 1½ cups water
- ½ teaspoon dried sage
- ½ cup dried lentils
- 2 teaspoons balsamic vinegar
- 1 teaspoon flaxseed oil
- ¼ teaspoon fine sea salt
- ½ teaspoon ground black pepper
- 2 tablespoons chopped fresh flat-leaf parsley
- 12 multigrain crispbreads (14 grams each)

1. In a medium heavy-bottom pot over medium heat, warm the olive oil. Cook the onions, the 3 tablespoons water, and the sage, stirring occasionally, for 15 minutes, or until the onions are just golden.

2. Add the lentils and the 1½ cups water. Reduce the heat to low, cover, and cook, stirring occasionally, for 30 minutes, or until the lentils are very tender.

3. Stir in the vinegar, flaxseed oil, salt, and pepper. Increase the heat to medium and cook, uncovered, for 5 minutes, or until the mixture is thick.

4. Remove from the heat, stir in the parsley, and let cool.

5. Spread evenly on the crispbreads and serve.

PER SERVING: 95 calories, 4 g protein, 17 g carbohydrates, 4 g fiber, 2 g total sugar, 1 g fat, 0 g saturated fat, 116 mg sodium

NOTES: *Cool the spread and refrigerate in a tightly sealed container for up to 1 week, or freeze for up to 1 month. This spread is also great on whole wheat pita chips or with sticks of broccoli stalks for dipping.*

Make it ahead! **CHICKPEA DIP WITH BABY CARROTS**

Makes 8 servings

PREP TIME: 5 MINUTES | TOTAL TIME: 5 MINUTES

1 can (15–19 ounces) chickpeas, rinsed and drained

1/2 cup chopped tomato

1 tablespoon freshly squeezed lime juice

1 tablespoon chopped fresh cilantro

2 teaspoons olive oil

1/2 teaspoon curry powder

1/4 teaspoon ground cumin

Hot-pepper sauce (optional)

2 cups baby carrots, halved

1. Set aside ¼ cup of the chickpeas.

2. In a medium bowl, combine the tomato, lime juice, cilantro, oil, curry powder, cumin, a few dashes of the hot-pepper sauce (if desired), and the remaining chickpeas. With a potato masher, squash the mixture into a paste. Add a few teaspoons of water, if needed, to make a softer mixture. Stir in the reserved chickpeas.

3. Serve with the baby carrots for dipping.

PER SERVING: 57 calories, 2 g protein, 8 g carbohydrates, 2 g fiber, 2 g total sugar, 2 g fat, 0 g saturated fat, 112 mg sodium

NOTES: *Refrigerate the dip in a tightly sealed container for up to 1 week, or freeze for up to 1 month. You can also serve the dip with multigrain tortilla chips instead of carrots.*

BEAN AND OLIVE BRUSCHETTA

Makes 4 servings

PREP TIME: 10 MINUTES | TOTAL TIME: 15 MINUTES

½ cup chopped plum tomatoes

2 teaspoons extra virgin olive oil

1 teaspoon flaxseed oil

1 clove garlic, crushed

⅛ teaspoon fine sea salt

⅛ teaspoon ground black pepper

1¼ cups canned white beans, rinsed and drained

2 tablespoons chopped fresh flat-leaf parsley

6 kalamata olives, sliced

4 slices crusty whole grain bread

1. In a medium bowl, combine the tomatoes, oils, garlic, salt, and pepper. Stir vigorously until the tomatoes release their juice. Add the beans, parsley, and olives.

2. Toast or grill the bread until lightly brown and crisp. Top with the bean mixture and any juices. Cut in half and serve.

PER SERVING: 214 calories, 10 g protein, 30 g carbohydrates, 6 g fiber, 2 g total sugar, 6 g fat, 1 g saturated fat, 271 mg sodium

SALSA FRESCA

Makes 20 servings

Make it ahead!

PREP TIME: 10 MINUTES | TOTAL TIME: 10 MINUTES + STANDING

- **4 cups finely chopped plum tomatoes**
- **1/2 cup finely chopped red onion**
- **1/2 cup chopped fresh cilantro**
- **2 jalapeño chile peppers or serrano chile peppers, seeded and finely chopped, or more to taste (wear plastic gloves when handling)**
- **1 tablespoon freshly squeezed lime juice**
- **2 cloves garlic, minced**
- **1/8 teaspoon fine sea salt**

In a glass jar or plastic storage container, combine the tomatoes, onion, cilantro, peppers, lime juice, garlic, and salt. Serve right away or let stand for at least 30 minutes to allow the flavors to blend.

PER SERVING: 7 calories, 0 g protein, 2 g carbohydrates, 0 g fiber, < 1 g total sugar, 0 g fat, 0 g saturated fat, 17 mg sodium

NOTE: *The salsa can be refrigerated for up to 1 week.*

SESAME CHICKEN SKEWERS

Make it ahead!

Makes 12 servings

PREP TIME: 10 MINUTES | TOTAL TIME: 25 MINUTES + MARINATING

¼ cup finely chopped scallions

2 teaspoons soy sauce

2 teaspoons toasted sesame oil

2 teaspoons flaxseed oil

2 teaspoons grated fresh ginger

2 cloves garlic, minced

1½ pounds boneless, skinless chicken breasts, cut into ½"-wide strips

2 tablespoons sesame seeds

1. In a large resealable plastic bag, combine the scallions, soy sauce, oils, ginger, and garlic. Add the chicken. Seal the bag and squeeze gently to coat the chicken with the marinade. Refrigerate for at least 15 minutes.

2. Coat a broiler-pan rack with cooking spray. Preheat the broiler.

3. Drain the chicken. Discard the marinade. Thread the chicken strips on 24 bamboo skewers (6" long) in loose S shapes. Sprinkle with the sesame seeds.

4. Broil the skewers 4" from the heat for 3 minutes. Turn over and broil for 3 to 5 minutes, or until the chicken is no longer pink and completely cooked through.

PER SERVING: 89 calories, 12 g protein, 1 g carbohydrates, 4 g fiber, < 1 g total sugar, 4 g fat, 1 g saturated fat, 115 mg sodium

NOTE: *Cool the skewers after cooking and refrigerate in an airtight container for up to 3 days. The chicken is delicious at room temperature.*

CHICKEN AND AVOCADO "QUESADILLAS"

Makes 4 servings

PREP TIME: 10 MINUTES | TOTAL TIME: 25 MINUTES

2 whole wheat tortillas (8" diameter)

1 cup shredded cooked chicken breast

1 tablespoon chopped fresh cilantro

1 avocado, sliced

½ cup baby spinach, shredded

1. Arrange the tortillas on a work surface. Top the lower half of each tortilla with ½ cup chicken, ½ tablespoon cilantro, half of the avocado slices, and ¼ cup spinach. Fold the top half of each tortilla over the filling to form a half moon. Brush one side of the tortillas with olive oil.

2. In a large nonstick skillet over medium heat, cook the quesadillas for 4 minutes on each side, or until lightly browned and the filling is hot.

3. Transfer to a cutting board. Let stand 1 minute. Cut each into 4 wedges and serve.

PER SERVING: 205 calories, 14 g protein, 16 g carbohydrates, 5 g fiber, < 1 g total sugar, 10 g fat, 2 g saturated fat, 195 mg sodium

SEAFOOD ANTIPASTO

Make it ahead!

Makes 6 servings

PREP TIME: 10 MINUTES | TOTAL TIME: 15 MINUTES

1 tablespoon balsamic vinegar

2 teaspoons extra virgin olive oil

1 bulb fennel, thinly sliced (about 1 cup) + fronds for garnish

¼ red or yellow bell pepper, thinly sliced

¼ small red onion, thinly sliced

1 can (3.75 ounces) water-packed sardines, drained and patted dry

1 can (5 ounces) wild-caught water-packed tuna, drained

Ground black pepper

In a medium bowl, whisk together the vinegar and oil. Add the fennel, bell pepper, onion, sardines, and tuna. Toss gently. Season to taste with the black pepper. Serve garnished with fennel fronds.

PER SERVING: 107 calories, 10 g protein, 4 g carbohydrates, 1 g fiber, < 1 g total sugar, 6 g fat, 1 g saturated fat, 245 mg sodium

NOTES: *Refrigerate the antipasto in a tightly sealed container for up to 3 days. You can replace the fennel with 4 sliced celery ribs.*

Make it ahead!

CURRIED LENTIL AND SPINACH SOUP

Makes 6 servings

PREP TIME: 10 MINUTES | TOTAL TIME: 55 MINUTES

1 tablespoon extra virgin olive oil

1 large onion, chopped

3 cloves garlic, minced

1 tablespoon curry powder

1 tablespoon grated fresh ginger

4 cups reduced-sodium vegetable broth

4 cups water

2 cups dried lentils

1 package (6 ounces) baby spinach

2 tablespoons white wine vinegar or red wine vinegar

¼ teaspoon fine sea salt

½ teaspoon ground black pepper

6 tablespoons 2% plain Greek yogurt

1. In a large heavy-bottom pot over medium-high heat, warm the oil. Cook the onion and garlic, stirring frequently, for 10 minutes, or until golden. Stir in the curry powder and ginger.

2. Add the broth, water, and lentils. Increase the heat to high and bring to a boil. Reduce the heat to medium-low, and simmer, uncovered, for 25 minutes, or until the lentils are tender.

3. Transfer 2 cups of the soup to a food processor or a blender. Process or blend until smooth and return to the pot. Add the spinach, vinegar, salt, and pepper. Simmer for 5 minutes, or until heated through.

4. Ladle the soup into bowls. Top each serving with 1 tablespoon of the yogurt.

PER SERVING: 299 calories, 19 g protein, 48 g carbohydrates, 22 g fiber, 4 g total sugar, 3 g fat, 1 g saturated fat, 252 mg sodium

NOTE: *Cool the soup and refrigerate in a tightly sealed container for up to 1 week, or freeze for up to 1 month.*

Make it ahead! **CREOLE CAULIFLOWER SOUP**

Makes 4 servings

PREP TIME: 15 MINUTES | TOTAL TIME: 55 MINUTES

1 teaspoon coconut oil or extra virgin olive oil

2 teaspoons Creole or Cajun seasoning

1 onion, halved and sliced

2 cloves garlic, minced

2 tablespoons + 2 cups water

1 cup reduced-sodium vegetable broth

1/2 head cauliflower, cut into small florets

2 cups thinly sliced mustard greens

1. In a large saucepan over medium heat, warm the oil. Stir in the seasoning and reduce the heat to medium-low. Add the onion, garlic, and the 2 tablespoons water. Cook, stirring occasionally, for 8 minutes, or until the onion is soft and translucent.

2. Add the broth, cauliflower, and the 2 cups water. Increase the heat to high and bring to a boil. Reduce the heat to medium and simmer, covered, for 25 minutes, or until cooked through.

3. Stir in the mustard greens and cook for 2 minutes, or until wilted.

PER SERVING: 55 calories, 3 g protein, 9 g carbohydrates, 3 g fiber, 3 g total sugar, 2 g fat, 0 g saturated fat, 68 mg sodium

NOTE: *The cooled soup can be refrigerated in a tightly sealed container for up to 5 days. Reheat and add additional water, if needed, to thin the soup.*

MEDITERRANEAN SEAFOOD SOUP

Make it ahead!

Makes 4 servings

PREP TIME: 15 MINUTES | TOTAL TIME: 45 MINUTES

1 tablespoon extra virgin olive oil

1/2 onion, chopped

1/2 red bell pepper, chopped

2 cloves garlic, minced

1 can (14.5 ounces) reduced-sodium vegetable broth

1 cup water

1/2 cup canned diced tomatoes

2 tablespoons white wine vinegar

1/8 teaspoon fine sea salt

8 littleneck clams, scrubbed

1/2 pound sea scallops, muscle removed

1/2 pound medium peeled and deveined shrimp

2 tablespoons finely chopped fresh flat-leaf parsley, for garnish

1. In a large pot over medium heat, warm the oil. Cook the onion, pepper, and garlic, stirring occasionally, for 5 minutes, or until softened. Add the broth, water, tomatoes, vinegar, and salt. Cover and bring almost to a boil. Reduce the heat to medium-low and simmer for 10 minutes to allow the flavors to blend.

2. Add the clams. Increase the heat to medium-high, cover, and cook for 5 minutes, or until the clams open. Stir in the scallops and shrimp. Cover and cook for 5 minutes, or until the scallops and shrimp are opaque. Discard any unopened clams. Stir in the parsley, if desired.

PER SERVING: 150 calories, 17 g protein, 8 g carbohydrates, 1 g fiber, 3 g total sugar, 5 g fat, 1 g saturated fat, 822 mg sodium

NOTE: *The cooled soup can be refrigerated in a tightly sealed container for up to 3 days.*

CURRIED QUINOA VEGETABLE SOUP

Makes 4 servings

PREP TIME: 10 MINUTES | TOTAL TIME: 30 MINUTES

2 teaspoons olive oil

½ cup quinoa

1 pound butternut squash, peeled, seeded, and cubed (3 cups)

2 large carrots, chopped

½ teaspoon curry powder

½ teaspoon fine sea salt

4 cups reduced-sodium vegetable broth

½ cup 2% plain Greek yogurt

1. In a nonstick saucepan over medium heat, warm the oil. Stir in the quinoa, squash, carrots, curry powder, and salt. Cover and cook, stirring occasionally, for 5 minutes, or until the quinoa is golden in color.

2. Add the broth. Reduce the heat to low and cook for 15 minutes, or until the quinoa is tender.

3. Transfer the soup to a blender or food processor. Blend or process until smooth.

4. Divide the soup among 4 bowls. Stir 2 tablespoons of the yogurt into each serving.

PER SERVING: 200 calories, 7 g protein, 34 g carbohydrates, 5 g fiber, 7 g total sugar, 4 g fat, 1 g saturated fat, 475 mg sodium

GREEK VEGETABLE OPEN-FACED SANDWICHES

Make it ahead!

Makes 4 servings

PREP TIME: 10 MINUTES | TOTAL TIME: 35 MINUTES

1 small eggplant (1/2 pound), cut into 8 slices

1 red onion, cut into 4 thick slices

1 red bell pepper, cut into 4 quarters

2 teaspoons extra virgin olive oil

1/8 teaspoon fine sea salt

1/4 teaspoon ground black pepper

1 cup canned white beans, rinsed and drained

1 tablespoon freshly squeezed lemon juice

1 teaspoon flaxseed oil

4 slices sprouted grain bread (such as Ezekiel 4:9 Sprouted Whole Grain Bread)

8 leaves romaine

2 tablespoons crumbled feta cheese

1. Coat a grill rack with cooking spray. Preheat the grill to medium-high.

2. Lightly brush the eggplant, onion, and bell pepper with the olive oil. Sprinkle with the salt and black pepper. Grill the eggplant for 4 to 5 minutes per side, or until tender and well marked. Grill the onion and bell pepper for 6 to 7 minutes per side, or until tender and well marked. Separate the onion slices into rings and slice the bell pepper into strips.

3. Meanwhile, in a small bowl, lightly mash the beans, lemon juice, and flaxseed oil with a fork until combined.

4. Toast or grill the bread. Spread each slice with one-quarter of the bean mixture. Top each slice with 2 romaine leaves, 2 eggplant slices, one-quarter of the onion rings and pepper strips, and one-quarter of the cheese.

PER SERVING: 248 calories, 12 g protein, 40 g carbohydrates, 10 g fiber, 6 g total sugar, 5 g fat, 1 g saturated fat, 214 mg sodium

NOTE: *The eggplant, onion, and bell pepper can be grilled, cooled, and refrigerated in a tightly sealed container for up to 5 days. The bean mixture can also be refrigerated for up to 5 days. To make the sandwiches, pick up the recipe at Step 4.*

TURKEY AND RED CABBAGE SLAW SANDWICH

Make it ahead!

Makes 1 serving

PREP TIME: 10 MINUTES | TOTAL TIME: 15 MINUTES

1 teaspoon extra virgin olive oil

2 teaspoons white wine vinegar

1/2 teaspoon dried thyme

1/2 cup finely shredded red cabbage

1 carrot, shredded

1 slice seeded whole grain rye bread

Stone-ground mustard (optional)

2 ounces roasted turkey breast, thinly sliced

Ground black pepper

1. In a medium bowl, whisk together the oil, vinegar, and thyme. Add the cabbage and carrot and toss to coat.

2. Toast the bread. Spread lightly with the mustard, if desired. Top with the turkey and slaw. Season with the pepper to taste. Serve right away.

PER SERVING: 237 calories, 21 g protein, 24 g carbohydrates, 5 g fiber, 5 g total sugar, 6 g fat, 1 g saturated fat, 291 mg sodium

NOTE: *The slaw can be refrigerated in a tightly sealed container for up to 3 days before making the sandwich. For a brown-bag lunch that won't get soggy, pack the slaw in a resealable plastic bag and top the sandwich with it just before eating.*

CHICKEN GYROS WITH CUCUMBER-YOGURT SAUCE

Makes 4 servings

PREP TIME: 15 MINUTES | TOTAL TIME: 30 MINUTES

½ pound boneless, skinless chicken breast halves

1 teaspoon extra virgin olive oil

½ teaspoon dried oregano

⅛ teaspoon ground black pepper

2 100% whole grain pitas

½ cup chopped romaine lettuce

1 plum tomato, chopped

¼ small red onion, thinly sliced

2 tablespoons crumbled feta cheese

½ cup 2% plain Greek yogurt

¼ cucumber, peeled and chopped

½ clove garlic, minced

1. Heat a grill pan coated with cooking spray over medium-high heat. In a medium bowl, combine the chicken, oil, oregano, and pepper. Grill for 5 to 6 minutes per side, or until a thermometer inserted in the thickest portion registers 165°F and the juices run clear. Transfer to a cutting board and cut into thin slices.

2. Meanwhile, cut the pitas in half and open to form a pocket.

3. Fill each pita half with equal amounts of lettuce, tomato, onion, cheese, and chicken.

4. In a small bowl, combine the yogurt, cucumber, and garlic. Spoon over the chicken.

PER SERVING: 175 calories, 18 g protein, 16 g carbohydrates, 2 g fiber, 3 g total sugar, 5 g fat, 2 g saturated fat, 249 mg sodium

CHICKEN FAJITAS

Makes 2 servings

1 boneless, skinless chicken breast half (6 ounces), cut into thin strips

½ small onion, sliced

½ small red bell pepper, sliced

1 teaspoon chopped garlic

½ cup water

½ teaspoon ground cumin

½ teaspoon chili powder

Dash of fine sea salt

2 whole grain tortillas (7" diameter)

½ cup canned black beans, rinsed and drained

½ cup shredded Cheddar cheese

¼ cup chopped avocado

2% plain Greek yogurt (optional)

1. In a medium skillet coated with cooking spray over medium heat, cook the chicken, onion, pepper, and garlic for 3 to 5 minutes, or until the chicken is no longer pink and the vegetables are tender.

2. Add the water, cumin, chili powder, and salt. Cook, stirring occasionally, for 5 minutes, or until the liquid has evaporated and the chicken is cooked through.

3. Meanwhile, place the tortillas between 2 sheets of paper towels. Microwave on high power for 15 seconds, or until softened. Place on serving plates.

4. Divide the chicken mixture, beans, cheese, and avocado between the 2 tortillas. Serve with the yogurt, if desired.

PER SERVING: 473 calories, 35 g protein, 41 g carbohydrates, 11 g fiber, 4 g total sugar, 19 g fat, 8 g saturated fat, 915 mg sodium

TURKEY-MUSHROOM BURGERS

Makes 4 servings

PREP TIME: 10 MINUTES | TOTAL TIME: 30 MINUTES

8 ounces button mushrooms, finely chopped

1/2 pound extra-lean ground turkey breast

1 egg

1 small onion, finely chopped

3 cloves garlic, finely chopped

1 teaspoon Worcestershire sauce

1/4 teaspoon salt

1/4 teaspoon ground black pepper

2 whole wheat pitas

4 leaves lettuce, optional

4 slices tomato, optional

1. In a large bowl, combine the mushrooms, turkey, egg, onion, garlic, and Worcestershire sauce. Shape into 4 equal patties.

2. In a large skillet coated with cooking spray over medium heat, cook the burgers for 12 to 15 minutes, turning once, or until a thermometer inserted in the center registers 165°F and the meat is no longer pink.

3. Cut the pitas in half and open to form a pocket. Place the burgers in the pitas. Add the lettuce and tomato, if desired.

PER SERVING: 212 calories, 17 g protein, 22 g carbohydrates, 3 g fiber, 2 g total sugar, 7 g fat, 2 g saturated fat, 362 mg sodium

ZESTY PORK TENDERLOIN WRAP

Makes 1 serving

PREP TIME: 5 MINUTES | TOTAL TIME: 5 MINUTES

1 corn tortilla (6" diameter)

5 thin slices roasted pork tenderloin (2 ounces), cut into strips

1 thin slice red onion, separated into rings

1 leaf red oak lettuce, shredded

1 tablespoon Salsa Fresca (page 346) or jarred salsa

1. Place the tortilla on a microwaveable plate and cover with waxed paper. Microwave on medium power for 30 seconds, or until hot and steaming.

2. Arrange the pork, onion rings, lettuce, and salsa on top. Roll into a wrap.

PER SERVING: 145 calories, 16 g protein, 13 g carbohydrates, 1 g fiber, < 1 g total sugar, 3 g fat, 0.5 g saturated fat, 46 mg sodium

VEGETARIAN SLOPPY JOES IN ROMAINE WRAPS

Makes 4 servings

PREP TIME: 10 MINUTES | TOTAL TIME: 45 MINUTES

2 cups (12 ounces) vegetarian meat crumbles

1 onion, finely chopped

2 cups no-salt-added tomato sauce

1 cup dried lentils

2 tablespoons tomato paste

1 tablespoon Worcestershire sauce

¼ teaspoon fine sea salt

¼ teaspoon ground black pepper

¼ teaspoon red-pepper flakes

8 leaves romaine lettuce

1. In a large nonstick skillet coated with cooking spray over medium-high heat, brown the vegetarian meat crumbles and onion, stirring often, for 5 to 7 minutes.

2. Stir in the tomato sauce, lentils, tomato paste, Worcestershire sauce, salt, black pepper, and red-pepper flakes. Reduce the heat to low, cover, and cook for 30 minutes, or until the lentils are soft and the flavors are blended.

3. Place the romaine leaves on 4 serving plates. Top each with the meat mixture and roll up wrap-style.

PER SERVING: 331 calories, 35 g protein, 54 g carbohydrates, 24 g fiber, 5 g total sugar, 2 g fat, 0 g saturated fat, 680 mg sodium

FAST AND FRESH SALAD
Makes 4 servings

PREP TIME: 5 MINUTES | TOTAL TIME: 5 MINUTES

2 teaspoons extra virgin olive oil

1 teaspoon flaxseed oil

2 teaspoons red wine vinegar or white wine vinegar

1 bag (10 ounces) prewashed salad greens with carrots and radicchio

1 cup grape tomatoes

3 scallions, sliced

Ground black pepper

In a large bowl, whisk together the oils and vinegar. Add the greens, tomatoes, and scallions. Toss to coat. Season to taste with the pepper.

PER SERVING: 53 calories, 1 g protein, 5 g carbohydrates, 2 g fiber, 3 g total sugar, 3 g fat, 0.5 g saturated fat, 12 mg sodium

SPINACH AND STRAWBERRY SALAD WITH MUSTARD DRESSING
Makes 4 servings

PREP TIME: 10 MINUTES | TOTAL TIME: 10 MINUTES

1 tablespoon extra virgin olive oil

1 tablespoon white wine vinegar

1 tablespoon freshly squeezed lemon juice

1 teaspoon Dijon mustard

8 cups torn spinach

1 cup sliced strawberries

2 tablespoons chopped toasted pecans

In a large bowl, whisk together the oil, vinegar, lemon juice, and mustard. Add the spinach and strawberries and toss to coat. Transfer to salad plates and sprinkle on the pecans.

PER SERVING: 77 calories, 2 g protein, 5 g carbohydrates, 2 g fiber, 2 g total sugar, 6 g fat, 0.5 g saturated fat, 59 mg sodium

ASPARAGUS AND BARLEY SALAD WITH DILL DRESSING

Makes 4 servings

PREP TIME: 10 MINUTES | TOTAL TIME: 1 HOUR 20 MINUTES + CHILLING

3 cups water

1 bunch asparagus, tough ends trimmed, cut diagonally into 2" pieces

2/3 cup barley (not pearled)

3/4 cup 2% plain yogurt

2 teaspoons extra virgin olive oil

1 teaspoon flaxseed oil

3 tablespoons chopped fresh dill

2 tablespoons freshly squeezed lemon juice

1 clove garlic, minced

1/4 teaspoon ground black pepper

1/8 teaspoon salt

3 scallions, thinly sliced

1. In a large saucepan over high heat, bring the water to a boil. Add the asparagus. Cook, stirring occasionally, for 3 to 5 minutes, or until tender-crisp. With a skimmer or slotted spoon, transfer the asparagus to a colander and rinse briefly under cold running water. Drain. Cover and refrigerate until ready to assemble the salad.

2. To the same water, add the barley and return to a boil. Reduce the heat to low, cover, and simmer for 45 minutes, or until the barley is tender. Drain in a colander. Place a piece of waxed paper on top of the barley and let it stand for 15 minutes, or until lukewarm.

3. In a large bowl, stir together the yogurt, oils, dill, lemon juice, garlic, pepper, and salt. Add the scallions, asparagus, and barley and toss gently to mix well. Cover and chill until ready to serve.

PER SERVING: 189 calories, 8 g protein, 33 g carbohydrates, 8 g fiber, 6 g total sugar, 4 g fat, 0.5 g saturated fat, 104 mg sodium

COUSCOUS-BEAN SALAD

Make it ahead!

Makes 4 servings

1¼ cups water

¾ cup whole wheat couscous

½ cup canned red kidney beans, rinsed and drained

2 stalks broccoli (8 ounces), peeled and chopped

½ red bell pepper, chopped

¼ red onion, chopped

¼ cup crumbled feta cheese

2 tablespoons thinly sliced fresh basil

2 tablespoons freshly squeezed lemon juice or white wine vinegar

2 teaspoons flaxseed oil

1 teaspoon extra virgin olive oil

¼ teaspoon ground black pepper

⅛ teaspoon fine sea salt

1. In a medium saucepan over medium-high heat, bring the water to a boil. Stir in the couscous and return to a boil. Reduce the heat to low, cover, and simmer for 2 minutes. Remove from the heat and let stand for 5 minutes. Fluff with a fork and cool, uncovered, for 5 minutes.

2. Meanwhile, in a large bowl, combine the beans, broccoli, bell pepper, onion, cheese, and basil. Add the couscous and toss well.

3. In a small bowl, combine the lemon juice or vinegar, oils, black pepper, and salt. Pour over the couscous-bean salad and toss well.

PER SERVING: 250 calories, 11 g protein, 41 g carbohydrates, 9 g fiber, 4 g total sugar, 6 g fat, 2 g saturated fat, 199 mg sodium

NOTES: *This salad is great for brown-bag lunches. It can be refrigerated in a tightly sealed container for up to 5 days.*

BROWN RICE ASPARAGUS SALAD

Makes 4 servings

PREP TIME: 5 MINUTES | TOTAL TIME: 40 MINUTES

1 cup brown rice

1 bunch thin asparagus, trimmed and cut into pieces

3 tablespoons freshly squeezed lemon juice

2 tablespoons olive oil

½ clove garlic, minced

3 scallions, chopped

1. Cook the rice according to package directions.

2. Steam the asparagus for 6 to 8 minutes, or until tender-crisp (for steaming instructions, see page 362).

3. In a large bowl, combine the lemon juice, oil, and garlic. Add the rice, asparagus, and scallions. Toss to coat well. Serve immediately or refrigerate to serve chilled.

PER SERVING: 261 calories, 6 g protein, 42 g carbohydrates, 4 g fiber, 3 g total sugar, 8 g fat, 1 g saturated fat, 6 mg sodium

QUINOA-CHICKPEA SALAD WITH TOMATO AND KALE

Makes 4 servings

PREP TIME: 10 MINUTES | TOTAL TIME: 30 MINUTES

1 cup quinoa

¼ teaspoon fine sea salt

2 tablespoons white wine vinegar

1 tablespoon olive oil

2 cups chopped tomatoes or cherry tomatoes, halved

1 cup baby kale

½ cup canned chickpeas, rinsed and drained

1. Prepare the quinoa according to package directions. Remove from the heat, add the salt, and let stand for 5 minutes.

2. Meanwhile, in a large bowl, whisk together the vinegar and oil. Add the quinoa, tomatoes, kale, and chickpeas. Toss to coat well. Serve warm or at room temperature.

PER SERVING: 233 calories, 8 g protein, 36 g carbohydrates, 4 g fiber, 4 g total sugar, 7 g fat, 1 g saturated fat, 205 mg sodium

CRUNCHY CHINESE SLAW

Makes 4 servings

PREP TIME: 15 MINUTES | TOTAL TIME: 15 MINUTES

2 tablespoons rice vinegar or white wine vinegar

2 teaspoons soy sauce

2 teaspoons sesame oil

1 teaspoon grated fresh ginger

½ head Napa cabbage, shredded

2 carrots, shredded

3 scallions, sliced

½ red bell pepper, thinly sliced

2 tablespoons chopped fresh cilantro

2 teaspoons toasted sesame seeds

In a large bowl, combine the vinegar, soy sauce, oil, and ginger. Add the cabbage, carrots, scallions, pepper, and cilantro. Toss to coat. Sprinkle each serving with the sesame seeds.

PER SERVING: 75 calories, 2 g protein, 11 g carbohydrates, 4 g fiber, 5 g total sugar, 3 g fat, 0.5 g saturated fat, 188 mg sodium

TEMPEH SALAD WITH SESAME-GARLIC DRESSING

Makes 4 servings

PREP TIME: 15 MINUTES | TOTAL TIME: 25 MINUTES

2 teaspoons + 1 tablespoon toasted sesame oil

1 package (8 ounces) tempeh, cut into 1" cubes

2 tablespoons soy sauce

2 tablespoons freshly squeezed lemon juice

1 clove garlic, minced

1/2 teaspoon red-pepper flakes

1 pound Napa cabbage, sliced (5 cups)

1 carrot, shredded

1/4 cup fresh cilantro, finely chopped

1/4 cup sliced almonds

1. In a large nonstick skillet over medium heat, warm the 2 teaspoons of oil. Cook the tempeh, stirring occasionally, for 5 to 7 minutes, or until browned on all sides.

2. In a large bowl, whisk together the soy sauce, lemon juice, garlic, red-pepper flakes, and the remaining 1 tablespoon oil.

3. Add the tempeh, cabbage, and carrot. Toss to coat well.

4. Divide the salad among 4 plates and sprinkle evenly with the cilantro and almonds.

PER SERVING: 247 calories, 11 g protein, 20 g carbohydrates, 7 g fiber, 3 g total sugar, 13 g fat, 1.5 g saturated fat, 472 mg sodium

CHICKEN OVER WILTED KALE SALAD

Makes 4 servings

PREP TIME: 15 MINUTES | TOTAL TIME: 40 MINUTES

2 boneless, skinless chicken breast halves (4 ounces each)

2 onions, cut into wedges

2 large apples, cored and cut into wedges

2 tablespoons olive oil, divided

2 cloves garlic, finely chopped

1 teaspoon dried thyme

3/4 teaspoon fine sea salt, divided

1/2 pound kale, stems removed and chopped (4 cups)

1-2 tablespoons apple cider vinegar

1. Preheat the oven to 375°F. Coat a roasting pan with cooking spray.

2. Arrange the chicken, onions, and apples in the pan. Drizzle with 1 tablespoon of the oil. Sprinkle on the garlic, thyme, and ½ teaspoon of the salt.

3. Bake for 20 minutes, or until a thermometer inserted in the thickest portion of the chicken registers 165°F and the juices run clear. Keep warm.

4. Meanwhile, in a large nonstick skillet over medium heat, warm the remaining 1 tablespoon oil. Cook the kale, tossing, for 3 to 4 minutes, or until wilted. Remove from the heat, drizzle with the vinegar, and sprinkle with the remaining ¼ teaspoon salt. Toss to combine.

5. Divide the kale among 4 plates. Slice each breast in half. Set one half on each plate along with equal portions of the onions and apples.

PER SERVING: 253 calories, 18 g protein, 27 g carbohydrates, 5 g fiber, 14 g total sugar, 9 g fat, 1.5 g saturated fat, 403 mg sodium

CHICKEN AND RICE SALAD WITH WALNUTS

Makes 4 servings

PREP TIME: 10 MINUTES | TOTAL TIME: 10 MINUTES

- ⅓ cup 2% plain Greek yogurt
- 1 teaspoon grated orange peel
- 3 tablespoons orange juice
- ¼ teaspoon fine sea salt
- ¼ teaspoon ground black pepper
- 2 cups chopped cooked boneless, skinless chicken breast
- 1 cup cooked brown basmati rice
- ¼ cup chopped walnuts
- 6 scallions, sliced
- 1 rib celery with leaves, finely chopped
- 2 cups torn red romaine lettuce leaves

In a large bowl, whisk together the yogurt, orange peel, orange juice, salt, and pepper. Add the chicken, rice, walnuts, scallions, and celery and toss well. Divide the lettuce among 4 serving plates and top with the chicken mixture.

PER SERVING: 180 calories, 26 g protein, 22 g carbohydrates, 3 g fiber, 4 g total sugar, 8 g fat, 1 g saturated fat, 228 mg sodium

GRILLED STEAK SALAD WITH ARTICHOKES AND MUSHROOMS

Makes 1 serving

PREP TIME: 10 MINUTES | TOTAL TIME: 25 MINUTES

2 ounces lean, grass-fed flank steak

¼ teaspoon fine sea salt

¼ teaspoon ground black pepper

1 small heart romaine lettuce, chopped (4 cups)

2 marinated artichoke hearts, coarsely chopped

1 cup white mushrooms, sliced

¼ small red onion, thinly sliced

2 tablespoons red wine vinegar

1 tablespoon fresh basil, chopped

1 tablespoon olive oil

1. Preheat the grill or broiler to high heat.

2. Sprinkle the steak with the salt and pepper. Grill or broil for 3 to 5 minutes per side. Let rest for 5 minutes. Thinly slice the steak against the grain.

3. Meanwhile, in a large bowl, toss the lettuce, artichokes, mushrooms, and onion. In a small bowl, whisk together the vinegar, basil, and oil. Add to the salad mixture and toss to coat well.

4. Place the salad on a plate and top with the sliced steak.

PER SERVING: 288 calories, 17 g protein, 14 g carbohydrates, 3 g fiber, 7 g total sugar, 19 g fat, 3 g saturated fat, 737 mg sodium

SHRIMP AND RASPBERRY SALAD WITH PITA WEDGES

Makes 1 serving

PREP TIME: 10 MINUTES | TOTAL TIME: 10 MINUTES

2 cups mixed baby greens

4 large peeled and deveined cooked shrimp

1 cup raspberries

¼ small red onion, sliced

1 tablespoon freshly squeezed lemon juice

1 tablespoon olive oil

¼ avocado, chopped

1 whole wheat pita, cut into wedges and toasted

1. Place the greens on a plate. Top with the shrimp, raspberries, and onion.

2. In a small bowl, whisk together the lemon juice and oil. Drizzle over the salad. Top with the avocado.

3. Serve with the pita wedges.

PER SERVING: 502 calories, 19 g protein, 63 g carbohydrates, 17 g fiber, 7 g total sugar, 22 g fat, 3 g saturated fat, 793 mg sodium

VEGGIE SKILLET

Makes 2 servings

PREP TIME: 15 MINUTES | TOTAL TIME: 20 MINUTES

2 carrots, cut into matchsticks

1 cup broccoli florets

1 small red onion, thinly sliced

⅛ teaspoon fine sea salt

In a large skillet coated with cooking spray over medium-high heat, cook the carrots, broccoli, onion, and salt, stirring often, for 4 minutes, or until tender-crisp.

PER SERVING: 49 calories, 2 g protein, 11 g carbohydrates, 3 g fiber, 4 g total sugar, 0 g fat, 0 g saturated fat, 201 mg sodium

MASHED CAULIFLOWER WITH PARMESAN

Makes 6 servings

PREP TIME: 10 MINUTES | TOTAL TIME: 40 MINUTES

1 head cauliflower, cut into large florets

2 cans (15–19 ounces each) cannellini beans, rinsed and drained

3 cloves garlic, finely chopped

1 teaspoon fine sea salt

¼ teaspoon ground black pepper

¾ cup 2% plain Greek yogurt

¼ cup grated Parmesan cheese

1. In a large saucepan over high heat, combine the cauliflower, beans, garlic, salt, pepper, and enough water to cover. Bring to a boil. Reduce the heat to medium-low, cover, and cook for 25 to 30 minutes, or until the cauliflower is tender.

2. Drain and return to the saucepan, off the heat. Add the yogurt and cheese. With an electric mixer at low speed, whip until well mixed.

PER SERVING: 142 calories, 12 g protein, 22 g carbohydrates, 6 g fiber, 5 g total sugar, 2 g fat, 1 g saturated fat, 604 mg sodium

ROASTED BROCCOLI AND CAULIFLOWER

Makes 4 servings

PREP TIME: 10 MINUTES | TOTAL TIME: 30 MINUTES

2 pounds broccoli

2 pounds cauliflower

1 tablespoon extra virgin olive oil

⅛ teaspoon fine sea salt

⅛ teaspoon ground black pepper

2 teaspoons flaxseed oil

2 teaspoons freshly grated lemon peel

1. Preheat the oven to 450°F. Coat a large baking sheet with cooking spray.

2. Peel the broccoli stalks. Cut the stalks and florets into bite-size pieces. Trim the cauliflower. Cut into bite-size pieces.

3. In a large bowl, toss the broccoli and cauliflower with the olive oil, salt, and pepper. Spread over the baking sheet.

4. Roast, stirring occasionally, for 20 minutes, or until tender-crisp and slightly browned. Return to the large bowl and toss with the flaxseed oil and lemon peel.

PER SERVING: 186 calories, 11 g protein, 27 g carbohydrates, 11 g fiber, 8 g total sugar, 7 g fat, 1 g saturated fat, 216 mg sodium

ROASTED SQUASH WITH RED ONION AND ARUGULA

Makes 4 servings

PREP TIME: 10 MINUTES | TOTAL TIME: 35 MINUTES

- 1 pound winter squash (butternut, delicata, or kabocha), peeled, seeded, and cubed
- 1 red onion, cut into eighths
- 2 tablespoons apple cider vinegar
- ¼ teaspoon fine sea salt
- 2 tablespoons olive oil, divided
- 1 bag (5 ounces) arugula (8 cups)
- 2 tablespoons lemon juice
- ½ cup walnuts, toasted and chopped

1. Preheat the oven to 375°F.

2. In a large bowl, toss the squash and onion with the vinegar, salt, and 1 tablespoon of the oil. Spread the mixture on a baking sheet.

3. Roast for 15 to 20 minutes, or until just tender. Set aside to cool for 10 minutes.

4. Meanwhile, in the same bowl, combine the arugula, lemon juice, and the remaining 1 tablespoon oil. Toss well.

5. Divide the arugula among 4 plates. Top each with the squash and onion mixture. Sprinkle with the walnuts.

PER SERVING: 215 calories, 5 g protein, 19 g carbohydrates, 4 g fiber, 5 g total sugar, 15 g fat, 2 g saturated fat, 168 mg sodium

TURKEY MEAT LOAF

Make it ahead!

Makes 6 servings

PREP TIME: 15 MINUTES | TOTAL TIME: 1 HOUR 15 MINUTES + COOLING AND STANDING

1 sweet potato (8 ounces), peeled and cut into ½" cubes

2 slices multigrain bread

1½ cups quick-cooking oats or regular oats

2 tablespoons ground flaxseed

½ cup 2% milk or plant-based milk

1 pound ground turkey breast

1 small onion, chopped

½ cup tomato puree, divided

¼ cup chopped fresh flat-leaf parsley

½ teaspoon fine sea salt

¼ teaspoon ground black pepper

1. Preheat the oven to 350°F. Coat a baking sheet with cooking spray.

2. Place the potato in a small saucepan with enough water to cover by 2". Bring to a boil over high heat and cook for 5 to 6 minutes, or until fork-tender but still firm. Drain and let cool for 5 minutes.

3. Meanwhile, in a food processor, pulse the bread into bread crumbs. Transfer to a large bowl and stir in the oats, flaxseed, and milk. Let stand for 5 minutes, or until softened.

4. Add the turkey, onion, 3 tablespoons of the tomato puree, the parsley, salt, pepper, and potato to the bread crumb mixture. Lightly mix with your hands until the ingredients come together. Transfer the mixture to the baking sheet and form into a 9" × 4" loaf. Spread the top with the remaining 5 tablespoons tomato puree.

5. Bake for 1 hour, or until a thermometer inserted into the thickest part of the loaf registers 165°F and the meat is no longer pink. Remove and let stand for 10 minutes before cutting into 12 slices.

PER SERVING: 288 calories, 21 g protein, 32 g carbohydrates, 6 g fiber, 6 g total sugar, 9 g fat, 2 g saturated fat, 401 mg sodium

NOTE: *To save time and work, double the recipe and bake 2 meat loaves. Tightly wrap leftover slices and refrigerate for up to 3 days, or freeze for up to 1 month. Use in brown-bag sandwiches or salads.*

KIDNEY BEAN AND TURKEY CHILI

Make it ahead!

Makes 4 servings

PREP TIME: 8 MINUTES | TOTAL TIME: 35 MINUTES

1 teaspoon extra virgin olive oil

1 onion, chopped

1 green bell pepper, chopped

2 cloves garlic, minced

1 jalapeño chile pepper, finely chopped (wear plastic gloves
    when handling)

1 tablespoon dried oregano

1 tablespoon chili powder

¼ pound ground turkey breast

1 can (28 ounces) no-salt-added diced tomatoes

1 can (15 ounces) tomato sauce

2 cups water

½ cup bulgur

2 cans (15–19 ounces each) red kidney beans, rinsed and drained

Hot-pepper sauce (optional)

1. In a Dutch oven over medium heat, warm the oil. Cook the onion, bell pepper, garlic, chile pepper, oregano, and chili powder, stirring occasionally, for 5 minutes, or until softened. Crumble in the turkey. Cook, stirring occasionally, for 2 minutes, or until the turkey is no longer pink.

2. Add the tomatoes, tomato sauce, and water. Increase the heat to medium-high and cook, stirring occasionally, for 5 minutes. Stir in the bulgur and beans. Reduce the heat to medium and cook for 15 minutes, or until thickened. Season with the hot-pepper sauce, if desired.

PER SERVING: 330 calories, 19 g protein, 57 g carbohydrates, 15 g fiber, 15 g total sugar, 4 g fat, 1 g saturated fat, 959 mg sodium

NOTE: *A great way to tone down the heat of your favorite chili is by pairing it with cooling condiments. Terrific low-fat chili toppers and add-ons include fat-free sour cream, fat-free plain yogurt, low-fat shredded cheese, lime wedges, chopped fresh cilantro, chopped fresh flat-leaf parsley, celery sticks, and carrot sticks.*

ARROZ CON POLLO

Make it ahead!

Makes 4 servings

PREP TIME: 20 MINUTES | TOTAL TIME: 1 HOUR + STANDING

2 large boneless, skinless chicken thighs (4 ounces each), cut into ½"-wide strips

½ teaspoon fine sea salt, divided

¼ teaspoon ground black pepper, divided

1 teaspoon extra virgin olive oil

1 large onion, chopped

2 cloves garlic, minced

1 red bell pepper, chopped

1 cup medium-grain brown rice

2 teaspoons ground cumin

1 can (14.5 ounces) diced tomatoes

2 cups vegetable broth

2 cups frozen edamame

Red-pepper flakes

1. Sprinkle the chicken with ¼ teaspoon of the salt and ⅛ teaspoon of the black pepper. In a large nonstick pot over medium-high heat, warm the oil. Cook the chicken for 2 minutes per side, or until browned. Transfer to a plate and set aside.

2. In the same pot, cook the onion, garlic, and bell pepper, stirring occasionally, for 4 minutes, or until the vegetables start to soften. Stir in the rice, cumin, and the remaining salt and pepper. Cook, stirring, for 1 minute.

3. Add the tomatoes, broth, and reserved chicken. Bring to a boil. Reduce the heat to medium-low, cover, and simmer for 30 minutes, or until the liquid has been absorbed and the rice is tender. Stir in the edamame and cook for 2 minutes, or until heated through.

4. Remove from the heat and let stand for 5 minutes. Serve with the red-pepper flakes.

PER SERVING: 409 calories, 25 g protein, 56 g carbohydrates, 8 g fiber, 8 g total sugar, 9 g fat, 1.5 g saturated fat, 656 mg sodium

NOTE: *Refrigerate leftovers in a tightly sealed container for up to 5 days. To reheat, transfer to a pot and heat gently over medium heat.*

ORANGE CHICKEN AND BROCCOLI STIR-FRY

Makes 4 servings

PREP TIME: 20 MINUTES | TOTAL TIME: 29 MINUTES

⅓ cup freshly squeezed orange juice

1 tablespoon soy sauce

2 teaspoons cornstarch

2 teaspoons coconut oil

1 pound chicken tenders, trimmed and cut into 1" pieces

3 scallions, sliced

3 large cloves garlic, minced

1 tablespoon grated fresh ginger

⅓ cup fat-free chicken broth

1½ pounds broccoli, stems trimmed and thinly sliced and florets cut into bite-size pieces

1 red bell pepper, thinly sliced

1 navel orange, peeled, pith completely removed, and cut into small chunks

2 teaspoons flaxseed oil

1. In a small bowl, stir together the orange juice, soy sauce, and cornstarch until blended. Set aside.

2. In a wok or large nonstick skillet over high heat, warm the coconut oil. Cook the chicken, stirring frequently, for 2 to 3 minutes, or until opaque and cooked through. Add the scallions, garlic, and ginger and stir to combine. With a slotted spoon, transfer the chicken to a plate.

3. Reduce the heat to medium, add the broth and broccoli, cover, and cook for 2 minutes. Increase the heat to high and add the pepper. Cook, stirring frequently, for 2 minutes, or until the broth evaporates and the vegetables are tender-crisp.

4. Stir the reserved orange mixture and add to the wok or skillet along with the chicken. Cook, stirring constantly, for 1 to 2 minutes, or until the sauce thickens and the chicken is hot. Stir in the orange and flaxseed oil.

PER SERVING: 254 calories, 32 g protein, 23 g carbohydrates, 6 g fiber, 9 g total sugar, 6 g fat, 2 g saturated fat, 405 mg sodium

Make it ahead!

OVEN-FRIED ROSEMARY CHICKEN BREASTS

Makes 4 servings

PREP TIME: 5 MINUTES | TOTAL TIME: 20 MINUTES + STANDING

4 boneless, skinless chicken breasts (4 ounces each)

1 tablespoon dried rosemary, crumbled

1 tablespoon ground flaxseed

1 tablespoon extra virgin olive oil

1 large clove garlic, minced

⅛ teaspoon fine sea salt

Balsamic vinegar (optional)

1. Preheat the oven to 475°F. Make several shallow, diagonal cuts in the smoother, rounder side of each chicken breast.

2. In a small bowl, combine the rosemary, flaxseed, oil, garlic, and salt. Rub the mixture on all sides of the chicken.

3. In an ovenproof skillet coated with cooking spray over high heat, cook the chicken for 5 minutes. Flip the chicken. Place the skillet in the oven and bake for 10 minutes, or until a thermometer inserted in the thickest portion registers 165°F and the juices run clear. Allow to stand for 5 minutes.

4. Cut the chicken diagonally into slices. Serve with a drizzle of the vinegar, if desired.

PER SERVING: 169 calories, 23 g protein, 1 g carbohydrates, 1 g fiber, 0 g total sugar, 7 g fat, 1.5 g saturated fat, 128 mg sodium

NOTE: *Extra cooked chicken may be wrapped tightly and refrigerated for up to 3 days. Use to garnish a main-dish salad or in a sandwich or wrap.*

SWEET-AND-SOUR RED CABBAGE WITH SAUSAGE

Makes 4 servings

PREP TIME: 5 MINUTES | TOTAL TIME: 40 MINUTES

1 tablespoon extra virgin olive oil or coconut oil, divided

½ onion, chopped

4 cups shredded red cabbage

1 can (15 ounces) sliced beets, rinsed, drained, and cut into sticks

2 tablespoons red wine vinegar

1 tablespoon agave nectar or honey

2 bay leaves

Ground black pepper

4 sweet Italian–flavored chicken sausage links (3 ounces each),
butterflied lengthwise

1. In a large pot over medium-low heat, warm 2 teaspoons of the oil. Cook the onion for 3 minutes, or until it sizzles. Do not brown.

2. Add the cabbage, beets, vinegar, agave or honey, and bay leaves. Cook, stirring occasionally, for 2 minutes, or until sizzling.

3. Cover and cook, stirring occasionally, for 30 minutes, or until the cabbage is very tender. Remove and discard the bay leaves. Season to taste with the pepper.

4. Meanwhile, in a large skillet over medium heat, warm the remaining 1 teaspoon oil. Cook the sausage, cut side down, for 3 minutes, or until golden. Flip and cook for 3 minutes, or until golden brown and cooked through.

5. Serve the cabbage with the sausage on top.

PER SERVING: 93 calories, 16 g protein, 18 g carbohydrates, 3 g fiber, 13 g total sugar, 10 g fat, 2 g saturated fat, 676 mg sodium

Make it ahead!

BEEF AND VEGETABLE STEW

Makes 4 servings

PREP TIME: 15 MINUTES | TOTAL TIME: 8 HOURS 20 MINUTES

1 teaspoon olive oil

8 ounces lean grass-fed beef stew meat, cubed

1 clove garlic, minced

2 onions, chopped

1½ cups frozen corn

1 can (14.5 ounces) vegetable broth

1 can (14.5 ounces) diced tomatoes

4 carrots, sliced

2 tablespoons tomato paste

1 teaspoon dried oregano

3 cups cooked brown rice

1. In a medium skillet over medium-high heat, warm the oil. Sear the beef cubes until browned on all sides. Add the garlic and cook for 1 minute, or until fragrant.

2. In a slow cooker, combine the beef, garlic, onions, corn, broth, tomatoes, carrots, tomato paste, and oregano. Cover and cook on low for 6 to 8 hours or on high for 3 to 4 hours.

3. Serve over the brown rice.

PER SERVING: 378 calories, 20 g protein, 64 g carbohydrates, 8 g fiber, 12 g total sugar, 6 g fat, 2 g saturated fat, 635 mg sodium

BRAISED BEEF WITH MUSHROOMS
Makes 8 servings

PREP TIME: 10 MINUTES | TOTAL TIME: 2 HOURS + SOAKING

¼ ounce dried wild mushrooms (2 tablespoons)

½ cup boiling-hot water

2 pounds 95% lean boneless top round or sirloin, cut into 1½" cubes

½ teaspoon fine sea salt

¼ teaspoon ground black pepper

2 tablespoons extra virgin olive oil

10 ounces portobello mushrooms, gills removed and quartered

1 onion, chopped

1 clove garlic, minced

2 tablespoons whole wheat flour

1¼ cups dry red wine or low-fat, reduced-sodium beef broth

1 cup water, divided

½ teaspoon dried thyme or oregano

1. Preheat the oven to 350°F.

2. In a bowl, soak the dried wild mushrooms in the boiling-hot water for 20 minutes, or until softened. Using tongs, pluck out the mushrooms and reserve the soaking water. Trim away dirty sections and chop any large pieces.

3. Meanwhile, trim the meat of any visible fat. Season with the salt and pepper. In a large ovenproof pot over medium-high heat, warm the oil. Working in batches, cook the meat for 12 to 15 minutes, or until browned, removing pieces to a plate as they are done.

4. Reduce the heat to medium and add the wild and portobello mushrooms, onion, and garlic. Cook, stirring occasionally, for 2 minutes. Return the meat to the pot, sprinkle with the flour, and cook, stirring, for 1 minute. Carefully pour in the reserved soaking water, leaving behind any grit. Add the wine or broth and ½ cup of the water. If the mixture is too thick, add up to ½ cup more water. Bring to a boil and add the thyme or oregano.

5. Cover, place in the oven, and bake for 1½ hours, or until the meat is tender.

PER SERVING: 240 calories, 27 g protein, 6 g carbohydrates, 1 g fiber, 2 g total sugar, 8 g fat, 2 g saturated fat, 221 mg sodium

PAPRIKA-RUBBED PORK LOIN

Makes 6 servings

PREP TIME: 10 MINUTES | TOTAL TIME: 50 MINUTES

1 red onion, thickly sliced

1¼ pounds boneless center-cut pork loin, trimmed

1 teaspoon minced garlic

½ teaspoon paprika

½ teaspoon fine sea salt

1 cup reduced-sodium vegetable broth

1. Preheat the oven to 350°F. Coat a roasting pan with cooking spray.

2. Arrange the onion slices in a single layer in the pan. Rub the loin with the garlic, paprika, and salt. Place the rubbed loin on top of the onion slices. Pour the broth around the pork.

3. Roast for 30 minutes, or until a thermometer inserted in the center reaches 145°F. Let stand for 10 minutes before slicing.

PER SERVING: 117 calories, 20 g protein, 2 g carbohydrates, 0 g fiber, 1 g total sugar, 2 g fat, 1 g saturated fat, 271 mg sodium

SALMON WITH SWISS CHARD

Make it ahead!

Makes 4 servings

PREP TIME: 10 MINUTES | TOTAL TIME: 28 MINUTES

1 pound Swiss chard, stalks and leaves, thinly sliced

¼ cup water

4 scallions, thinly sliced

2 cloves garlic, minced

¼ teaspoon ground black pepper

4 skinless wild-caught salmon fillets (4–5 ounces each), 1½" thick

1 teaspoon lemon-pepper seasoning

4 lemon wedges (optional)

1. In a large, deep nonstick skillet over high heat, cook the chard, water, scallions, and garlic for 4 minutes, or until the mixture boils. Stir and reduce the heat to medium. Cover and cook for 2 minutes, or until the chard leaves are wilted. Season with the pepper.

2. Meanwhile, rub the fillets with the seasoning. Set them atop the chard mixture, adding up to ¼ cup water if the liquid has evaporated. Increase the heat to medium-high, cover, and cook for 10 to 12 minutes, or until the salmon is opaque.

3. Transfer the fillets to 4 plates. Increase the heat to high and cook off any remaining liquid. Spoon the chard next to each fillet. Serve with the lemon wedges, if desired.

PER SERVING: 230 calories, 31 g protein, 6 g carbohydrates, 2 g fiber, 2 g total sugar, 9 g fat, 1 g saturated fat, 337 mg sodium

NOTE: *Refrigerate leftover individual portions for a quick brown-bag lunch salad. Combine the salmon and chard with ½ cup cooked brown rice, whole wheat couscous, or other cooked whole grain. Drizzle with balsamic vinegar to taste. Season with red-pepper flakes, if desired.*

ROASTED SALMON, CARROTS, AND LEEKS WITH PENNE

Makes 4 servings

PREP TIME: 25 MINUTES | TOTAL TIME: 1 HOUR 10 MINUTES

1¹/2 pounds leeks, white part only, rinsed well and cut crosswise into 2" pieces and quartered lengthwise

3 carrots, thinly sliced

¼ cup vegetable broth

1 tablespoon extra virgin olive oil, divided

2 teaspoons dried thyme

¼ teaspoon ground black pepper

1 pound skinless wild-caught salmon fillet

2 cups whole wheat penne (8 ounces)

1. Preheat the oven to 400°F.

2. In a 9" x 13" baking dish, combine the leeks, carrots, broth, 2 teaspoons of the oil, the thyme, and pepper. Cover with foil and bake for 15 minutes.

3. Add the salmon to the baking dish and drizzle with the remaining 1 teaspoon oil. Cover and bake for 30 minutes, or until the salmon is opaque and the vegetables are tender.

4. Meanwhile, prepare the pasta according to package directions. Place the penne or rice in a large serving bowl. Break the salmon into bite-size pieces and add to the penne with the vegetables and pan juices.

PER SERVING: 458 calories, 30 g protein, 57 g carbohydrates, 8 g fiber, 10 g total sugar, 12 g fat, 1.5 g saturated fat, 131 mg sodium

NOTE: *You can replace the penne with 2 cups cooked brown rice.*

PECAN-CRUSTED ROASTED SALMON

Makes 4 servings

PREP TIME: 5 MINUTES | TOTAL TIME: 17 MINUTES

2 tablespoons finely chopped pecan halves

1 large clove garlic, finely chopped

1 teaspoon olive oil

⅛ teaspoon fine sea salt

1 pound skinless wild-caught salmon fillet, cut in 4 equal pieces

Ground black pepper

1. Preheat the oven to 425°F. Coat a baking sheet with cooking spray.

2. In a small bowl, stir together the pecans, garlic, oil, and salt to make a paste. Rub on the salmon. Place the salmon on the baking sheet.

3. Roast for 10 to 12 minutes, or until just opaque. Season to taste with the pepper.

PER SERVING: 193 calories, 23 g protein, 1 g carbohydrates, 0 g fiber, < 1 g total sugar, 11 g fat, 1 g saturated fat, 124 mg sodium

GRILLED TROUT WITH SCALLION AND DILL SAUCE

Makes 4 servings

PREP TIME: 5 MINUTES | TOTAL TIME: 15 MINUTES

2/3 cup vegetable broth

1 tablespoon minced scallion greens

1 tablespoon finely chopped fresh dill or 1 teaspoon dried

1 teaspoon stone-ground mustard

2 teaspoons extra virgin olive oil

4 rainbow trout fillets (4–5 ounces each), skin on

1. Coat a grill rack with cooking spray. Preheat the grill to medium-high.

2. In a medium skillet over high heat, bring the broth, scallions, dill, and mustard to a boil, whisking frequently. Continue to boil and whisk for 3 minutes, or until the sauce has been reduced to half of its volume. Keep warm over very low heat.

3. Rub the oil over the surface of each fillet. Set on the grill rack, skin side down, and cook for 4 to 5 minutes per side, or until the fish is opaque.

4. Transfer the fish to 4 plates. Drizzle with the sauce.

PER SERVING: 160 calories, 23 g protein, 1 g carbohydrates, 0 g fiber, 0 g total sugar, 6 g fat, 1 g saturated fat, 75 mg sodium

MACKEREL AND SPINACH IN SPICY TOMATO SAUCE

Makes 6 servings

PREP TIME: 5 MINUTES | TOTAL TIME: 25 MINUTES

2 teaspoons extra virgin olive oil

2 large cloves garlic, minced

1 can (14.5 ounces) diced tomatoes

1 cup water

1 teaspoon dried oregano

1/2 teaspoon red-pepper flakes (optional)

6 mackerel fillets (4 ounces each), skin on

1 bag (6 ounces) baby spinach

1. In a large skillet over medium heat, warm the oil. Cook the garlic for 2 minutes, or until fragrant. Add the tomatoes, water, oregano, and red-pepper flakes (if desired). Increase the heat to high and bring to a boil. Reduce the heat to medium-high and briskly simmer for 8 minutes, or until the mixture thickens.

2. Place the fish, skin side down, in the skillet. Press lightly to submerge in the sauce. Cover and cook for 8 minutes, or until the fish flakes easily. Transfer the fish to pasta bowls.

3. Increase the heat to high and add the spinach to the skillet. Cook, stirring occasionally, for 2 minutes, or until the spinach is wilted. Spoon the spinach mixture over the fish.

PER SERVING: 276 calories, 22 g protein, 7 g carbohydrates, 2 g fiber, 2 g total sugar, 17 g fat, 4 g saturated fat, 301 mg sodium

LEMON SNAPPER WITH CURRY-GARLIC CAULIFLOWER

Makes 4 servings

PREP TIME: 10 MINUTES | TOTAL TIME: 30 MINUTES

½ small head cauliflower, cut into small florets (3 cups)

4 teaspoons olive oil, divided

2 teaspoons curry powder

¼ teaspoon garlic powder

¼ teaspoon ground ginger

½ teaspoon fine sea salt, divided

1 pound red snapper fillet, cut in 4 equal pieces

2 tablespoons freshly squeezed lemon juice

1. Preheat the oven to 450°F.

2. On a baking sheet, toss the cauliflower with 2 teaspoons of the oil, the curry powder, garlic powder, ginger, and ¼ teaspoon of the salt. Spread in a single layer and bake, stirring once, for 10 minutes.

3. Meanwhile, brush both sides of the snapper with the remaining 2 teaspoons oil. Sprinkle with the lemon juice and the remaining ¼ teaspoon salt. Add the fillets to the pan and bake for 5 to 7 minutes, or until the fish is cooked through.

PER SERVING: 179 calories, 25 g protein, 5 g carbohydrates, 2 g fiber, 2 g total sugar, 6 g fat, 1 g saturated fat, 392 mg sodium

Make it ahead!

SHRIMP WITH ORZO AND EDAMAME
Makes 4 servings

PREP TIME: 7 MINUTES | TOTAL TIME: 22 MINUTES

1½ cups whole wheat orzo or other small pasta (6 ounces)

1 teaspoon extra virgin olive oil

1 onion, finely chopped

2 cloves garlic, minced

½ pound medium shrimp, peeled, deveined, and halved lengthwise

1 cup frozen shelled edamame, thawed

¾ cup dry white wine or vegetable broth

⅛ teaspoon fine sea salt

¼ teaspoon ground black pepper

¼ cup finely chopped fresh flat-leaf parsley

1. Cook the orzo or other small pasta according to package directions. Drain well.

2. In a medium nonstick skillet over medium-high heat, warm the oil. Cook the onion and garlic, stirring frequently, for 5 minutes, or until the onion is soft but not browned. Add the shrimp and edamame. Cook for 1 minute. Turn and cook for 1 minute, or until the shrimp are opaque.

3. Add the wine or broth, salt, and pepper. Bring to a boil. Reduce the heat to medium and cook for 2 to 3 minutes, or until the liquid is reduced by half.

4. Add the orzo and parsley. Toss well.

PER SERVING: 300 calories, 19 g protein, 28 g carbohydrates, 9 g fiber, 3 g total sugar, 4 g fat, 0 g saturated fat, 401 mg sodium

NOTE: *Refrigerate leftover individual portions for brown-bag lunches. The pasta is delicious at room temperature drizzled with a little lemon juice or white wine vinegar. Or reheat in a microwave with 2 teaspoons water on medium-high power for 2 minutes, or until heated through.*

SHRIMP SCAMPI

Makes 4 servings

PREP TIME: 10 MINUTES | TOTAL TIME: 45 MINUTES

1 cup brown rice

1 tablespoon extra virgin olive oil

8 scallions, trimmed and cut into ½" pieces

4 cloves garlic, minced

1 pound extra-large peeled and deveined shrimp

½ cup freshly squeezed lemon juice

½ cup finely chopped fresh flat-leaf parsley

¼ teaspoon ground black pepper

1. Cook the rice according to package directions. Set aside and keep warm.

2. In a large nonstick skillet over medium-high heat, warm the oil for 1 minute. Cook the scallions and garlic for 1 minute, or until fragrant. Add the shrimp and cook for 2 to 3 minutes, or until they start to turn opaque.

3. Add the lemon juice, parsley, and pepper and bring to a brisk simmer for 2 minutes, or until the shrimp are opaque.

4. Serve hot over the reserved rice.

PER SERVING: 307 calories, 20 g protein, 43 g carbohydrates, 3 g fiber, 2 g total sugar, 6 g fat, 1 g saturated fat, 654 mg sodium

ITALIAN ROASTED VEGETABLE LASAGNA

Makes 4 servings

PREP TIME: 20 MINUTES | TOTAL TIME: 1 HOUR 45 MINUTES

4 ounces sliced mixed mushrooms

1 small zucchini, sliced

1 onion, chopped

1 teaspoon olive oil

1/2 teaspoon fine sea salt

1/4 teaspoon ground black pepper

1 cup ricotta cheese or mashed tofu

2 tablespoons chopped fresh basil

2 tablespoons chopped fresh flat-leaf parsley

1 clove garlic, chopped

1 cup marinara sauce

6 whole wheat no-boil (oven-ready) lasagna noodles

1/4 cup Parmesan cheese

1. Preheat the oven to 400°F.

2. On a baking sheet, toss the mushrooms, zucchini, and onion with the oil and salt and pepper. Spread in a single layer and roast for 20 minutes, tossing the vegetables once. Remove from the oven. Reduce the heat to 350°F.

3. Meanwhile, in a food processor or blender, combine the ricotta or tofu, basil, parsley, and garlic. Blend or process until smooth.

4. To assemble the lasagna, spread 1/4 cup of the marinara sauce in an 8" x 8" baking dish. Top with 2 of the lasagna noodles. Layer half of the roasted vegetables over the noodles. Dollop half of the cheese mixture evenly over the vegetables.

5. Repeat the layering with 2 noodles, half of the remaining marinara sauce, the remaining vegetables, and the remaining cheese mixture. Top with the 2 remaining noodles and the remaining sauce. Sprinkle with the Parmesan. Cover the dish with foil.

6. Bake for 40 minutes, or until heated through. Remove the foil and bake for 5 to 10 minutes, or until the cheese is slightly browned. Let stand for 10 minutes before cutting and serving.

PER SERVING: 282 calories, 15 g protein, 35 g carbohydrates, 5 g fiber, 3 g total sugar, 10 g fat, 4 g saturated fat, 614 mg sodium

BROCCOLI, MUSHROOM, AND TOFU
STIR-FRY WITH WALNUTS
Makes 4 servings

PREP TIME: 10 MINUTES | TOTAL TIME: 40 MINUTES

½ cup brown rice

1 tablespoon extra virgin olive oil, divided

8 ounces portobello mushrooms, gills removed and sliced

4 cups broccoli florets

1 bunch scallions, thinly sliced

1 large clove garlic, minced

1 package (14 ounces) tofu, drained and cubed

2 teaspoons soy sauce

¼ cup chopped walnuts

1. Cook the rice according to package directions.

2. When the rice is almost done, in a wok or large skillet over medium-high heat, warm 1 teaspoon of the oil. Cook the mushrooms, covered, for 1 minute, or until they start to sizzle. Stir and cook, covered, for 4 minutes, or until the mushrooms give off their liquid. Add the broccoli, scallions, and garlic. Cover and cook for 2 minutes, or until the broccoli is bright green. Transfer the broccoli-mushroom mixture to a plate.

3. In the same wok or skillet on medium-high heat, warm the remaining 2 teaspoons oil. Cook the tofu, stirring constantly, for 5 minutes, or until golden. Return the broccoli-mushroom mixture to the wok or skillet. Add the soy sauce. Cook, stirring, for 2 minutes to blend the flavors. Sprinkle on the walnuts.

4. Serve each portion with ½ cup of the brown rice.

PER SERVING: 298 calories, 16 g protein, 31 g carbohydrates, 6 g fiber, 2 g total sugar, 4 g fat, 2 g saturated fat, 178 mg sodium

TOFU-STUFFED PEPPERS

Makes 2 servings

½ cup quick-cooking brown rice

2 red bell peppers, tops cut off and seeds scooped out

1 tablespoon olive oil, divided

½ cup shredded carrots

¼ cup marinara sauce

¼ teaspoon fine sea salt

8 ounces crumbled tofu

¼ cup shredded mozzarella cheese

1. Prepare the brown rice according to package directions. Preheat the oven to 350°F.

2. Fill a medium saucepan halfway up with water and bring to a boil over high heat. Cook the peppers for 2 to 3 minutes, or until softened but still able to hold their shape. Drain and run under cold water. Pat the peppers dry with a paper towel. Rub the outside of the peppers with ½ teaspoon of the oil.

3. In a large nonstick skillet over medium heat, warm the remaining 2½ teaspoons oil. Stir in the cooked rice, carrots, marinara, and salt and heat for 1 minute.

4. Fill the peppers with the rice mixture. Top each evenly with the tofu and cheese. Place the filled peppers in a baking dish and bake for 20 minutes, or until heated through and the cheese is melted.

PER SERVING: 418 calories, 25 g protein, 35 g carbohydrates, 7 g fiber, 6 g total sugar, 21 g fat, 4 g saturated fat, 561 mg sodium

NOTE: *You can replace the tofu with 2 cups cooked lentils.*

Make it ahead!

BEANS IN TOMATO-BASIL SAUCE

Makes 4 servings

PREP TIME: 10 MINUTES | TOTAL TIME: 25 MINUTES

2 teaspoons extra virgin olive oil

1 onion, sliced

2 large cloves garlic, thinly sliced

1 small zucchini (6 ounces), cut into ¼" chunks

¼ teaspoon fine sea salt

¼ teaspoon ground black pepper

1 can (14.5 ounces) diced tomatoes

1 tablespoon ground flaxseed

1 can (15–19 ounces) white beans, rinsed and drained

2 tablespoons chopped fresh basil

1. In a large nonstick skillet over medium heat, warm the oil. Cook the onion and garlic, stirring often, for 5 minutes, or until tender. Add the zucchini and sprinkle with the salt and pepper. Stir to blend well.

2. Add the tomatoes and flaxseed and bring to a simmer. Cook, stirring occasionally, for 6 to 8 minutes, or until the zucchini is tender-crisp. Add the beans. Cover and cook for 2 to 3 minutes, or just until heated through. Sprinkle with the basil.

PER SERVING: 131 calories, 6 g protein, 20 g carbohydrates, 5 g fiber, 6 g total sugar, 3 g fat, 0 g saturated fat, 562 mg sodium

NOTE: *The beans can be refrigerated in a tightly sealed container for up to 1 week or frozen for up to 1 month.*

Make it ahead!

DARK CHOCOLATE-RASPBERRY PATTIES

Makes 6 servings

PREP TIME: 5 MINUTES | TOTAL TIME: 15 MINUTES + CHILLING

4 ounces 70% chocolate, chopped

½ teaspoon vanilla extract

36 raspberries

1. In a small heavy-bottom saucepan over very low heat, melt the chocolate, stirring frequently. (Or microwave on low power for 90 seconds, stirring frequently.) Stir in the vanilla.

2. Spoon the chocolate onto a foil-lined plate in 12 patties. Press 3 raspberries into each patty. Refrigerate for 1 hour, or until the chocolate is set.

PER SERVING: 120 calories, 2 g protein, 10 g carbohydrates, 3 g fiber, 5 g total sugar, 8 g fat, 4.5 g saturated fat, 4 mg sodium

Make it ahead!

BAKED PEARS WITH CREAMY LEMON SAUCE

Makes 4 servings

PREP TIME: 5 MINUTES | TOTAL TIME: 35 MINUTES

4 tablespoons water

2 teaspoons extra virgin olive oil

4 small ripe pears, peeled, halved, and cored

1 tablespoon freshly squeezed lemon juice

2 teaspoons freshly grated lemon peel

1 cup 2% plain Greek yogurt

1. Preheat the oven to 375°F.

2. In a 9" × 13" baking dish, stir together the water and oil with a fork or flat whisk. Place the pears in the baking dish and turn in the mixture until coated. Turn the pears cut side up, making sure some of the liquid is in the cavities. Bake for 15 to 20 minutes, or until the pears are very tender when pierced with a fork.

3. In a small bowl, whisk together the lemon juice, lemon peel, and yogurt.

4. Allow the pears to cool in the baking dish for 10 minutes. Transfer 2 halves to each of 4 dessert dishes. Spoon some of the pan juices and ¼ cup of the lemon sauce over each.

PER SERVING: 144 calories, 5 g protein, 25 g carbohydrates, 4 g fiber, 17 g total sugar, 4 g fat, 1 g saturated fat, 20 mg sodium

NOTE: *You can double this recipe. Cool the leftover pears and refrigerate with the cooking sauce in a tightly sealed container for up to 1 week.*

BLUEBERRY-RICOTTA SUNDAE

Makes 4 servings

PREP TIME: 5 MINUTES | TOTAL TIME: 15 MINUTES + CHILLING

2 cups frozen blueberries

1 tablespoon chia seeds

2 teaspoons freshly squeezed lemon juice

1/2 cup part-skim ricotta cheese

1/2 cup 2% plain Greek yogurt

1 1/2 teaspoons vanilla extract

Dash of ground cinnamon

2 tablespoons chopped almonds

1. In a small saucepan over medium-high heat, cook the blueberries, chia seeds, and lemon juice, stirring occasionally, for 5 minutes, or until the sauce thickens slightly. Transfer to a large bowl, cover, and refrigerate for at least 1 hour, or until chilled.

2. In a blender or food processor, combine the ricotta, yogurt, vanilla, and cinnamon. Blend or process until smooth. Spoon into 4 dessert bowls. Spoon on the blueberry sauce and top with the almonds.

PER SERVING: 138 calories, 7 g protein, 14 g carbohydrates, 3 g fiber, 8 g total sugar, 6 g fat, 2 g saturated fat, 50 mg sodium

NOTE: *You can replace the blueberries with strawberries or raspberries.*

WARM GLAZED ORANGES WITH WALNUTS
Makes 4 servings

PREP TIME: 10 MINUTES | TOTAL TIME: 15 MINUTES

4 navel oranges

2 tablespoons agave nectar or honey*

1 tablespoon water

1 teaspoon coconut oil or olive oil

¼ cup chopped walnuts

1. Grate the peel from 2 of the oranges into a large nonstick skillet. Add the agave or honey, water, and oil. Set over low heat.

2. Peel the oranges and slice into rounds. Place in the skillet and cook, shaking the pan occasionally, for 3 minutes, or until the oranges are glazed.

3. Spoon the oranges and pan juices onto 4 dessert plates. Sprinkle on the walnuts.

PER SERVING: 156 calories, 2 g protein, 27 g carbohydrates, 4 g fiber, 20 g total sugar, 6 g fat, 1.5 g saturated fat, 2 mg sodium

*REMOVE FOR THE JUMPSTART PROTOCOL

STRAWBERRY SORBET
Makes 4 servings

PREP TIME: 5 MINUTES | TOTAL TIME: 10 MINUTES

1 pound frozen unsweetened strawberries

½ cup fat-free plain yogurt or silken tofu

1. In a food processor, combine the strawberries and yogurt or tofu. Process until creamy, stopping to scrape down the sides of the bowl as needed. If the fruit doesn't break down completely, gradually add cold water through the feed tube, 1 or 2 tablespoons at a time, being careful not to process the sorbet into liquid.

2. Serve immediately or transfer to an airtight container to freeze. To serve later, allow 10 to 15 minutes for the sorbet to soften at room temperature.

PER SERVING: 52 calories, 2 g protein, 13 g carbohydrates, 2 g fiber, 7 g total sugar, 0 g fat, 0 g saturated fat, 19 mg sodium

NOTE: *You can replace the strawberries with frozen mixed berries.*

CINNAMON-CHOCOLATE ICE POPS

Make it ahead!

Makes 4 servings

PREP TIME: 5 MINUTES | TOTAL TIME: 10 MINUTES + FREEZING TIME

4 ounces 85% chocolate, finely chopped

2 tablespoons packed light brown sugar*

¼ teaspoon ground cinnamon

1 cup unsweetened almond milk

½ teaspoon vanilla extract

1. In a medium glass bowl, combine the chocolate, sugar, and cinnamon.

2. In a small saucepan over medium heat, bring the milk to just a simmer. Pour over the chocolate mixture and stir until the chocolate is melted and the mixture is well blended. Add the vanilla.

3. Pour the mixture evenly into ice pop molds (or ice cube trays) and insert ice pop sticks in the center of each. Freeze for 6 to 8 hours, or until firm.

4. To remove the pops, run warm water over the outside of the mold for 10 seconds, or until you can gently pull the pops out by their sticks.

PER SERVING: 201 calories, 4 g protein, 18 g carbohydrates, 5 g fiber, 10 g total sugar, 14 g fat, 8 g saturated fat, 47 mg sodium

*REMOVE FOR THE JUMPSTART PROTOCOL

Make it ahead!

CHOCOLATE-PEANUT BUTTER SQUARES

Makes 10 servings

PREP TIME: 5 MINUTES | TOTAL TIME: 10 MINUTES + COOLING

3/4 cup smooth, unsalted peanut butter

1/2 cup honey*

1 tablespoon vanilla protein powder

4 cups puffed brown rice cereal

1/2 cup 70% chocolate chips or chunks

1. Coat an 11½" x 8" pan with cooking spray.

2. In a large pot over low heat, cook the peanut butter, honey, and protein powder, stirring often, for 2 minutes, or until smooth.

3. When melted, remove the mixture from the heat. Add the rice cereal and chocolate chips. Stir well.

4. Press the mixture into the pan. Cool completely before cutting into 10 pieces.

PER SERVING: 263 calories, 6 g protein, 32 g carbohydrates, 3 g fiber, 18 g total sugar, 13 g fat, 3 g saturated fat, 54 mg sodium

*REMOVE FOR THE JUMPSTART PROTOCOL

CINNAMON-APPLE YOGURT WITH PITA DIPPERS

Makes 1 serving

PREP TIME: 5 MINUTES | TOTAL TIME: 10 MINUTES

1/2 cup 2% plain Greek yogurt

1/4 cup chopped apple

2 teaspoons chopped pecans or almonds

1 small whole wheat pita (4" diameter)

1½ teaspoons olive oil

1/4 teaspoon ground cinnamon

1. In a small bowl, mix together the yogurt, apple, and nuts.

2. Toast the pita. Brush on the oil, sprinkle with the cinnamon, and cut into wedges.

3. Use the wedges to scoop the yogurt mixture.

PER SERVING: 258 calories, 13 g protein, 25 g carbohydrates, 4 g fiber, 8 g total sugar, 13 g fat, 3 g saturated fat, 162 mg sodium

CARAMEL BANANA DESSERT

Makes 2 servings

PREP TIME: 5 MINUTES | TOTAL TIME: 10 MINUTES

1 tablespoon butter

1 tablespoon packed light brown sugar

1 tablespoon rum or ¼ teaspoon rum extract

1 large firm-ripe banana, sliced diagonally into ½" pieces

1 tablespoon finely chopped pecans

¼ cup 2% vanilla Greek yogurt

1. In a small nonstick skillet over medium heat, melt the butter. Add the sugar and rum and cook, stirring constantly, for 1 minute, or until the sugar dissolves.

2. Stir in the banana. Cook for 2 minutes, carefully turning over once, or until the banana is browned and caramelized.

3. Divide the banana between 2 dessert plates. Drizzle with the rum sauce. Top evenly with the pecans and yogurt.

PER SERVING: 207 calories, 3 g protein, 27 g carbohydrates, 2 g fiber, 19 g total sugar, 9 g fat, 4 g saturated fat, 68 mg sodium

DOUBLE CHOCOLATE PUDDING

Make it ahead!

Makes 4 servings

PREP TIME: 5 MINUTES | TOTAL TIME: 30 MINUTES + COOLING

- 6 tablespoons unsweetened cocoa powder
- 2 tablespoons cornstarch
- 1 teaspoon instant coffee powder
- 2 cups 2% milk
- ¼ cup agave nectar or honey*
- 1 ounce unsweetened chocolate, finely chopped
- 2 teaspoons vanilla extract

1. In a medium saucepan, whisk together the cocoa, cornstarch, and coffee powder until blended. Gradually whisk in the milk and agave or honey.

2. Place over medium heat and cook, stirring constantly, for 10 minutes, or until the pudding thickens and comes to a boil. Reduce the heat to low and add the chocolate. Cook, stirring constantly, for 1 minute, or until the chocolate melts. Remove from the heat and stir in the vanilla.

3. Allow to cool, stirring constantly, for 15 minutes. Pour the pudding into 4 custard cups. Serve warm, or cover with plastic wrap and refrigerate for at least 2 hours, or until cold.

PER SERVING: 209 calories, 6 g protein, 31 g carbohydrates, 3 g fiber, 22 g total sugar, 8 g fat, 4 g saturated fat, 60 mg sodium

*REMOVE FOR JUMPSTART PROTOCOL

Food Shopping Guide

These comprehensive lists are the cornerstones of the eating plan, to be used in conjunction with the Meal Builder template (page 173). Each category of food includes healthy brand options and their nutritionals.

Here, dietitian Andie Schwartz, RD, lists many of her favorite products. If choosing your own, be careful to eyeball grams of sugar and fiber per serving, and steer clear of packaged foods that contain artificial flavors, sweeteners, or preservatives, high fructose corn syrup, and trans fats.

Whole Grains

BREADS

- **Ezekiel 4:9 7 Sprouted Grains Bread** (1 slice): 80 calories, 3 g fiber, 1 g sugar
- **Ezekiel 4:9 Sprouted Corn Tortillas** (2 tortillas): 120 calories, 3 g fiber, 1 g sugar
- **Ezekiel 4:9 Gluten Free Brown Rice English muffins** (1 muffin): 110 calories, 2 g fiber, 3 g sugar
- **Rudi's Organic Bakery 7 Grain with Flax** (1 slice): 90 calories, 3 g fiber, 2 g sugar
- **Van's 8 Whole Grains GMO-Free Waffle** (1 waffle): 75 calories, 3.5 g fiber, 1 g sugar
- **Van's 8 Whole Grains GMO-Free Pancake** (1 pancake): 80 calories, 2.5 g fiber, 2.5 g sugar
- **Arrowhead Mills Organic Sprouted Grain Pancake Mix** (¼ cup): 120 calories, 3 g fiber, 2 g sugar

CEREALS

Cold

- **Post Shredded Wheat Cereal** (1 cup): 170 calories, 6 grams fiber, 0 g sugar
- **Uncle Sam Original Flakes** (¾ cup): 190 calories, 10 g fiber, 1 g sugar
- **Erewhon Crispy Brown Rice— Gluten Free Cereal** (1 cup): 110 calories, 0 g fiber, 1 g sugar
- **Food for Life Ezekiel 4:9 Sprouted Whole Grain Cereal, Almond flavor** (½ cup): 200 calories, 6 g fiber, 1 g sugar
- **Two Moms in the Raw Plain Grain-Free Cereal** (½ cup): 250 calories, 6 g fiber, 6 g sugar

Hot

- **Bob's Red Mill Organic Scottish Oatmeal** (¼ cup, cooked): 140 calories, 4 g fiber, 0 g sugar
- **Trader Joe's Gluten-Free Rolled Oats** (½ cup, uncooked): 150 calories, 4 g fiber, 1 g sugar
- **Bob's Red Mill Creamy Brown Rice Farina Hot Cereal** (¼ cup, uncooked): 140 calories, 2 g fiber, 0 g sugar

CRACKERS

- **Mary's Gone Crackers** (13 crackers): 140 calories, 3 g fiber, 0 g sugar
- **Wasa Multigrain Crispbread** (2 slices): 120 calories, 4 g fiber, 0 g sugar
- **Lundberg Thin Stackers Brown Rice** (4 cakes): 100 calories, 2 g fiber, 0 g sugar
- **Lundberg Brown Rice Cakes** (2 cakes): 120 calories, 2 g fiber, 0 g sugar

PASTA

- **Ezekiel 4:9 Sprouted Whole Grain Elbow Pasta** (2-ounce serving): 210 calories, 7 g fiber, 0 g sugar
- **Explore Asian Gluten-Free Organic Thai Brown Rice Penne Pasta** (2-ounce serving): 200 calories, 1.5 g fiber, 0 g sugar
- **Explore Asian Organic Black Bean Spaghetti** (2 ounces dry): 180 calories, 12 g fiber, 5 g sugar
- **King Soba Organic 100% Buckwheat Noodles** (1.9-ounce serving): 170 calories, 5 g fiber, 1 g sugar

Lean Proteins

CANNED FISH

- **Wild Planet Wild Pacific Sardines in Extra Virgin Olive Oil** (2 ounces): 110 calories, 10 g protein
- **Crown Prince Wild Caught Skinless and Boneless Sardines** (3.75 ounces): 170 calories, 21 g protein
- **Bar Harbor Skinless, Boneless Smoked Sardine Fillets** (55 grams): 110 calories, 11 g protein

PLANT PROTEINS

- **Hilary's Adzuki Bean Burger** (1 burger): 190 calories, 5 g protein, 0 g sugar
- **Beyond Meat's Beefy Crumble** (½ cup): 100 calories, 13 g protein, 1 g sugar

PROTEIN POWDERS

- **Garden of Life Raw Protein, vanilla flavor** (1 level scoop): 90 calories, 3 g fiber, >1 g sugar
- **Tera's Organic Whey, all flavors** (2 scoops): 110 calories, 0 g fiber, 3 g sugar
- **Nutria Hemp Protein, vanilla or chocolate** (3 tablespoons): 120 calories, 5 g fiber, 10 g protein, 7 g sugar

Can't Do Dairy at All?

WHETHER YOU'RE LACTOSE-INTOLERANT OR SIMPLY TRYING to limit your intake of animal protein, dairy-free alternatives fill the gap. They contain fewer calories and less dietary cholesterol and saturated fat—unhealthy fats you don't need to worry about with dairy yogurt.

CHEESE ALTERNATIVES

- Cabot: Their aged cheddar is lactose-free (cabotcheese.coop/lactose-free-cheese).
- Daiya: Their products are sold at Whole Foods; check the Web site for store locations (us.daiyafoods.com).

LACTOSE-FREE YOGURT

- Green Valley Organics Lactose-Free Yogurt
- So Delicious Almond Milk Plain Greek Yogurt
- Wholesoy Soy Yogurt, Unsweetened Plain

Plant-Based Milks

- **Silk Almond Milk, shelf-stable or refrigerated**: 15 calories, 0 g sugar
- **So Delicious Dairy Free Unsweetened Coconut Milk, refrigerated**: 45 calories, 0 g sugar
- **Rice Dream Organic Classic Original, shelf-stable**: 60 calories, 5.5 g sugar
- **Westsoy Organic Unsweetened Plain Soy Milk, shelf-stable**: 45 calories, >1 g sugar

Dark Chocolate

BARS

- **Baker's unsweetened, 100% cocoa baking chocolate** (2 pieces): 90 calories, 3 g fiber, 0 g sugar (15 milligrams flavanols per gram)
- **Ghirardelli Twilight Delight 72% cocoa** (3 squares): 200 calories, 4 g fiber, 10 g sugar (9.3 milligrams flavanols per gram)

COCOA POWDER (TO STIR INTO COCOA, SMOOTHIES, AND YOGURT)

- **Cocoapro unsweetened stick packs** (1 stick): 25 calories, 1 g fiber, 0 g sugar

Packaged Snacks

- **G.H. Cretors Organic Extra Virgin Olive Oil Popped Corn** (3.5 cups): 140 calories, 3 g fiber, 0 g sugar
- **Mary's Gone Crackers Hot 'n Spicy Jalapeno Crackers** (13 crackers): 130 calories, 3 g fiber, 0 g sugar
- **Chic-a-Peas Crunchy Falafel Chickpeas** (1 ounce): 110 calories, 5 g fiber, 3 g sugar
- **Kind Dark Chocolate Nuts and Sea Salt** (1 bar): 200 calories, 7 g fiber 5 g sugar

Desserts

- **Luna & Larry's Organic Coconut Bliss Non-Dairy Frozen Dessert, Dark Chocolate flavor** (½ cup): 200 calories, 2 g fiber, 15 g sugar
- **Luna & Larry's Organic Coconut Bliss Non-Dairy Frozen Dessert, Cappuccino flavor** (½ cup): 210 calories, 1 g fiber, 13 g sugar
- **Alter Eco Dark Organic Chocolate Bar with Quinoa** (3 sections): 132 calories, 1.8 g fiber, 12 g sugar
- **Siggi's Icelandic Style Skyr Strained Non-Fat Yogurt, Pomegranate & Passion Fruit,** 1 container (5.3 ounces): 100 calories, 0 g fiber, 9 g sugar

Product Guide

The following products are recommended by our GLOW experts. All are available through the manufacturers' Web sites and in well-stocked drugstores or beauty chains as well as online retail outlets. The products marked with a blue asterisk* are winners of *Prevention* magazine's Beauty Awards or are recommended by the *Prevention* editors. All prices are approximate and may change, depending on the source.

First you'll treat your skin with Dr. Jeannette Graf's suggested skin-care products that were used by the panelists in this book. You may also browse Dr. Graf's own line of skin-care products on www.hsn.com under Dr. Jeannette Graf.

Beauty products including hair care and makeup from Eva Scrivo can be found on evascrivo.com.

Dr. Jeannette Graf's Skin-Care Plan

CLEANSER
- **Avène Micellar Lotion Cleanser and Make-Up Remover** ($20)
- **Cetaphil Daily Facial Cleanser** (for normal-to-oily skin) ($10)
- **Benzac Skin Balancing Foaming Cleanser** (for oily skin) ($12)
- **Shu Uemura Cleansing Oils** ($67–$90)

SERUM
- **Neutrogena Ageless Intensives Deep Wrinkle Serum** ($20)
- **Olay Regenerist Micro-Sculpting Serum** ($26)

FACIAL MOISTURIZER
- **Avène Hydrance Optimale Light Hydrating Cream** ($32)

FACIAL MOISTURIZER (CONT.)

- Neutrogena Healthy Defense Daily Moisturizer Broad Spectrum SPF 50—Sensitive Skin ($14)
- Aveeno Positively Radiant Daily Moisturizer Broad Spectrum SPF 30 ($17)
- Derma e Deep Wrinkle Peptide Moisturizer ($35)

FACIAL SUNSCREEN

- EltaMD UV Clear ($32)
- Avène High Protection Tinted Compact SPF 50 ($36)

RETINOID

- RoC Retinol Correxion Sensitive Night Cream ($22)
- Avène RetrinAL 0.1 Intensive Cream ($69)

EYE CREAM

- Roc Retinol Correxion Sensitive Eye Cream ($23)

FADE CREAM FOR AGE SPOTS

- Glytone Fading Lotion ($52)
- Glyquin ($55, prescription only)
- Tri-Luma ($100, prescription only)
- Lustra-AF ($140, prescription only)

HAND CREAM

- Eucerin Intensive Repair Extra-Enriched Hand Crème ($5)
- Neutrogena Hand Cream Fragrance-Free ($5)

MISCELLANEOUS

- Avène Thermal Spring Water ($14)

OTHER BOOKS BY DR. GRAF

- *Stop Aging, Start Living: The Revolutionary 2-Week pH Diet That Erases Wrinkles, Beautifies Skin, and Makes You Feel Fantastic*

Eva Scrivo's Hair-Care Routine

PROFESSIONAL SALON COLOR

Demi-Permanent

- Colorance by Goldwell (goldwell.us/salonfinder/ for salon locator)
- Dia Richesse by L'Oreal Professional (lorealprofessionnel.com/index.aspx for salon locator)

Permanent

- Topchic by Goldwell (goldwell.us/salonfinder/ for salon locator)

SHAMPOO

- Bumble and Bumble Sunday Shampoo ($25)
- Dove Intensive Repair Shampoo ($8)*

CONDITIONING

- L'Huile de Leonor Greyl Pre-Shampoo Oil Treatment ($59)
- Pantene Pro-V Expert Collection Age Defy Conditioner ($6)*

HAIRBRUSH

- Janeke Medium Mixed Bristle Brush ($48)

VOLUMIZING MOUSSE

- Mousse au Lotus Volumatrice by Leonor Greyl ($46)
- Mousse Bouffante by Kerastase ($37)

SMOOTHING LOTION

- Goldwell Elixir Oil ($38)

HAIR SERUM
- Fibre Architecte Serum by Kerastase ($43)

HAIR-LOSS PRODUCTS
- Densifique Minoxidil by Kerastase ($35)
- Women's Rogaine 2% Minoxidil Topical Solution ($40)
- 5% Minoxidil Topical Foam ($40)*
- Complexe Énergisant by Leonor Greyl ($56)
- Keranique's Instant FX 100% Natural Hair Fibers ($40)

- MegaFood Skin, Nails and Hair supplement (starting at $35)

HAIR EXTENSIONS
- Invisi-Tab (www.invisitab.com/index.php/find-a-salon/ for salon locator)

SMOOTHING TREATMENT
- Kerasilk by Goldwell (goldwell.us/salonfinder/ for salon locator)

Eva Scrivo's Beauty Routine

MAKEUP APPLICATORS
- Alcone Non-Latex Sponges (1 dozen, $24)
- Make Up For Ever HD Microfinish Puff ($10)
- T. LeClerc makeup brushes ($22–$58)

PRIMER
Water-based
- Smashbox Photo Finish Primer Water ($32)

Silicone-based
- Nars Light Optimizing Primer Broad Spectrum SPF 15 ($35)
- Hydrating Fluid Foundation T. LeClerc ($54)
- Jane Iredale Amazing Base loose mineral powder ($44)

Oil-Free, Water Based or Liquid (for combination skin)
- Jane Iredale Smooth Affair for Oily Skin ($48)

Fragrance-Free Liquid or Tinted Moisturizer (for sensitive skin)
- LORAC CC cream ($30)

CONCEALER
- T. LeClerc Corrector Fluid Concealer ($38)
- Japonesque Velvet Touch Concealer ($20)*

LOOSE POWDER
- Chantecaille Talc-Free Loose Powder ($65)

EYEBROW PENCIL
- T. LeClerc Eyebrow Pencil ($24)
- Maybelline New York Brow Precise Shaping Pencil ($8)*

EYE SHADOW
- Laura Mercier Artists Palette for Eyes and Cheeks ($55)

LIQUID LINER
- T. LeClerc Eyeliner ($30)

EYELASH CURLER
- Shu Uemura Eyelash Curler ($20)

MASCARA
- Thickening mascara: Dior Show by Christian Dior ($28)
- Lengthening mascara: Hypnôse Volumizing Mascara by Lancome ($28)

LIP PENCIL
- T. LeClerc Lip Pencil ($23)

LIP COLOR
- YSLRouge Pur Couture ($36)
- BareMinerals Marvelous Moxie Lipstick ($18)*

BLUSH
- Nars Blush ($30)
- Elizabeth Arden Beautiful Color Radiance Blush ($26)*

HIGHLIGHTER
- High Beam Liquid Skin Highlighter by Benefit Cosmetics ($26)

FOR HANDS
- Strivectin Volumizing Hand Treatment ($29)

FOR LEGS
- Clarins Body Lift Cellulite Control ($70)
- Dermablend Leg and Body Cover ($31)
- Clarins Delicious Self Tanning Cream ($44)

OTHER BOOKS BY EVA SCRIVO
- *Eva Scrivo on Beauty: The Tools, Techniques, and Insider Knowledge Every Woman Needs to Be Her Most Beautiful, Confident Self*

ENDNOTES

EAT

Health Benefits of a Plant-Based Diet

Marta Crous-Bou et al., "Mediterranean Diet and Telomere Length in Nurses' Health Study: Population Based Cohort Study," *BMJ* 349 (2014): g6674.

D. L. Katz and S. Meller, "Can We Say What Diet Is Best for Health?" *Annual Review of Public Health* 35 (March 2014): 83–103.

Physicians Committee for Responsible Medicine, "A Plant-Based Diet Causes Weight Loss, According to New Mega-Study," news release, January 22, 2015, www.pcrm.org/media/news/a-plant-based-diet-causes-weight-loss.

A. Vang et al., "Meats, Processed Meats, Obesity, Weight Gain and Occurrence of Diabetes among Adults: Findings from Adventist Health Studies," *Annals of Nutrition and Metabolism* 52, no. 2 (2008): 96–104.

American Heart Association, "Semi-Veggie Diet Effectively Lowers Heart Disease, Stroke Risk," press release, March 5, 2015, http://newsroom.heart.org/news/semi-veggie-diet-effectively-lowers-heart-disease-stroke-risk.

"UCL Study Finds New Evidence Linking Fruit and Vegetable Consumption with Lower Mortality," University College London, April 1, 2014, www.ucl.ac.uk/news/news-articles/0414/010413-fruit-veg-consumption-death-risk.

Oyinlola Oyebode et al., "Fruit and Vegetable Consumption and All-Cause, Cancer and CVD Mortality: Analysis of Health Survey for England Data," *Journal of Epidemiology and Community Health* 68 (2014): 856–62.

"Defining Vegetarian Diets," Oldways, accessed December 29, 2015, http://oldwayspt.org/resources/heritage-pyramids/vegetarian-diet-pyramid/defining-vegetarian-diets.

Karen Leibowitz et al., "What Do Vegetarian Groups Consider Vegetarian & Vegan?" The Vegetarian Resource Group, www.vrg.org/journal/vj2014issue2/2014_issue2_what_do_consider.php.

Jennifer Di Noia, "Defining Powerhouse Fruits and Vegetables: A Nutrient Density Approach," *Preventing Chronic Disease* 11 (2014): 130390.

Martha Clare Morris et al., "MIND Diet Associated with Reduced Incidence of Alzheimer's Disease," *Alzheimer's & Dementia* 11, no. 9 (September 2015): 1007–14.

Benefits of Eating Organic

K. L. Bassil et al., "Cancer Health Effects of Pesticides: Systematic Review," *Canadian Family Physician* 53, no. 10 (2007): 1704–11.

"Industrial Agriculture," Union of Concerned Scientists, accessed December 29, 2015, www.ucsusa .org/our-work/food-agriculture/our-failing-food-system/industrial-agriculture#. ViXAXcuFOM8.

Jayson Beckman, "U.S. Beef Exports to the EU Grow Despite Trade Barriers," U.S. Department of Agriculture, April 6, 2015, www.ers.usda.gov/amber-waves/2015-april/us-beef-exports-to-the -eu-grow-despite-trade-barriers.aspx#.ViXRZ8uFOM9.

"Food & Agriculture," Union of Concerned Scientists, accessed December 29, 2015, www.ucsusa.org/ food_and_agriculture#.ViXMnMuFOM9.

Marcin Barański et al., "Higher Antioxidant and Lower Cadmium Concentrations and Lower Incidence of Pesticide Residues in Organically Grown Crops: A Systematic Literature Review and Meta-Analyses," *British Journal of Nutrition* 112 (2014): 794–811.

"EWG's Shopper's Guide to Pesticides in Produce," Environmental Working Group, accessed December 29, 2015, www.ewg.org/foodnews/summary.php.

Maximizing Nutrition in Vegetables through Cooking

Diane M. Barrett, "Maximizing the Nutritional Value of Fruits and Vegetables," *Food Technology* 61, no. 4 (2007): 40–44.

A. M. Jiménez-Monreal et al., "Influence of Cooking Methods on Antioxidant Activity of Vegetables," *Journal of Food Science* 74, no. 3 (April 2009): H97–H103.

Home Cooking and Eating Habits

J. A. Wolfson and S. N. Bleich, "Is Cooking at Home Associated with Better Diet Quality or Weight-Loss Intention?" *Public Health Nutrition* 18, no. 8 (June 2015): 1397–406.

Collin Payne et al., "Serve It Here; Eat It There: Serving off the Stove Results in Less Food Intake Than Serving off the Table," Food and Brand Lab, Cornell University, http://foodpsychology.cornell .edu/images/posters/serveofftable.pdf.

Health Consequences of Added Sugars

James J. DiNicolantonio and Sean C. Lucan, "Sugar Season. It's Everywhere, and Addictive," *New York Times*, December 22, 2014, www.nytimes.com/2014/12/23/opinion/sugar-season-its -everywhere-and-addictive.html?_r=1.

Q. Yang et al., "Added Sugar Intake and Cardiovascular Diseases Mortality among US Adults," *JAMA Internal Medicine* 174, no. 4 (April 2014): 516–24.

Cindy W. Leung et al., "Soda and Cell Aging: Associations between Sugar-Sweetened Beverage Consumption and Leukocyte Telomere Length in Healthy Adults from the National Health and Nutrition Examination Surveys," *American Journal of Public Health* 104, no. 12 (December 2014): 2425–31.

S. H. Ahmed, K. Guillem, and Y. Vandaele, "Sugar Addiction: Pushing the Drug-Sugar Analogy to the Limit," *Current Opinion in Clinical Nutrition and Metabolic Care* 16, no. 4 (July 2013): 434–39.

Health Benefits of Dark Chocolate

Thozhukat Sathyapalan et al., "High Cocoa Polyphenol Rich Chocolate May Reduce the Burden of the Symptoms in Chronic Fatigue Syndrome," *Nutrition Journal* 9 (2010): 55.

Will Clower, *Eat Chocolate, Lose Weight* (Emmaus, PA: Hearst Magazines, Inc. 2014), 148.

Beatrice A. Golomb, Sabrina Koperski, and Halbert L. White, "Association between More Frequent Chocolate Consumption and Lower Body Mass Index," *Archives of Internal Medicine* 172, no. 6 (March 26, 2012): 519–21.

American Chemical Society, "The Precise Reason for the Health Benefits of Dark Chocolate: Mystery Solved," press release, March 18, 2014, www.acs.org/content/acs/en/pressroom/ newsreleases/2014/march/the-precise-reason-for-the-health-benefits-of-dark-chocolate-mystery-solved.html.

Alexander N. Sokolov et al., "Chocolate and the Brain: Neurobiological Impact of Cocoa Flavanols on Cognition and Behavior," *Neuroscience & Biobehavioral Reviews* 37, no. 10, part 2 (December 2013): 2445–53.

Astrid Nehlig, "The Neuroprotective Effects of Cocoa Flavanol and Its Influence on Cognitive Performance," *British Journal of Clinical Pharmacology* 75, no. 3 (March 2013): 716–27.

G. Desideri et al., "Benefits in Cognitive Function, Blood Pressure, and Insulin Resistance through Cocoa Flavanol Consumption in Elderly Subjects with Mild Cognitive Impairment: The Cocoa, Cognition, and Aging (CoCoA) Study," *Hypertension* 60 (2012): 794–801.

Daniela Mastroiacovo et al., "Cocoa Flavanol Consumption Improves Cognitive Function, Blood Pressure Control, and Metabolic Profile in Elderly Subjects: The Cocoa, Cognition, and Aging (CoCoA) Study—A Randomized Controlled Trial," *American Journal of Clinical Nutrition* 101, no. 3 (March 2015): 538–48.

Science of Gut Health

"Everything You Always Wanted to Know about the Gut Microbiotia," Gut Microbiota Worldwatch, accessed December 29, 2015, www.gutmicrobiotawatch.org/gut-microbiota-info/.

Meghan Jardine, "Seven Foods to Supercharge Your Gut Bacteria," Physicians Committee for Responsible Medicine, accessed December 29, 2015, www.pcrm.org/media/online/sept2014/seven-foods-to-supercharge-your-gut-bacteria.

Francesca De Filippis et al., "High-Level Adherence to a Mediterranean Diet Beneficially Impacts the Gut Microbiota and Associated Metabolome," *Gut* (September 2015), http://gut.bmj.com/content/early/2015/09/03/gutjnl-2015-309957.abstract.

Jonathan Vernon, "Mediterranean Diet Best for a Healthy Gut, Study Finds," *Medical News Today*, September 29, 2015, www.medicalnewstoday.com/articles/300073.php.

Joanne Slavin, "Fiber and Prebiotics: Mechanisms and Health Benefits," *Nutrients* 5, no. 4 (2013): 1417–35.

Helene Ragovin, "What's So Great about Yogurt?" TuftsNow, January 29, 2015, http://now.tufts.edu/articles/whats-so-great-about-yogurt.

Mu Chen et al., "Dairy Consumption and Risk of Type 2 Diabetes: 3 Cohorts of US Adults and an Updated Meta-Analysis," *BMC Medicine* 12 (2014): 215.

Huifen Wang et al., "Yogurt Consumption, Blood Pressure, and Incident Hypertension: A Longitudinal Study in the Framingham Heart Study," *Hypertension* 60 (2012): A188.

Huifen Wang et al., "Longitudinal Association between Dairy Consumption and Changes of Body Weight and Waist Circumference: The Framingham Heart Study," *International Journal of Obesity* 38, no. 2 (February 2014): 299–305.

Paul F. Jacques and Huifen Wang, "Yogurt and Weight Management," *American Journal of Clinical Nutrition* 99, no. 5 (2014): S1229–S1234.

Health Benefits of Certain Beverages

Lawrence E. Armstrong et al., "Mild Dehydration Affects Mood in Healthy Young Women," *Journal of Nutrition* 142, no. 2 (February 1, 2012): 382–88.

Virginia Tech News, "Clinical Trial Confirms Effectiveness of Simple Appetite Control Method," press release, August 23, 2010, www.vtnews.vt.edu/articles/2010/08/082310-cals-davy.html.

Michael R. Simpson and Tom Howard, *Selecting and Effectively Using Hydration for Fitness* (Indianapolis: American College of Sports Medicine, 2011), https://www.acsm.org/docs/brochures/selecting-and-effectively-using-hydration-for-fitness.pdf.

Jackilen Shannon et al., "Relationship of Food Groups and Water Intake to Colon Cancer Risk," *Cancer Epidemiology Biomarkers and Prevention* 5 (July 1996): 495–502.

Dominique S. Michaud et al., "Total Fluid and Water Consumption and the Joint Effect of Exposure to Disinfection By-Products on Risk of Bladder Cancer," *Environmental Health Perspectives* 115, no. 11 (2007): 1569–72.

Drexel University College of Nursing and Health Professions, "Green Tea: The Fountain of Youth," April 19, 2013, news release, www.drexel.edu/cnhp/news/current/archive/2013/April/2013-04 -19-Green-Tea-The-Fountain-of-Youth/.

Andre Schmidt et al., "Green Tea Extract Enhances Parieto-Frontal Connectivity during Working Memory Processing," *Psychopharmacology* 231, no. 19 (2014): 3879–88.

S. K. Bøhn et al., "Effects of Tea and Coffee on Cardiovascular Disease Risk," *Food and Function* 3, no. 6 (June 2012): 575–91.

Sarah Nechuta et al., "Prospective Cohort Study of Tea Consumption and Risk of Digestive System Cancers: Results from the Shanghai Women's Health Study," *American Journal of Clinical Nutrition* 96, no. 5 (November 2012): 1056–63.

"Green Tea Protects Brain Cells," *Tufts University Health & Nutrition Letter*, June 2013, www .nutritionletter.tufts.edu/issues/9_6/current-articles/Green-Tea-Protects-Brain-Cells_999-1.html.

Shinichi Kuriyama et al., "Green Tea Consumption and Cognitive Function: A Cross-Sectional Study from the Tsurugaya Project," *American Journal of Clinical Nutrition* 83, no. 2 (February 2006): 355–61.

Neal D. Freedman et al., "Association of Coffee Drinking with Total and Cause-Specific Mortality," *New England Journal of Medicine* 366 (2012): 1891–904.

Francesca Bravi et al., "Coffee Reduces Risk for Hepatocellular Carcinoma: An Updated Meta-Analysis," *Clinical Gastroenterology and Hepatology* 11, no. 11 (November 2013): 1413–21.

Chuanhai Cao et al., "Caffeine Synergizes with Another Coffee Component to Increase Plasma GCSF: Linkage to Cognitive Benefits in Alzheimer's Mice," *Journal of Alzheimer's Disease* 25, no. 2 (2011): 323–35.

Michael Lucas et al., "Coffee, Caffeine, and Risk of Depression among Women," *Archives of Internal Medicine* 171, no. 17 (September 26, 2011): 1571–78.

R. C. Gliottoni et al., "Effect of Caffeine on Quadriceps Muscle Pain during Acute Cycling Exercise in Low versus High Caffeine Consumers," *International Journal of Sport Nutrition and Exercise Metabolism* 19, no. 2 (April 2009): 150–61.

Dietary Importance of and Guidelines for Protein Consumption

Russell J. de Souza et al., "Intake of Saturated and Trans Unsaturated Fatty Acids and Risk of All Cause Mortality, Cardiovascular Disease, and Type 2 Diabetes: Systematic Review and Meta-Analysis of Observational Studies," *BMJ* 351 (2015): h3978.

"Jury Still Out on Whether Saturated Fat Is Bad for You, Researchers Say," University of Utah Health Care, August 11, 2015, http://healthcare.utah.edu/healthlibrary/related/doc.php?type =6&id=702234.

Morgan E. Levine et al., "Low Protein Intake Is Associated with a Major Reduction in IGF-1, Cancer, and Overall Mortality in the 65 and Younger but Not Older Population," *Cell Metabolism* 19, no. 3 (March 4, 2014): 407–17.

Thomas L. Halton et al., "Low-Carbohydrate-Diet Score and the Risk of Coronary Heart Disease in Women," *New England Journal of Medicine* 355 (2006): 1991–2002.

Dariush Mozaffarian et al., "Changes in Diet and Lifestyle and Long-Term Weight Gain in Women and Men," *New England Journal of Medicine* 364 (2011): 2392–404.

Scientific Report of the 2015 USDA Dietary Guidelines Advisory Committee, USDA, February 2015, www.health.gov/dietaryguidelines/2015-scientific-report/PDFs/Scientific-Report-of-the-2015 -Dietary-Guidelines-Advisory-Committee.pdf.

Rex Barnes, "Eggstra! Eggstra! Learn All About Them," USDA Blog, April 6, 2012, http://blogs.usda .gov/2012/04/06/eggstra-eggstra-learn-all-about-them/.

Mario Kratz, Ton Baars, and Stephan Guyenet, "The Relationship between High-Fat Dairy Consumption and Obesity, Cardiovascular, and Metabolic Disease," *European Journal of Nutrition* 52, no. 1 (February 2013): 1–24.

"The Protein Myth," Physicians Committee for Responsible Medicine, accessed December 29, 2015, www.pcrm.org/health/diets/vegdiets/how-can-i-get-enough-protein-the-protein-myth.

Nuts and Appetite Suppression

S. Y. Tan and R. D. Mattes, "Appetitive, Dietary and Health Effects of Almonds Consumed with Meals or as Snacks: A Randomized, Controlled Trial," *European Journal of Clinical Nutrition* 67 (2013): 1205–14.

Maira Bes-Rastrollo et al., "Nut Consumption and Weight Gain in a Mediterranean Cohort: The SUN Study," *Obesity* 15, no. 1 (January 2007): 107.

Health Benefits of Fish

Cyrus A. Raji et al., "Regular Fish Consumption and Age-Related Brain Gray Matter Loss," *American Journal of Preventive Medicine* 47, no. 4 (October 2014): 444–51.

Sharon G. Curhan et al., "Fish and Fatty Acid Consumption and the Risk of Hearing Loss in Women," *American Journal of Clinical Nutrition* 100 (November 2014): 1371–77.

Michael J. Orlich et al., "Vegetarian Dietary Patterns and the Risk of Colorectal Cancers," *JAMA Internal Medicine* 175, no. 5 (2015): 767–76.

"What You Need to Know about Mercury in Fish and Shellfish (Brochure)," U.S. Food and Drug Administration, March 2004, www.fda.gov/food/resourcesforyou/consumers/ucm110591.htm.

Jennifer K. Nelson, "Which Fish to Pick—Farmed or Wild?" *Nutrition-Wise Blog* (Mayo Clinic), July 9, 2015, www.mayoclinic.org/healthy-lifestyle/nutrition-and-healthy-eating/expert-blog/farmed -vs-wild-fish/bgp-20146479.

"Keeping Seafood Safe and Plentiful," National Oceanic and Atmospheric Administration, accessed December 29, 2015, www.noaa.gov/features/resources_0908/safeseafood.html.

"Commercial Aquaculture: Potential Environmental Issues," Sustainable Seafood Coalition, accessed December 29, 2015, http://sustainableseafoodcoalition.org/commercial-aquaculture-potential -environmental-issues/.

"Sardines," The World's Healthiest Foods, accessed December 29, 2015, http://www.whfoods.com/ genpage.php?tname=foodspice&dbid=147.

"Seafood and Your Health," Monterey Bay Aquarium Seafood Watch, accessed December 29, 2015, www.seafoodwatch.org/consumers/seafood-and-your-health.

"Eat Sardines!" *Tufts University Health & Nutrition Letter*, March 21, 2014, www.nutritionletter.tufts .edu/news/-1444-1.html.

"4 Reasons Sardines Are Great—And 2 Recipes to Convince You," Bastyr University, August 22, 2011, www.bastyr.edu/node/868.

Health Benefits of Mushrooms

"Vitamin D," MedlinePlus, U.S. National Library of Medicine, reviewed March 26, 2015, https://www .nlm.nih.gov/medlineplus/vitamind.html.

"Vitamin D Fact Sheet for Health Professionals," National Institutes of Health, November 10, 2014, https://ods.od.nih.gov/factsheets/VitaminD-HealthProfessional/#h7.

Joshua W. Miller et al., "Vitamin D Status and Rates of Cognitive Decline in a Multiethnic Cohort of Older Adults," *JAMA Neurology* 72, no. 11 (November 2015): 1295–303.

"Ingredient of the Month: Mushrooms," ACFEF Chef & Child Foundation and Clemson University, October 2011, www.clemson.edu/cafls/cuchefs/files/mushrooms.pdf.

Myrdal Miller et al., "Flavor-Enhancing Properties of Mushrooms in Meat-Based Dishes in Which Sodium Has Been Reduced and Meat Has Been Partially Substituted with Mushrooms," *Journal of Food Science* 79, no. 9 (September 1979): S1795–S1804.

Jean-Xavier Guinard and Amy Myrdal Miller, "Using Mushrooms to Improve the Nutrition Properties and Consumer Appeal of Popular Meat-Based Dishes," Mushroom & Health Summit, http:// mushroominfo.com/wp-content/uploads/2013/09/Mushroom-Summit-Lunch-Educational -Activity.pdf.

"What Is Umami?" Umami Information Center, accessed December 29, 2015, www.umamiinfo .com/2011/02/What-exactly-is-umami.php.

Jane Black, "The Meat-Mushroom Blend Makes Sense," *Washington Post*, August 1, 2014, www
.washingtonpost.com/lifestyle/food/the-meat-mushroom-blend-makes-sense/2014/08/01
/769884e6-0e9b-11e4-b8e5-d0de80767fc2_story.html.

Nozomi Hishikawa et al., "Effects of Turmeric on Alzheimer's Disease with Behavioral and
Psychological Symptoms of Dementia," *Ayu* 33, no. 4 (October–December 2012): 499–504.

Spices and Weight Loss

Vilai Kuptniratsaikul et al., "Efficacy and Safety of *Curcuma domestica* Extracts in Patients with Knee
Osteoarthritis," *Journal of Alternative and Complementary Medicine* 15, no. 8 (August 2009): 891–97.

R. Zare et al., "Effect of Cumin Powder on Body Composition and Lipid Profile in Overweight and
Obese Women," *Complementary Therapies in Clinical Practice* 20, no. 4 (November 2014): 297–301.

MOVE

Exercise and Antiaging

Lynn F. Cherkas et al., "The Association between Physical Activity in Leisure Time and Leukocyte
Telomere Length," *Archives of Internal Medicine* 168, no. 2 (2008): 154–58.

"Exercise and Age," MedlinePlus, U.S. National Library of Medicine, updated May 6, 2013, https://
www.nlm.nih.gov/medlineplus/ency/article/002080.htm.

Marla Paul, "Morning Rays Keep Off the Pounds," Northwestern University, April 2, 2014, www
.northwestern.edu/newscenter/stories/2014/04/morning-rays-keep-off-the-pounds.html.

Kathryn J. Reid et al., "Timing and Intensity of Light Correlate with Body Weight in Adults," *PLoS
ONE* 9, no. 4 (2014): e92251.

Cardiovascular Exercise and Endurance

"Oxygen Consumption—VO2," UC Davis Sports Medicine, accessed December 29, 2015, www.ucdmc
.ucdavis.edu/sportsmedicine/resources/vo2description.html.

Richard Weil, "Aerobic Exercise," MedicineNet, reviewed January 26, 2015, www.medicinenet.com/
aerobic_exercise/article.htm.

Mark Hamer et al., "Physical Activity and Inflammatory Markers Over 10 Years," *Circulation* 126
(2012): 928–33.

"THRIVE Week 10: How F.A.R. Can You Go? F.A.C.E Your Future," *Dr. Vonda Wright MD: Fortify, Achieve,
Revive* (blog), April 5, 2013, www.drvondawright.com/how-far-can-you-go-face-your-future/.

Kristian Karstoft et al., "Mechanisms behind the Superior Effects of Interval vs Continuous Training
on Glycaemic Control in Individuals with Type 2 Diabetes: A Randomised Controlled Trial,"
Diabetologia 57, no. 10 (October 2014): 2081–93.

Mayo Clinic Staff, "Exercise Intensity: How to Measure It," Mayo Clinic, February 5, 2014, www
.mayoclinic.org/healthy-lifestyle/fitness/in-depth/exercise-intensity/art-20046887.

Vonda Wright and Ruth Winter, *Fitness after 40: How to Stay Strong at Any Age* (New York: AMACOM,
2009), 77.

Benefits of Strength Training

Wright and Winter, *Fitness after 40*, 94.

Office of the Surgeon General (US), "Determinants of Bone Health," chap. 6 in *Bone Health and
Osteoporosis: A Report of the Surgeon General* (Rockville, MD: Office of the Surgeon General [US],
2004).

"Why Strength Training?" Centers for Disease Control and Prevention, reviewed February 24, 2011,
www.cdc.gov/physicalactivity/growingstronger/why/index.html.

C. Rosa et al., "Order Effects of Combined Strength and Endurance Training on Testosterone, Cortisol, Growth Hormone, and IGF-1 Binding Protein 3 in Concurrently Trained Men, *Journal of Strength and Conditioning Research* 29, no. 1 (January 2015): 74–79.

"Exercise and Physical Activity: Your Everyday Guide from the National Institute on Aging," National Institute on Aging, updated January 22, 2015, https://www.nia.nih.gov/health/publication/exercise-physical-activity/sample-exercises-strength.

J. Carson Smith et al., "Physical Activity Reduces Hippocampal Atrophy in Elders at Genetic Risk for Alzheimer's Disease," *Frontiers in Aging Neuroscience* 6 (2014): 61.

Sandra B. Chapman et al., "Shorter Term Aerobic Exercise Improves Brain, Cognition, and Cardiovascular Fitness in Aging," *Frontiers in Aging Neuroscience* 5 (2013): 75.

Importance of Flexibility

Can-Fit-Pro, "The Importance and Purpose of Flexibility," in *Foundations of Professional Personal Training* (Champaign, IL: Human Kinetics Publishers, 2012).

Balance and Aging

"Balance Problems," HealthinAging.org, updated March 2012, www.healthinaging.org/aging-and -health-a-to-z/topic:balance-problems/.

Wright and Winter, *Fitness after 40*, 126.

"Exercise & Physical Activity," https://www.nia.nih.gov/health/publication/exercise-physical -activity/sample-exercises-balance.

Walking and Creativity

Marily Oppezzo and Daniel L. Schwartz, "Give Your Ideas Some Legs: The Positive Effect of Walking on Creative Thinking," *Journal of Experimental Psychology: Learning, Memory, and Cognition* 40, no. 4 (July 2014): 1142–52.

Benefits of Foam Rolling

"Why You Should Be Foam Rolling," American Council on Exercise, October 3, 2013, www.acefitness .org/acefit/healthy-living-article/60/3543/why-you-should-be-foam-rolling/.

"Foam Rollers Can Help Ease Aches and Pains from Exercise, a Desk Job," Indiana University News Room, accessed December 29, 2015, http://newsinfo.iu.edu/web/page/normal/18180.html.

Wright and Winter, *Fitness after 40*, 47.

ENGAGE

Sleep Hygiene and Health

"Sleep Hygiene," National Sleep Foundation, spring 2003, https://sleepfoundation.org/ask-the -expert/sleep-hygiene.

Optimism and Well-Being

Hilary A. Tindle et al., "Optimism, Cynical Hostility, and Incident Coronary Heart Disease and Mortality in the Women's Health Initiative," *Circulation* 120 (2009): 656–62.

J. W. Schooler et al., "The Pursuit and Assessment of Happiness May Be Self-Defeating," in *The Psychology of Economic Decisions,* ed. J. Carrillo and I. Brocas (Oxford: Oxford University Press, 2003), 41–70.

Lise Solberg Nes, Suzanne C. Segerstrom, and Sandra E. Sephton, "Engagement and Arousal: Optimism's Effects during a Brief Stressor," *Personality & Social Psychology Bulletin* 31, no. 1 (January 2005): 111–20.

M. E. Seligman et al., "Positive Psychology Progress: Empirical Validation of Interventions," *The American Psychologist* 60, no. 5 (July–August 2005): 410–21.

Stress and Effects on Health

"What Is Stress?" The American Institute of Stress, accessed December 29, 2015, www.stress.org/what-is-stress/.

"Six Myths about Stress," American Psychological Association, accessed December 29, 2015, www.apa.org/helpcenter/stress-myths.aspx.

"Stress," University of Maryland Medical Center, reviewed January 30, 2013, http://umm.edu/health/medical/reports/articles/stress.

"Stress and Insomnia," National Sleep Foundation, accessed December 29, 2015, http://sleepfoundation.org/ask-the-expert/stress-and-insomnia.

"Stress," American Diabetes Association, reviewed June 7, 2013, www.diabetes.org/living-with-diabetes/complications/mental-health/stress.html.

Kirstin Aschbacher et al., "Chronic Stress Increases Vulnerability to Diet-Related Abdominal Fat, Oxidative Stress, and Metabolic Risk," *Psychoneuroendocrinology* 46 (August 2014): 14–22.

"Stress and Heart Health," American Heart Association, reviewed June 2014, www.heart.org/HEARTORG/GettingHealthy/StressManagement/HowDoesStressAffectYou/Stress-and-Heart-Health_UCM_437370_Article.jsp.

National Institutes of Health, "First Sister Study Results Reinforce the Importance of Healthy Living," news release, March 16, 2009, www.nih.gov/news/health/mar2009/niehs-16.htm.

"Stress Tip Sheet," American Psychological Association, accessed December 29, 2015, www.apa.org/helpcenter/stress-tips.aspx.

N. Uedo et al., "Reduction in Salivary Cortisol Level by Music Therapy during Colonoscopic Examination," *Hepato-Gastroenterology* 51, no. 56 (March–April 2004): 451–53.

Alexander Samel et al., "Sleep Deficit and Stress Hormones in Helicopter Pilots on 7-Day Duty for Emergency Medical Services," *Aviation, Space, and Environmental Medicine* 75, no. 11 (November 2004): 935–40.

A. N. Vgontzas et al., "Daytime Napping after a Night of Sleep Loss Decreases Sleepiness, Improves Performance, and Causes Beneficial Changes in Cortisol and Interleukin-6 Secretion," *American Journal of Physiology; Endocrinology and Metabolism* 292, no. 1 (January 2007): E253–E261.

Andrew Steptoe et al., "The Effects of Tea on Psychophysiological Stress Responsivity and Post-Stress Recovery: A Randomised Double-Blind Trial," *Psychopharmacology* 190, no. 1 (January 2007): 81–89.

P. A. Boelens et al., "A Randomized Trial of the Effect of Prayer on Depression and Anxiety," *International Journal of Psychiatry in Medicine* 39, no. 4 (2009): 377–92.

Social Ties and Health

Debra Umberson and Jennifer Karas Montez, "Social Relationships and Health: A Flashpoint for Health Policy," *Journal of Health and Social Behavior* 51, no. S1 (November 2010): S54–S66.

Julianne Holt-Lunstad, Timothy B. Smith, and J. Bradley Layton, "Social Relationships and Mortality Risk: A Meta-Analytic Review," *PLoS Medicine* 7, no. 7 (July 27, 2010): e1000316.

Ye Luo et al., "Loneliness, Health, and Mortality in Old Age: A National Longitudinal Study," *Social Science & Medicine* 74, no. 6 (March 2012): 907–14.

Harry T. Reis et al., "Familiarity Does Indeed Promote Attraction in Live Interaction," *Journal of Personality and Social Psychology* 101, no. 3 (September 2011): 557–70.

Christopher M. Masi et al., "A Meta-Analysis of Interventions to Reduce Loneliness," *Personality and Social Psychology Review* 15, no. 3 (August 2011): 219–66.

Anna Miller, "Friends Wanted," *Monitor on Psychology* 45, no. 1 (January 2014): 54.

S. B. Algoe, B. L. Fredrickson, and S. L. Gable, "The Social Functions of the Emotion of Gratitude via Expression," *Emotion* 13, no. 4 (August 2013): 605–9.

Resilience and Its Origins

"The Road to Resilience," American Psychological Association, accessed December 29, 2015, www
.apa.org/helpcenter/road-resilience.aspx.

Dilip V. Jeste et al., "Association between Older Age and More Successful Aging: Critical Role of
Resilience and Depression," *American Journal of Psychiatry* 170, no. 2 (February 2013): 188–96.

Harry Mills and Mark Dombeck, "Defining Resilience," MentalHelp.net, June 25, 2005, https://www
.mentalhelp.net/articles/defining-resilience/.

Turhan Canli et al., "An fMRI Study of Personality Influences on Brain Reactivity to Emotional
Stimuli," *Behavioral Neuroscience* 115, no. 1 (2001): 33–42.

Meditation and Its Health Benefits

National Center for Complementary and Integrative Health, "Nationwide Survey Reveals Widespread
Use of Mind and Body Practices," news release, February 10, 2015, https://nccih.nih.gov/news/
press/02102015mb.

John W. Thomas and Marc Cohen, "A Methodological Review of Meditation Research," *Frontiers in
Psychiatry* 5 (2014): 74.

"Meditation: What You Need to Know," National Center for Complementary and Integrative Health,
updated November 2014, https://nccih.nih.gov/health/meditation/overview.htm.

L. S. Colzato, A. Ozturk, and B. Hommel, "Meditate to Create: The Impact of Focused-Attention and
Open-Monitoring Training on Convergent and Divergent Thinking," *Frontiers in Psychology* 3
(2012): 116.

E. Luders, N. Cherbuin, and F. Kurth, "Forever Young(er): Potential Age-Defying Effects of Long-Term
Meditation on Gray Matter Atrophy," *Frontiers in Psychology* 5 (2015): 1551.

C. Y. Fang et al., "Enhanced Psychosocial Well-Being Following Participation in a Mindfulness-Based
Stress Reduction Program Is Associated with Increased Natural Killer Cell Activity," *Journal of
Alternative and Complementary Medicine* 16, no. 5 (May 2010): 531–38.

T. L. Jacobs et al., "Intensive Meditation Training, Immune Cell Telomerase Activity, and Psychological
Mediators," *Psychoneuroendocrinology* 36, no. 5 (June 2011): 664–81.

L. J. Kelly, "New to Meditation: One Breath at a Time," New York Insight Meditation Center, April
2001, www.nyimc.org/how-to-meditate/.

M. Hirano and S. Yukawa, "The Impact of Mindfulness Meditation on Anger," abstract, *Shinrigaku
Kenkyu* 84, no. 2 (June 2013): 93–102, www.ncbi.nlm.nih.gov/pubmed/23847996.

Cary Barbor, "The Science of Meditation," PsychologyToday.com, reviewed April 10, 2013, https://
www.psychologytoday.com/articles/200105/the-science-meditation.

"The Monkey Mind," Guide to Buddhism A to Z, accessed December 29, 2015,

www.buddhisma2z.com/content.php?id=274.

Judson A. Brewer et al., "Meditation Experience Is Associated with Differences in Default Mode
Network Activity and Connectivity," *PNAS* 108, no. 50 (2011): 20254–59.

Matthew Williams, "Neuroscience of Mindfulness: Default Mode Network, Meditation, and
Mindfulness," Mindfulness, MD, July 8, 2014, www.mindfulnessmd.com/2014/07/08/
neuroscience-of-mindfulness-default-mode-network-meditation-mindfulness/.

Matthew A. Killingsworth and Daniel T. Gilbert, "A Wandering Mind Is an Unhappy Mind," *Science*
330, no. 6006 (November 12, 2010): 932.

Volunteering and Health

M. A. Okun, E. W. Yeung, and S. Brown, "Volunteering by Older Adults and Risk of Mortality: A
Meta-Analysis," *Psychology and Aging* 28, no. 2 (2013): 564–77.

R. Ramos et al., "Busy Yet Socially Engaged: Volunteering, Work-Life Balance, and Health in the
Working Population," *Journal of Occupational and Environmental Medicine* 57, no. 2 (February 2015):
164–72.

E. J. Tan et al., "Volunteering: A Physical Activity Intervention for Older Adults—The Experience Corps Program in Baltimore," *Journal of Urban Health* 83, no. 5 (September 2006): 954–69.

Rodlescia S. Sneed and Sheldon Cohen, "A Prospective Study of Volunteerism and Hypertension Risk in Older Adults," *Psychology and Aging* 28, no. 2 (June 2013): 578–86.

M. A. Musick and J. Wilson, "Volunteering and Depression: The Role of Psychological and Social Resources in Different Age Groups," *Social Science and Medicine* 56, no. 2 (January 2003): 259–69.

Sara Konrath et al., "Motives for Volunteering Are Associated with Mortality Risk in Older Adults," *Health Psychology* 31, no. 1 (January 2012): 87–96.

Career, Aging, and Health

Amy Adkins, "Majority of U.S. Employees not Engaged Despite Gains in 2014," Gallup, January 28, 2015, www.gallup.com/poll/181289/majority-employees-not-engaged-despite-gains-2014.aspx.

Mark Miller, "5 Tips for Mid-Life Career Change," Salisbury University Career Services Alumni, accessed December 29, 2015, www.salisbury.edu/careerservices/alumni/Midlifealum.html.

"How to Find a Career Coach," *Wall Street Journal*, May 8, 2009, http://guides.wsj.com/careers/how-to-start-a-job-search/how-to-find-a-career-coach/.

J. R. Moon et al., "Transition to Retirement and Risk of Cardiovascular Disease: Prospective Analysis of the US Health and Retirement Study," *Social Science and Medicine* 75, no. 3 (August 2012): 526–30.

Institute of Economic Affairs, "Retirement Causes a Major Decline in Physical and Mental Health, New Research Finds," press release, May 16, 2013, www.iea.org.uk/in-the-media/press-release/retirement-causes-a-major-decline-in-physical-and-mental-health-new-resea.

Hugo Westerlund et al., "Self-Rated Health before and after Retirement in France (GAZEL): A Cohort Study," *The Lancet* 374, no. 9705 (December 2009): 1889–96.

Hobbies and Health

American Academy of Neurology, "Can Arts, Crafts and Computer Use Preserve Your Memory?" press release, April 8, 2015, https://www.aan.com/PressRoom/Home/PressRelease/1363.

Denise C. Park et al., "The Impact of Sustained Engagement on Cognitive Function in Older Adults: The Synapse Project," *Psychological Science* 25, no. 1 (January 2014): 103–12.

Effects of Nature on Mood

N. Weinstein, A. K. Przybylski, and R. M. Ryan, "Can Nature Make Us More Caring? Effects of Immersion in Nature on Intrinsic Aspirations and Generosity," *Personality and Social Psychology Bulletin* 35, no. 10 (October 2009): 1315–29.

Juyoung Lee et al., "Restorative Effects of Viewing Real Forest Landscapes, Based on a Comparison with Urban Landscapes," *Scandinavian Journal of Forest Research* 24, no. 3 (2009): 227–34.

Richard M. Ryan et al., "Vitalizing Effects of Being Outdoors and in Nature," *Journal of Environmental Psychology* 30, no. 2 (June 2010): 159–68.

Irving Biederman and Edward Vessel, "Perceptual Pleasure and the Brain," *American Scientist* 94, no. 3 (May–June 2006): 247.

Jo Barton and Jules Pretty, "What Is the Best Dose of Nature and Green Exercise for Improving Mental Health? A Multi-Study Analysis," *Environmental Science and Technology* 44, no. 10 (2010): 3947–55.

B. J. Park et al., "The Physiological Effects of Shinrin-yoku (Taking in the Forest Atmosphere or Forest Bathing): Evidence from Field Experiments in 24 Forests across Japan," *Environmental Health and Preventive Medicine* 15, no. 1 (January 2010): 18–26.

Sex and Aging

B. Whipple et al., "The Health Benefits of Sexual Expression," Planned Parenthood Federation of America white paper, July 2007, https://www.plannedparenthood.org/files/3413/9611/7801/Benefits_Sex_07_07.pdf.

"Aging Changes in the Female Reproductive System," MedlinePlus, U.S. National Library of Medicine, updated November 16, 2014, https://www.nlm.nih.gov/medlineplus/ency/article/004016.htm.

U.S. Food and Drug Administration, "FDA Approves Osphena for Postmenopausal Women Experiencing Pain during Sex," news release, February 26, 2013, www.fda.gov/NewsEvents/Newsroom/PressAnnouncements/ucm341128.htm.

Pet Ownership and Health

American Heart Association, "AHA Scientific Statement: Pet Ownership and Cardiovascular Risk," *Circulation* 127 (2013): 2353–63.

Karen Allen, Barbara E. Shykoff, and Joseph L. Izzo Jr., "Pet Ownership, but Not ACE Inhibitor Therapy, Blunts Home Blood Pressure Responses to Mental Stress," *Hypertension* 38 (2001): 815–20.

Allen R. McConnell et al., "Friends with Benefits: On the Positive Consequences of Pet Ownership," *Journal of Personality and Social Psychology* 101, no. 6 (December 2011): 1239–52.

E. Friedmann et al., "Animal Companions and One-Year Survival of Patients after Discharge from a Coronary Care Unit," *Public Health Reports* 95, no. 4 (July–August 1980): 307–12.

Screen Time and Health

Netflix, "Netflix Declares Binge Watching is the New Normal," press release, December 13, 2013, https://pr.netflix.com/WebClient/getNewsSummary.do?newsId=496.

J. Lennert Veerman et al., "Television Viewing Time and Reduced Life Expectancy: A Life Table Analysis," *British Journal of Sports Medicine* 46 (2012): 927–30.

University of Pittsburgh, "Each Hour Watching Television Increases Diabetes Risk, Pitt Public Health Finds," news release, April 1, 2015, www.upmc.com/media/NewsReleases/2015/Pages/rockette-kriska-television-diabetes.aspx.

Colin D. Chapman et al., "Watching TV and Food Intake: The Role of Content," *PLoS ONE* 9, no. 7 (July 1, 2014): e100602.

Impact of Awe on Stress

Jennifer E. Stellar et al., "Positive Affect and Markers of Inflammation: Discrete Positive Emotions Predict Lower Levels of Inflammatory Cytokines," *Emotion* 15, no. 2 (April 2015): 129–33.

GLOW

Aging and Environmental Effects on Skin

Suzan Obagi, "Why Does Skin Wrinkle with Age? What Is the Best Way to Slow or Prevent This Process?" *Scientific American*, September 26, 2005, www.scientificamerican.com/article/why-does-skin-wrinkle-wit/.

"What Causes Our Skin to Age?" American Academy of Dermatology, accessed December 29, 2015, https://www.aad.org/dermatology-a-to-z/health-and-beauty/every-stage-of-life/adult-skin/what-causes-aging-skin.

"Sun and UV Exposure," American Cancer Society, accessed December 29, 2015, www.cancer.org/cancer/cancercauses/sunanduvexposure/sun-and-uv-exposure-landing-page.

Andrea Vierkötter et al., "Airborne Particle Exposure and Extrinsic Skin Aging," *Journal of Investigative Dermatology* 130 (2010): 2719–26.

"Moisturizers: Options for Softer Skin," Mayo Clinic, February 1, 2014, www.mayoclinic.org/diseases-conditions/dry-skin/in-depth/moisturizers/art-20044232.

Effective Skin Care Ingredients

"Aging Skin and Skin Care Products," American Academy of Dermatology, December 29, 2015, https://www.aad.org/media-resources/stats-and-facts/cosmetic-treatments/aging-skin-and-skin-care-products.

Reza Kafi et al., "Improvement of Naturally Aged Skin with Vitamin A (Retinol)," *Archives of Dermatology* 143, no. 5 (2007): 606–12, http://archderm.jamanetwork.com/article.aspx?articleid=412795&resultClick=3.

Effects of Sun and UV Protection

"Understanding UVA and UVB," Skin Cancer Foundation, accessed December 29, 2015, www.skincancer.org/prevention/uva-and-uvb/understanding-uva-and-uvb.

Ian D. Stephen, Vinet Coetzee, and David I. Perrett, "Carotenoid and Melanin Pigment Coloration Affect Perceived Human Health," *Evolution and Human Behavior* 32, no. 3 (May 2011): 216–27.

"How Do I Protect Myself from UV Rays?" American Cancer Society, revised March 20, 2015, www.cancer.org/cancer/cancercauses/sunanduvexposure/skincancerpreventionandearlydetection/skin-cancer-prevention-and-early-detection-u-v-protection.

Stacy Simon, "Protect Your Skin from the Sun," American Cancer Society, May 11, 2015, www.cancer.org/cancer/news/features/stay-sun-safe-this-summer.

American Academy of Dermatology, "Study: Most Americans Don't Use Sunscreen," news release, May 19, 2015, https://www.aad.org/stories-and-news/news-releases/study-most-americans-don-t-use-sunscreen.

"Year-Round Sun Protection," Skin Cancer Foundation, accessed December 29, 2015, www.skincancer.org/prevention/sun-protection/prevention-guidelines/year-round-sun-protection.

Diet and Skin

Maeve C. Cosgrove et al., "Dietary Nutrient Intakes and Skin-Aging Appearance among Middle-Aged American Women," *American Journal of Clinical Nutrition* 86, no. 4 (October 2007): 1225–31.

Sleep and Skin

University Hospitals, "Estee Lauder Clinical Trial Finds Link between Sleep Deprivation and Skin Aging," news release, July 17, 2013, http://www.uhhospitals.org/about/media-news-room/current-news/2013/07/estee-lauder-clinical-trial-finds-link-between-sleep-deprivation-and-skin-aging.

Effectiveness of Noninvasive Surgical Procedures

U.S. Food and Drug Administration, "FDA Approves Treatment for Fat below the Chin," press release, April 29, 2015, www.fda.gov/NewsEvents/Newsroom/PressAnnouncements/ucm444978.htm.

"Injectable Fillers Guide," American Board of Cosmetic Surgery, accessed December 29, 2015, www.americanboardcosmeticsurgery.org/procedure-learning-center/non-surgical/injectable-fillers-guide/.

"MicroPen Elite Frequently Asked Questions," Eclipse MicroPen, accessed December 29, 2015, www.eclipsemicropen.com/faqs/.

How to Eat Clean & Green

WHOLE GRAINS

S. B. Patil and M. K. Khan, "Germinated Brown Rice as a Value Added Rice Product: A Review," *Journal of Food Science and Technology* 48, no. 6 (2011): 661–67.

EGGS

H. D. Karsten et al., "Vitamins A, E and Fatty Acid Composition of the Eggs of Caged Hens and Pastured Hens," *Renewable Agriculture and Food Systems* 25 (March 2010): 45–54.

PROTEIN AND MUSCLE

Madonna M. Mamerow et al., "Dietary Protein Distribution Positively Influences 24-H Muscle Protein Synthesis in Healthy Adults," *Journal of Nutrition* 144, no. 6 (June 2014): 876–80.

PREBIOTICS AND PROBIOTICS

"Diet & Gut Microbiota," Gut Microbiota Worldwatch, accessed December 29, 2015, www .gutmicrobiotawatch.org/en/diet-gut-microbiota/.

FISH

"Fish and Omega-3 Fatty Acids," American Heart Association, updated June 15, 2015, www.heart .org/HEARTORG/GettingHealthy/NutritionCenter/HealthyEating/Fish-and-Omega-3-Fatty -Acids_UCM_303248_Article.jsp.

"Seafood & Your Health," Monterey Bay Aquarium Seafood Watch, accessed December 29, 2015, www.seafoodwatch.org/consumers/seafood-and-your-health.

HEALTHY SMOOTHIES

"National Nutrient Database for Standard Reference Release 28: Basic Report 09093, Figs, Canned, Extra Heavy Syrup Pack, Solids and Liquids," U.S. Department of Agriculture, Agricultural Research Service, accessed December 29, 2015, http://ndb.nal.usda.gov/ndb/foods/ show/2205?manu=&fgcd=.

WATER

U.S. Institute of Medicine Panel on Dietary Reference Intakes for Electrolytes and Water, *Dietary Reference Intakes for Water, Potassium, Sodium, Chloride, and Sulfate* (Washington, DC: The National Academies Press, 2005).

COFFEE

"FDA to Investigate Added Caffeine," U.S. Food and Drug Administration, May 3, 2013, www.fda .gov/ForConsumers/ConsumerUpdates/ucm350570.htm.

Xinguo Su et al., "Polyphenolic Profile and Antioxidant Activities of Oolong Tea Infusion under Various Steeping Conditions," *International Journal of Molecular Sciences* 8, no. 12 (December 2007): 1196–205.

AVOCADOS

Michelle Wien et al., "A Randomized 3x3 Crossover Study to Evaluate the Effect of Hass Avocado Intake on Post-Ingestive Satiety, Glucose and Insulin Levels, and Subsequent Energy Intake in Overweight Adults," *Nutrition Journal* 12 (2013): 155.

Li Wang et al., "Effect of a Moderate Fat Diet with and without Avocados on Lipoprotein Particle Number, Size and Subclasses in Overweight and Obese Adults: A Randomized, Controlled Trial," *Journal of the American Heart Association* 4, no. 1 (January 2015): e001355.

Nuray Z. Unlu, "Carotenoid Absorption from Salad and Salsa by Humans Is Enhanced by the Addition of Avocado or Avocado Oil," *Journal of Nutrition* 135, no. 3 (March 1, 2005): 431–36.

NUTS

"Nuts: The Whole Truth and Nutting but the Truth," Cleveland Clinic, accessed December 29, 2015, http://my.clevelandclinic.org/services/heart/prevention/nutrition/food-choices/nuts.

Weeks 1–8

Risks of Water Retention

"Diseases and Conditions: Edema," Mayo Clinic, September 19, 2014, www.mayoclinic.org/diseases-conditions/edema/basics/symptoms/con-20033037.

Movement and Cravings

William D. S. Killgore et al., "Citicoline Affects Appetite and Cortico-Limbic Responses to Images of High Calorie Foods," *International Journal of Eating Disorders* 43, no. 1 (January 2010): 6–13.

Pep Talk and Exercise

Sanda Dolcos and Dolores Albarracin, "The Inner Speech of Behavioral Regulation: Intentions and Task Performance Strengthen When You Talk to Yourself as a You," *European Journal of Social Psychology* 44, no. 6 (October 2014): 636–42.

Music and Exercise Boost

Ju-Han Lin and Frank Jing-Horng Lu, "Interactive Effects of Visual and Auditory Intervention on Physical Performance and Perceived Effort," *Journal of Sports Science & Medicine* 12, no. 3 (September 2013): 388–93.

Dennis Y. Hsu et al., "The Music of Power: Perceptual and Behavioral Consequences of Powerful Music," *Social Psychological and Personality Science* 6, no. 1 (January 2015): 75–83.

Treating Lower Back Pain

"Low Back Pain," FamilyDoctor.org, updated March 2014, http://familydoctor.org/familydoctor/en/diseases-conditions/low-back-pain.printerview.all.html.

Tai Chi and Knee Pain

"Tai Chi as Effective as 'Standard' PT for Knee OA," Advance Healthcare Network News and Notes, November 16, 2015, http://physical-therapy.advanceweb.com/Northeast/News/Daily-News-Watch/Tai-Chi-As-Effective-as-Standard-PT-for-Knee-OA.aspx.

Ginger and Osteoarthritis Pain

Tessa Therkleson, "Ginger Compress Therapy for Adults with Osteoarthritis," *Journal of Advanced Nursing* 66, no. 10 (October 2010): 2225–33.

Tylenol and Osteoarthritis

Gustavo C. Machado et al., "Efficacy and Safety of Paracetamol for Spinal Pain and Osteoarthritis: Systematic Review and Meta-Analysis of Randomised Placebo Controlled Trials," *BMJ* 350 (March 31, 2015): h1225.

Treatments for Hot Flashes

"Health & Aging: Menopause," National Institute on Aging, updated July 20, 2015, www.nia.nih.gov/health/publication/menopause.

Nancy E. Avis et al., "Duration of Menopausal Vasomotor Symptoms over the Menopause Transition," *JAMA Internal Medicine* 175, no. 4 (2015): 531–39.

"Nonhormonal Management of Menopause-Associated Vasomotor Symptoms: 2015 Position Statement of The North American Menopause Society," *Menopause* 22, no. 11 (2015): 1155–74.

Asuka Hirose et al., "Tomato Juice Intake Increases Resting Energy Expenditure and Improves Hypertriglyceridemia in Middle-Aged Women: An Open-Label, Single-Arm Study," *Nutrition Journal* 14 (April 8, 2015): 34.

Treatments for Thinning Hair

"Telogen Effluvium Hair Loss," American Osteopathic College of Dermatology, accessed December 29, 2015, www.aocd.org/?page=TelogenEffluviumHa.

"Female Pattern Baldness," MedlinePlus, U.S. National Library of Medicine, updated February 25, 2014, https://www.nlm.nih.gov/medlineplus/ency/article/001173.htm.

"Hair Loss," MedlinePlus, U.S. National Library of Medicine, updated May 15, 2013, https://www.nlm.nih.gov/medlineplus/ency/article/003246.htm.

"Thinning Hair and Hair Loss: Could It Be Female Pattern Hair Loss?" American Academy of Dermatology, accessed December 29, 2015, https://www.aad.org/dermatology-a-to-z/health-and-beauty/hair-care/thinning-hair-and-hair-loss.

Caroline Le Floc'h et al., "Effect of a Nutritional Supplement on Hair Loss in Women," *Journal of Cosmetic Dermatology* 14, no. 1 (March 2015): 76–82.

Memory and Aging

"Memory," MedlinePlus, U.S. National Library of Medicine, reviewed April 24, 2014, www.nlm.nih.gov/medlineplus/memory.html.

E. M. Zelinski and S. T. Stewart, "Individual Differences in 16-Year Memory Changes," *Psychology and Aging* 13, no. 4 (December 1998): 622–30.

Robert A. Nash et al., "Does Rapport-Building Boost the Eyewitness Eyeclosure Effect in Closed Questioning?" *Legal and Criminological Psychology*, 2015, http://onlinelibrary.wiley.com/doi/10.1111/lcrp.12073/abstract.

Natural Ways to Lower Blood Pressure

"Prevention and Treatment of High Blood Pressure," American Heart Association, updated August 25, 2015, www.heart.org/HEARTORG/Conditions/HighBloodPressure/PreventionTreatmentofHighBloodPressure/Prevention-Treatment-of-High-Blood-Pressure_UCM_002054_Article.jsp.

Lee Hooper et al., "Effects of Chocolate, Cocoa, and Flavan-3-ols on Cardiovascular Health: A Systematic Review and Meta-Analysis of Randomized Trials," *American Journal of Clinical Nutrition* 95, no. 3 (March 2012): 740–51.

Y. Yokoyama et al., "Vegetarian Diets and Blood Pressure: A Meta-Analysis," *JAMA Internal Medicine* 174, no. 4 (April 2014): 577–87.

Haiou Yang et al., "Work Hours and Self-Reported Hypertension Among Working People in California," *Hypertension* 48 (2006): 744–50.

Dirk Taubert et al., "Effects of Low Habitual Cocoa Intake on Blood Pressure and Bioactive Nitric Oxide: A Randomized Controlled Trial," *JAMA* 298, no. 1 (July 4, 2007): 49–60.

Blood Pressure and Brain Health

Donald Liu et al., "UVA Irradiation of Human Skin Vasodilates Arterial Vasculature and Lowers Blood Pressure Independently of Nitric Oxide Synthase," *Journal of Investigative Dermatology* 134 (2014): 1839–46.

Majon Muller et al., "Joint Effect of Mid- and Late-Life Blood Pressure on the Brain," *Neurology* 82, no. 24 (June 17, 2014): 2187–95.

Balance and Aging

"Balance Problems," HealthinAging.org, updated March 2012, www.healthinaging.org/aging-and-health-a-to-z/topic:balance-problems/.

"About Balance Problems," NIH Senior Health, reviewed October 2014, http://nihseniorhealth.gov/balanceproblems/aboutbalanceproblems/01.html.

Hands and Skin Care

"Americans Get a 'B-' on Hand Hygiene," American Cleaning Institute—For Better Living, September 21, 2009, www.cleaninginstitute.org/clean_living/clean_hands_report_card.aspx.

N. Scheinfeld, M. J. Dahdah, and R. Scher, "Vitamins and Minerals: Their Role in Nail Health and Disease," *Journal of Drugs in Dermatology* 6, no. 8 (August 2007): 782–87.

Hearing Loss and Aging

"What Is Hearing Loss?" NIH Senior Health, accessed December 29, 2015, http://nihseniorhealth.gov/hearingloss/hearinglossdefined/01.html.

"Hearing Aids," National Institute on Deafness and Other Communication Disorders, updated September 2013, https://www.nidcd.nih.gov/health/hearing/pages/hearingaid.aspx.

Vision Loss and Aging

"The Burden of Vision Loss," Centers for Disease Control and Prevention, updated September 25, 2009, www.cdc.gov/visionhealth/basic_information/vision_loss_burden.htm.

Family Health Team, "How You Can Cope with Declining Senses as You Age," Cleveland Clinic, April 1, 2015, http://health.clevelandclinic.org/2015/04/how-you-can-cope-with-declining-senses-as-you-age/.

"Adult Vision: 41 to 60 Years of Age," American Optometric Association, accessed December 29, 2015, www.aoa.org/patients-and-public/good-vision-throughout-life/adult-vision-19-to-40-years-of-age/adult-vision-41-to-60-years-of-age?sso=y#1.

"Cataract," MedlinePlus, U.S. National Library of Medicine, updated November 6, 2015, www.nlm.nih.gov/medlineplus/cataract.html.

R. G. Cumming, P. Mitchell, and R. Lim, "Iris Color and Cataract: The Blue Mountains Eye Study," *American Journal of Ophthalmology* 130, no. 2 (August 2000): 237–38.

Food Allergies and Intolerances

"Is It Food Allergy or Food Intolerance?" National Institute of Allergy and Infectious Diseases, updated December 2, 2010, www.niaid.nih.gov/topics/foodAllergy/understanding/Pages/foodIntolerance.aspx.

James T. C. Li, "What's the Difference between a Food Intolerance and Food Allergy?" Mayo Clinic, October 10, 2014, www.mayoclinic.org/diseases-conditions/food-allergy/expert-answers/food-allergy/faq-20058538.

Atenodoro R. Ruiz Jr., "Lactose Intolerance," Merck Manual, accessed December 29, 2015, www.merckmanuals.com/home/digestive-disorders/malabsorption/lactose-intolerance.

J. R. Biesiekierski et al., "No Effects of Gluten in Patients with Self-Reported Non-Celiac Gluten Sensitivity after Dietary Reduction of Fermentable, Poorly Absorbed, Short-Chain Carbohydrates," *Gastroenterology* 145, no. 2 (August 2013): 320-8.e1-3.

"Irritable Bowel Syndrome," MedlinePlus, U.S. National Library of Medicine, updated September 30, 2015, https://www.nlm.nih.gov/medlineplus/irritablebowelsyndrome.html.

Remedies for Heartburn

"Heartburn," eMedicine Health, reviewed December 3, 2014. www.emedicinehealth.com/heartburn/article_em.htm#heartburn_definition.

"Understanding Heartburn—The Basics," WebMD, reviewed March 18, 2015, www.webmd.com/heartburn-gerd/guide/understanding-heartburn-basics.

Causes of and Solutions for Constipation

"Understanding Constipation," American Gastroenterological Association, accessed December 29, 2015, www.gastro.org/patient-center/Understanding_Constipation_Brochure_Jan_2013.pdf.

Norton J. Greenberger, "Constipation," Merck Manual, accessed December 29, 2015, www.merckmanuals.com/home/digestive-disorders/symptoms-of-digestive-disorders/constipation.

A. Attaluri et al., "Randomised Clinical Trial: Dried Plums (Prunes) versus Psyllium for Constipation," *Alimentary Pharmacology and Therapeutics* 33, no. 7 (April 2011): 822–28.

Alayne D. Markland et al., "Associations of Low Dietary Intake of Fiber and Liquids with Constipation: Evidence from the National Health and Nutrition Examination Survey," *American Journal of Gastroenterology* 108 (2013): 796–803.

Jill Jin, "Over-the-Counter Laxatives," *JAMA* 312, no. 11 (2014): 1167.

"Concerned about Constipation?" National Institute on Aging, updated December 22, 2015, https://www.nia.nih.gov/health/publication/concerned-about-constipation.

"Irritable Bowel Syndrome," National Institute of Diabetes and Digestive and Kidney Diseases, NIH-Publication No. 13-693, September 2013, www.niddk.nih.gov/health-information/health-topics/digestive-diseases/irritable-bowel-syndrome/Documents/ibs_508.pdf.

Causes of and Solutions for Gas and Bloating

"Small Bowel Bacterial Overgrowth," MedlinePlus, U.S. National Library of Medicine, updated May 15, 2014, https://www.nlm.nih.gov/medlineplus/ency/article/000222.htm.

"What Do I Need to Know about Gas?" National Institute of Diabetes and Digestive and Kidney Diseases, NIH Publication No. 12-4156, October 2011, page updated July 31, 2013, www.niddk.nih.gov/health-information/health-topics/digestive-diseases/gas/Pages/ez.aspx.

Gut Bacteria and Home Environment

Robert R. Dunn et al., "Home Life: Factors Structuring the Bacterial Diversity Found within and between Homes," *PLoS ONE* 8, no. 5 (2013): e64133.

Pelvic Floor Disorder Causes and Remedies

"Frequently Asked Questions about Pelvic Floor Disorders," University of Chicago Medicine, accessed December 29, 2015, www.uchospitals.edu/specialties/pelvic/faq/pelvic-floor-disorders.html.

Alison J. Huang et al., "A Group-Based Yoga Therapy Intervention for Urinary Incontinence in Women: A Pilot Randomized Trial," *Female Pelvic Medicine & Reconstructive Surgery* 20, no. 3 (May–June 2014): 147–54.

Adult Acne Causes and Treatments

"Adult Acne," American Academy of Dermatology, accessed December 29, 2015, https://www.aad.org/dermatology-a-to-z/health-and-beauty/every-stage-of-life/adult-skin/adult-acne.

"All about Rosacea," National Rosacea Society, www.rosacea.org/patients/allaboutrosacea.php.

"What Is Rosacea?" University of Rochester Medical Center Health Encyclopedia, accessed December 29, 2015, https://www.urmc.rochester.edu/encyclopedia/content.aspx?ContentTypeID=85&ContentID=P00311.

Savoring and Happiness

Paul E. Jose, Bee T. Lim, and Fred B. Bryant, "Does Savoring Increase Happiness?" *Journal of Positive Psychology* 7, no. 3 (2012): 176–87.

Housework and Happiness

D. E. Saxbe, R. L. Repetti, and A. P. Graesch, "Time Spent in Housework and Leisure: Links with Parents' Physiological Recovery from Work," *Journal of Family Psychology* 25, no. 2 (April 2011): 271–81.

Flow and Happiness

"Mihaly Csikszentmihalyi," The Pursuit of Happiness, accessed December 29, 2015, www.pursuit-of -happiness.org/history-of-happiness/mihaly-csikszentmihalyi/.

Meaning and the Immune System

Center for the Advancement of Health, "Searching for Meaning in Life May Boost Immune System," *ScienceDaily*, April 29, 2003, www.sciencedaily.com/releases/2003/04/030429083520.htm.

Experiences and Happiness

Darwin A. Guevarra and Ryan T. Howell, "To Have in Order to Do: Exploring the Effects of Consuming Experiential Products on Well-Being," *Journal of Consumer Psychology* 25, no. 1 (2015): 28–41.

INDEX

Underscored page references indicate boxed text. **Boldface** references indicate tables and illustrations.